Nutrition in Traditional Therapeutic Foods

– Volume 1 –

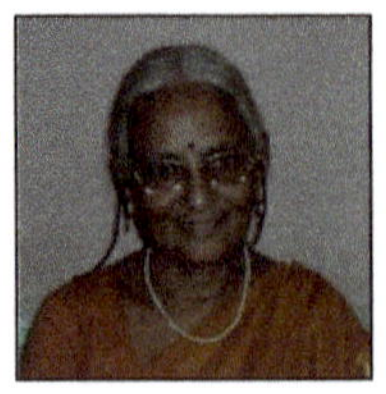

Dr. G. Subbulakshmi is an eminent nutritionist with over 45 years of teaching, research and administrative experience. She has a Ph.D in Food Science and Nutrition and has also worked as a post doctoral fellow in CFTRI, Mysore in early 1970s. She has worked as the First Principal of the S.M. Patel College of Home Science in Vallabh Vidyanagar, Gujarat and Indramani Mandelia College of Home Science in Pilani, Rajasthan. She has been instrumental in introducing internship for the students in Home Science colleges and Sports Nutrition and Food Science and Technology in the Nutrition curriculum.

She has published several research papers and her book on Food Processing and Preservation has been widely used in the colleges. She has guided more than 25 PhD students in Food Science and Nurition apart from more than 60 M.Sc. students in their Dissertations. She has published more than 70 Research Papers in National and International Journals. Dr. Subbulakshmi has worked towards the improvement of community Health and Nutrition. Having worked on research projects funded by National and International Agencies, she has prepared a number of booklets and pamphlets on nutrition related topics for educating the common man.

She has received Fulbright award for studying the college administration in USA, PL480 Research Scholarship for doing Ph.D., UGC's National Research Associateship award as well as Hari Om Ashram Prizes for 3 different best Research papers in Nutrition. The various awards received by Dr. Subbulakshmi speak of her abilities. She has been awarded M.L. Khurana Memorial Award –2002; T.K. Basu Award for excellent contributions to Nutritional Sciences from International College of Nutrition USA; Life Time Achievement Award from Alumni Association of the M.S. University of Baroda; Life Time Achievement Award from Nutrition Society of India, Mumbai Chapter.

She is an active life member of many Professional Organizations like Nutrition Society of India, Association of Food Scientists and Technologists of India, Indian Dietetic Association, Home Science Association of India, Association for Women Scientists, Indian Association for Preschool Education and many others.

Dr. Mandalika Subhadra is an expert in Food Science and Nutrition. She is a post graduate of Sri Satya Sai Institute of Higher Learning, Anantapur,(A.P., India) and awarded gold medal for securing first rank. She has received her PhD in Food Science and Nutrition from SNDT Women's University, Mumbai, India. She has contributed her valuable expertise to various institutions during her 20 years of service as an academician and researcher. Her contribution was appreciated with a best teacher award by the Rajamahendri Degree College for Women, Andhra Pradesh. She is also a recognised PhD guide of the University of Mumbai and selected as PhD referee by various other reputed Universities. She has been actively involved in teaching and research guidance at under graduate and post-graduate levels. She has guided around 25 post-graduate students and 6 PhD scholars on research topics from various branches of nutrition including Clinical Nutrition, Community Nutrition. Nutritional Food Product Development, Food Science and Technology, Biochemistry, Micronutrients, Antioxidants, Sports and exercise Nutrition. She has got several research publications to her credit in various peer reviewed journals and has been a co-editor of a book on Methodologies of Nutritional assessment. She has shared her research achievements in various national and international conferences. Her deep interest in research is evident through a Patency (No. 225689) she has Obtained on 'Antiestrogenic activity of phytosterols from fenugreekseeds'. She has coordinated major and minor research projects sponsored by DAE/BRNS, UGC, University of Mumbai, and reputed food industries.

Dr.Subhadra has been invited as a resource person at various seminars and conferences. She was honoured with an Ambassadorial Scholarship of Good Will by the Rotary International to take up an academic assignment at the University of Mauritius for 3 and half months in Mauritius which was highly appreciated. Besides being an academician, she is also actively involved in community outreach programmes. Currently she is working as a faculty of Home Science in the specialisation of Foods, Nutrition and Dietetics of College of Home Science, Nirmala Niketan, Mumbai.

Nutrition in Traditional Therapeutic Foods

– Volume 1 –

— Authors —

G. Subbulakshmi

Nutrition Consultant,
Former Director,
Department of PGSR in Home Science,
SNDT Women's University, Mumbai

and

M. Subhadra

Assistant Professor,
Department of Food, Nutrition and Dietetics,
College of Home Science, Nirmala Niketan, Mumbai

2013

Daya Publishing House®

A Division of

Astral International Pvt. Ltd.

New Delhi – 110 002

ISBN 9789351300786

Published by : **Daya Publishing House®**
A Division of
Astral International Pvt. Ltd.
– ISO 9001:2008 Certified Company –
4760-61/23, Ansari Road, Darya Ganj
New Delhi-110 002
Ph. 011-43549197, 23278134
E-mail: info@astralint.com
Website: www.astralint.com

Laser Typesetting : Classic Computer Services, Delhi - 110 035

Printed at : Salasar Imaging Systems, Delhi - 110 035

PRINTED IN INDIA

Acknowledgements

The globally renowned traditional therapeutic dietary practices are the strongest source of inspiration to the authors towards this endeavor. Our intense desire was to compile the available scientific evidence on these practices and present it in a nutshell for the benefit of future generation. Our heartfelt acknowledgement to all the students, friends and others who have directly or indirectly inspired us towards this effort.

We sincerely thank all the scientists for sharing the outcome of their excellent research through publications. We are also immensely thankful to all the web search engines for providing access to the authentic scientific information without which this venture would have been impossible. The valuable contribution of the scientists has been duly acknowledged in the text as well as in the references. The copy right of the sources of information remains with the original authors. However, if reference to any author/s is missing in book, it is purely inadvertent and unintentional .

We are grateful to Dr. B. Sesikeran, Former Director of National Institute of Nutrition, Hyderabad, India, for kindly writing the foreword for the book. We appreciate and acknowledge the help rendered by our beloved students Ms. Neha Vaidya, Ms. Minelly Rodrigues and Ms. Shagufta Sheikh.

G. Subbulakshmi

M. Subhadra

Foreword

This is going to be a really amazing book, one which has captured all the essence of traditional foods and food ingredients. A good amount of scientifically researched and published information on each of the traditional foods and food ingredients has been compiled to make this an excellent reference. Every food like Amla or Fenugreek or Ajwain is given in detail from its taxonomy to composition or nutrient content along with both traditional therapeutics and modern uses. The information at times is folklore but backed up with scientific reasoning. The book would be of immense utility to Nutritionists, Ayurvedic practitioners, Allopaths, scientists involved in research of traditional foods or food components in India, Pharmacologists or even for home use. Students would have a single source of this kind of information which would make their lives lot easier. Overall, this book has something for everyone as it is in a user friendly manner with scientific back up in the form of extensive cross references.

B. Sesikeran

Former Director,
National Institute of Nutrition,
Hyderabad

Preface

Globally several foods and food ingredients have been valued for their preventive/curative qualities in clinical conditions such as CVD, diabetes, cancers, ulcers etc. Dietary modification in the management of various diseases has been in vogue since time immemorial across the cultures in all systems of medicine. Interestingly, almost all the foods recommended traditionally for their therapeutic benefits are natural vegetarian foods. The scientific evidence established by modern research has indeed given a boost to these traditional therapeutic food practices, which are now termed as nutritional support.

The present book on *'Nutrition In Traditional Therapeutic Foods'* emphasizes the available scientific proof on the therapeutic role of various foods/food ingredients. This book is unique as it integrates the traditional wisdom with modern science and emphasizes the need to carry forward the traditional food research. Being a compilation of available research on the dietetic value of foods and herbs, it can serve as a reference book as well as a 'think tank' to nutrition enthusiasts and also trigger research interests in the minds of future scientists who intend to delve into the cultural practices. Several books are available in the market on clinical nutrition or Dietetics but this book gives due importance to dietetic value of specific foods and herbs and thereby enables dieticians/healthcare specialists to plan their dietary advice with strong scientific conviction and make it suitable to patients' own dietary practices and also to consider community oriented dietary approach wherever required. Students from the field of Nutrition and Dietetics would not only benefit from the information on therapeutic applications of various foods but also understand the scientific efforts/methods/techniques involved in establishing the same. Also the book would be useful for those who want to consider food based approach for health. Acadmicians, scientists, students, research scholars, and entrepreneurs could draw intellectual benefit from the Nutritional, Clinical, Microbiological, Biochemical and Nutraceutical aspects of various foods covered in the book.

The book comprises of 20 chapters. Each chapter covers information on details of the food / plant, Traditional usage and Overview of therapeutic benefits, Chemical and nutritional composition, Details of scientific evidence and Safety issues wherever applicable.

Dr. G. Subbulakshmi

Dr. M. Subhadra

Contents

Introduction

Food is an important part of religious observance for many different faiths, including Christianity, Judaism, Islam, Hinduism and Buddhism. Most religions include food observances as a vital part of their faith.

World over, different countries comprise of people from various religions and communities living together, preserving their customs and traditions that are thousands of years old, till date. Each religious community has its own food beliefs, medicinal and nutritional practices which are followed from generation to generation. What is intriguing is that the stem of these practices run throughout the world in spite of the vast differences and distances. This traditional knowledge, skills and practices are based on the theories of Ayurveda, beliefs and experiences indigenous to different cultures.

Ayurveda dates back to the period of the Indus Valley civilization (about 3000 BC) and has been passed on through generations by word of mouth. References to the herbal medicines of Ayurveda are found in all of the four Vedas, suggesting that Ayurveda predates the Vedas by at least several centuries. It was already in full practice at the time of Buddha (6th) century BC) and had produced two of the greatest physicians of ancient India, Charaka and Shushrutha who composed the basic texts of their trade, the Samhitas. The ancient ayurvedic scriptures depict the use of various natural foods for treatment of diseases. In fact, before the surge in allopathic medicine, these herbal therapeutic foods were the main alternative treatment for various illnesses and conditions. The major advantage of these therapeutic foods was easy availability.

Traditional therapeutic foods are wholesome, preventive/curative, natural and less processed with no proven side-effects. Interestingly, the three golden rules followed by the older generation for a healthy living were: 1. Eating garden fresh foods prepared and consumed fresh. 2. Inclusion of foods from each category such as cereals, pulses, vegetables, fruits etc. in the daily diet. (It is interesting to note that dairy products (though animal source) were a part of the daily diet in those days even among the vegetarians. It is only later that a scientific basis has been found that milk and milk products are the best quality protein sources for vegetarians). 3. "Mitahar" was the essence of their daily routine. 'Mita' means 'proportionate' or 'enough to nourish', and 'Ahar' means 'food'. "Mitahar" therefore means 'moderation in eating'.

But, it is a pity that this "orthodox wisdom" has been dying fast with the disappearance of the older generation because the present generation considers these practices as superstitions/blind faith/fads and fallacies etc. and demand a strong scientific proof for each of these practices through systematic research protocol. As rightly said by American editor and poet, T.S. Eliot, "a tradition without intelligence is not worth having", it is important to know the scientific reasons behind the use of certain natural foods as medicine and supplementing allopathy with nature cure. Therefore, the popular therapeutic habits and successes have to be retrieved and validated in order to use this information to develop new cost-effective, safe and efficacious system of medicine.

A national congress on traditional science and technologies of India was organized during 1993 specifically to comprehend and evaluate our traditions in diverse domains of knowledge and practice. This was considered an important step in our developmental efforts at the grassroot levels, as many of these living traditions have the potential to contribute to the well being of people. In the recent past, many pharmacological drugs are manufactured by extracting the vital ingredients of medicinal plants. For example: WHO reported that new anti-malarial drugs are developed from the discovery and isolation of artemisinin from *Artemisia annua* L., a plant used in China for almost 2000 years.

In Western culture, until recently the conventional medicine has largely rejected the use of such "alternative" therapeutic intervention. Based on an increasing database though, insight has been gained concerning the scientific validity of many previously established 'nutraceuticals' that are becoming more widely accepted as an adjunct to conventional therapies for enhancing general well-being.

US Patent has prompted us to get back to our roots

Interestingly, an awakening in the minds of scientists has strengthened the research efforts towards establishing scientific proof of traditional therapeutics and their safety issues. Studies all over the world have explored the anti-inflammatory, cholekinetic and anti-oxidant potentials of traditional foods with the recent investigations focusing on their preventive and curative effects.

Several foods have been identified with great therapeutic potential and spicesa occupy prime position among them. In India, spices are considered as "Spice for Life". Current biomedical efforts are focused on their scientific merits, to provide science-based evidence for the traditional uses and to develop either functional foods or nutraceuticals.

Among the spices, fenugreek seeds (*Trigonella foenumgraecum*), garlic (*Allium sativum*), onion (*Allium cepa*), and turmeric (*Curcuma longa*) have been experimentally documented to possess antidiabetic potential. The Indian traditional medical systems use turmeric for wound healing, rheumatic disorders, gastrointestinal symptoms, deworming, and as a cosmetic (Krishnaswamy, 2008). The nutrigenomic effect of turmeric is currently under investigation. In a limited number of studies, cumin seeds (*Cuminum cyminum*), ginger (*Zingiber officinale*), mustard (*Brassica nigra*), curry leaves (*Murraya koenigii*) and coriander (*Coriandrum sativum*) have been reported to be hypoglycaemic (Srinivasan 2005). Apart from these, bael (*Aegle marmelos*), garlic (*Allium sativum*) and jamun (*Eugenia jambolana*) also have been found to be useful in diabetes associated with ischemic heart disease (Dwivedi and Aggarwal, 2009). Their active biomolecules have been identified and also have been demonstrated to be safe for long-term use. In addition, the foods currently in focus today such as coarse grains (Barley, oats and flaxseeds), fruits (Figs, Amla, Olives and Dates) and Honey have also been extensively researched for their health benefits.

This book is a sincere attempt to compile most of the available documented scientific literature on various foods which have been traditionally believed to be preventive and/or curative of several clinical conditions.

References

Srinivasan, K. (2005). Plant foods in the management of diabetes mellitus: spices as beneficial antidiabetic food adjuncts. Int. J. Food Sci. Nutr. 56 (6): 399–414.

Krishnaswamy, K. (2008). Traditional Indian spices and their health significance. Asia Pac J Clin Nutr. 17 Suppl. 1: 265–68.

Dwivedi, S. and Aggarwal A. (2009). Indigenous drugs in ischemic heart disease in patients with diabetes. J. Altern. Complement. Med. 15 (11): 1215–21.

Chapter 1

Ajwain

(*Carum copticum/Trachyspermum ammi*)

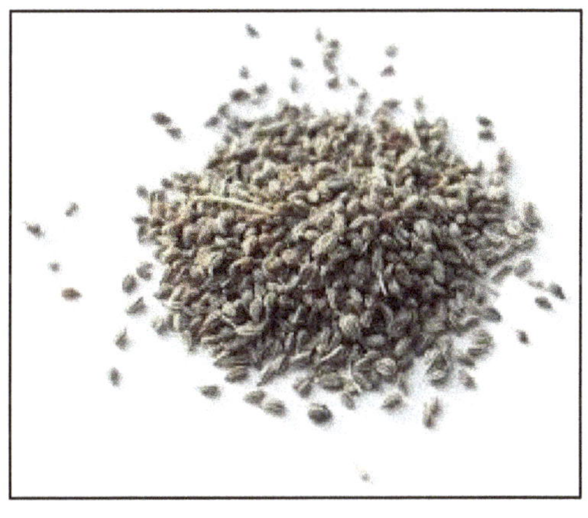

Omum, commonly known as ajowan, bishop's weed, ajwain, ajowan caraway, carom seeds, or thymol seeds etc. is popular in India and the Near East as a spice. Ajwain is believed to have originated from various parts of the globe such as the Middle East, Egypt, the Indian subcontinent, Iran and Afghanistan. The main areas of cultivation today are Persia and India, but the spice is of importance in global usage. In India, the major ajwain producing states are Rajasthan and Gujarat, where Rajasthan produces about 90 per cent of India's total production.

The plant has a similarity to parsley. Because of their seed like appearance, the fruit pods are sometimes called seeds; they are egg-shaped and grayish in colour. Raw ajwain smells almost exactly like thyme because it also contains thymol, (and hence, also called thymol seeds) but is more aromatic and less subtle in taste, as well as slightly pungent. Even a small amount of raw ajwain will completely dominate the flavour of a dish.

Ajwain is believed to be a cure in its raw powder form as well as water extract for digestive problems (colic, diarrhoea, dysentery and indigestion), blocked nose, common cold and rheumatic pain. The omum water is a household medicine not only in India but also in Srilanka, Malaysia and even in some Arabian countries. It is sometimes used as an ingredient in 'berbere', a spice mixture favoured in Ethiopia.

Nutritional and Chemical Constituents of Ajwain

Ajwain seeds contain moisture (8.9 per cent), fiber (11.9 per cent), carbohydrates (38.6 per cent), protein (15.4 per cent), fat (18.1 per cent), nicotinic acid, mineral matter (7.1 per cent) (Calcium, iron, Zinc, Copper and Phosphorus), and phytochemicals such as tannins, glycosides, saponins and flavones (Ishikawah *et al.*, 2001; Pruthi, 1992; Gupta *et al.*, 2003). The protein in ajwain showed abundant presence of amino acids–aspartine and glutamine. Devasankaraiah *et al.* (1974) confirmed the presence of acetylcholine (a neurotransmitter) and choline in the roasted omum seed extract by paper and gas chromatography.

Ajwain yields 2 to 4 per cent essential oil which is almost colourless to brownish with characteristic odor and a sharp pungent taste. Recently, 30 chemical compounds have been identified in the ajwain essential oil (AEO) using GC-MS by Paul and Kang (2011) with thymol as the major constituent (35 per cent to 60 per cent). It also contains 6-O-β-glucopyranosyloxythymol (Garg and Kumar, 1998) and 25 per cent oleoresin (Nagalakshmi *et al.*, 2000). According to Choudhury (1998) the other constituents in ajwain oil are carvone (46 per cent), limonene (38 per cent), and dillapiole (9 per cent). Singh *et al.* (2004) identified p-cymene (30.8 per cent), gamma-terpinene (23.2 per cent), beta-pinene (1.7 per cent) and terpinene-4-ol (0.8 per cent) in AEO. Acetone extract of ajwain seeds contain thymol as a major component (39.1 per cent) along with oleic acid (10.4 per cent), linoleic acid (9.6 per cent), gamma-terpinene (2.6 per cent), p-cymene (1.6 per cent), palmitic acid (1.6 per cent), and xylene (0.1 per cent). However, isothymol (50 per cent) was found to be the dominant constituent in the essential oil distilled from aerial parts (flowers, leaves) of ajwain grown in Algeria. But the name isothymol is not well defined and might refer to both 2-isopropyl-4-methylphenol and 3-isopropyl-6-methylphenol (carvacrol).

Nutritional value of Ajwain (per 100 g).

Nutrient	*Amount*	*Nutrient*	*Amount*
Energy (kcal)	363	Carbohydrates (g)	24.6
Dietary fiber (g)	21.2	Fat (g)	21.8
Protein (g)	17.1	Calcium (mg)	1525
Iron (mg)	12.5	Magnesium (mg)	141
Phosphorus (mg)	443	Zinc (mg)	4.52
Nutrient	Amount	Thiamine (Vit. B1) (mg)	0.21
Riboflavin (Vit.B2) (mg)	0.28	Niacin (Vit. B3) (mg)	2.1
Carotene (µg)	71		

Gopalan *et al.*, 2010.

Folkloric Beliefs

In Indian system of medicine, *ajwain* is administered for curing stomach disorders. A paste of crushed seeds is applied externally for relieving colic pains; and a hot and dry fomentation of the seeds is applied on chest for relief from asthma (Singh *et al.*, 2003). Surveys conducted among rural women of Punjab, Jammu and Madhya Pradesh (India), reported the use of ajwain by the local communities in stomach ailments, spasms and flatulence (Sidhu *et al.*, 2007; Dwivedi *et al.*, 2006). It is also thought to be carminative, stimulant, antiflatulent and antiemetic and hence consumed after meal to aid the digestion (Aggarwal and Kotwal, 2009). Similar practice of using ajwain in gastrointestinal disorders has been reported in Makkah al-Mukarramah (Bajrai, 2010) and Rawalpindi (Pakistan) (Hussain and Malik, 2008).

Therapeutic Benefits of Ajwain – The Scientific Evidence

Since ancient times, along with its culinary uses, ajwain has been used as a digestive stimulant, galactogogue, antispasmodic, antiinfective agent as well as a remedy for flatulence, atonic dyspepsia, diarrhea, abdominal tumours, abdominal pains, piles, bronchial problems, lack of appetite, asthma and amenorrhoea (Wadhwa *et al.*, 2010). Its medicinal properties have been attributed to the presence of biologically active compounds such as glycosides, saponins, phenolic compounds and volatile oils (thymol, daku-terpinene, para-cymene, and α- and β-pinene) (Bairwa *et al.*, 2012).

The total alcoholic extract and total aqueous extract of the ajwain seeds exhibited significant ($P<0.001$) anti-inflammatory activity in the animal models (Thangam and Dhananjayan, 2003). Gilani *et al.* (2005) rationalized some of the traditional uses of the aqueous-methanolic extract of ajwain as the antihypertensive (dose-dependent fall in arterial blood pressure in anaesthetized rats fed the extract), antispasmodic (inhibitory effect on the K^+-induced contractions in isolated rabbit aorta and jejunum preparations), bronchodilator (calcium channel blocking effect) and hepatoprotective agent (reduced serum alkaline phosphatase and aminotransferases and prevention of the CCl_4-induced prolongation in pentobarbital-induced sleeping time in mice).

Some of the prominent therapeutic benefits of ajwain are further enlisted below.

Antioxidant Potential

Zahin *et al.* (2010) reported that the methanol fraction showed the highest antioxidant activity by phosphomolybdenum (2087.7 micromol) and DPPH assay (90.2 per cent) followed by other fractions comparable to ascorbic acid and BHT. Pre-feeding of ajwain extract at 1 per cent level to rats injected with HCH (hexachlorocyclohexane) reverted the significant changes in catalase, G-6-Phosphate DH, GST and glutamyl transpeptidase. HCH-induced formation of micronuclei in femur bone marrow was also reduced significantly. At the same time there was a significant reduction in hepatic levels of HCH-induced rise in lipid peroxides (Anilakumar *et al.*, 2009). Due to the antioxidant potential, ajwain exerts several health benefits.

Antimicrobial Effect

Antibacterial efficacy shown by ajwain plant provides a scientific basis and thus, validates its traditional use as homemade remedy (Kaur and Arora, 2009). The Phenolic compounds, such as thymol and carvacrol, in AEO are known to be either bactericidal or bacteriostatic agents depending on the concentration used (Mayaud *et al.*, 2008; Singh *et al.*, 2002; Caccioni *et al.*, 2000). Saxena and Vyas (1986) and Wadhwa *et al.* (2010) reported the antimicrobial activity of ajwain against gram +ve bacteria such as *B. subtilis* and *S. aureus* and gram–ve bacteria such as *E. coli*. Dhiman and Choudhary (2012) also confirmed the inhibitory effects of ajwain extracts against *E. coli, S. aureus, P. aeruginosa* along with *S. typhi*. Similar observations were made by Tambekar and Dahikar (2011) on the methanol and acetone extracts of Ajmodadi churna, an ayurvedic herbal preparation made of ajwain thus confirming its beneficial role in treating enteric infections.

Isolation and purification of different phytochemicals form ajwain may further yield significant antibacterial agents. Javed *et al.* (2012) confirmed that the presence of ethanol in ajwain contributes to its antibacterial property while carvacrol to its antifungal property thus supporting the centuries old use of ajwain for gastro-intestinal disorders.

The volatile constituents of ajwain seeds were found to inhibit the growth of fungi *A. fusispora, F.chlamydosporum, F. poae, M. roridum, Papulaspora* sp., *A. grisea, A. tenuissima, D. tetramera,* and *R.solani* by 72-90 per cent (Singh *et al.*, 1979). The broad spectrum fungitoxic behaviour against *A. niger, A. flavus* (Singh *et al.*, 2000), *A. oryzae, A. ochraceus, F.monoliforme, F. graminearum, P. citrium, P. viridicatum, P. madriti,* and *C. lunata* through absolute mycelial zone inhibition at 6-µl. (Singh *et al.*, 2004; Rasooli *et al.*, 2008) was also reported. In addition, the essential oil has some use in the treatment of intestinal dysbiosis too. Its benefit comes from being able to inhibit the growth of undesired pathogens while not adversely affecting the beneficial flora (Hawrelak *et al.*, 2009).

Ajwain has been found to show Anthelmintic activity against specific helminths, *e.g.Ascaris lumbricoides* in humans and *Haemonchus contortus* in sheep (Kwon Park *et al.*, 2007) by interference with the energy metabolism of parasites through potentiation of ATPase activity (Kostyukovsky *et al.*, 2002). The plant has also been reported to possess cholinergic activity with peristaltic movements of the gut, thus helping in expulsion of intestinal parasites which might also be a contributory factor to its anthelmintic activity (Tamurab and Iwamoto, 2004; Jabbar *et al.*, 2006).

Lymphatic filariasis is caused by infection with the parasitic filarial nematodes *W. bancrofti, B. malayi* and *B. timori,* transmitted by mosquitoes. The lack of an adulticidal drug poses a challenge to filariasis elimination, hence it is essential to develop an effective anti-filarial drug which could either kill or permanently sterilize the adult worms. Mathew *et al.* (2008) found that the crude extract of ajwain showed significant activity against the adult S. digitata by both a worm motility and MTT [3-(4,5-dimethylthiazol-2-yl)-2,5-diphenyltetrazolium bromide] reduction assays. The isolated active principle was chemically characterized by IR, H-NMR and MS analysis and identified as a phenolic monoterpene. It was screened for *in vivo* anti-filarial activity against the human filarial worm *B. malayi* in Mastomys coucha rats. The findings thus provide a new lead for development of a macro-filaricidal drug from ajwain.

The emerging trends of multidrug resistance among several groups of micro-organisms against different classes of antibiotics led different researchers to develop efficient drugs from plant sources to counter multidrug resistant strains. Khan *et al.* (2010 a) investigated different solvent extracts of ajwain to determine the efficacy against multidrug resistant microbes. The petroleum ether fraction (least MIC- 625 μ/ml) showed best activity against multidrug resistant strains of *C. glabrata, E. coli* and reference strains of *S. mutans* and *S. bovis* when compared to its other fractions.

Khan *et al.* (2010 b) isolated and characterized a novel active compound, a naphthalene derivative (4aS, 5R, 8aS) 5, 8a-di-1-propyl-octahydronaphthalen-1-(2H) from ajwain seeds, which was found effective against adherent cells of S. mutans (a major causal organism of dental caries) by reducing water-insoluble glucan synthesis and inhibiting the reduction in pH. Thus a Ajwain exhibits great potential as a therapeutic agent against dental caries.

Cardioprotective Effect

Ajwain has been shown to possess hypolipidemic (Kumari and Prameela, 1992) and hyportensive (Gilani *et al.*, 2005) effects. An ether extract of omum was found to inhibit platelet aggregation induced by arachidonic acid (AA), epinephrine and collagen. But it was most effective against AA-induced aggregation. Effect of omum on platelet thromboxane production could be explained as (i) Reduced TxB2 formation in intact platelet preparations from added arachidonate, and (ii) Reduced formation of TxB2 from AA-labelled platelets after stimulation with Ca^{2+}-ionophore A23187 by a direct action on cyclooxygenase. Thus an increased formation of lipoxygenase-derived products from exogenous AA in omum-treated platelets was apparently due to redirection of AA from cyclooxygenase to the lipoxygenase pathway (Srivastava, 1988).

Methanol and petroleum ether extracts of ajwain equivalent to its powder (2 g/kg body weight) and simvastatin (0.6 mg/kg body weight) were equally effective in treating hyperlipidaemia in albino rabbits. In fact, petroleum ether extract appeared to be more potent than methanol extract on the basis of increasing the level of HDL-cholesterol and lowering the LDL-cholesterol more effectively. Petroleum ether extract reduced atherogenic index (total cholesterol/HDL-cholesterol) more effectively than methanol extract (Javed *et al.*, 2002; 2006) due to the significant increase in HDL-Cholesterol (42 per cent), which effect was non-significant ($P>0.05$) in case of methanol extract.

Anticarcinogenic and Antimutagenic Effect

Ajwain exhibited a significant reduction in the skin as well as the fore stomach tumour multiplicity with all doses (2 per cent, 4 per cent, and 6 per cent) of test diet as compared to the control group. Biochemical assays revealed a significant increase in the activities of phase I enzymes especially with 6 per cent test diet with a concomitant increase in the activities of the phase II enzymes and antioxidant enzymes observed in the other groups. Also a significant elevation in the reduced glutathione content and a significant reduction in the peroxidative damage along with lactate dehydrogenase activity were observed in all the groups. These findings were indicative of chemopreventive potential of ajwain seeds (Singh and Kale, 2010).

Antitussive (Cough suppressant) Effect

The aqueous and macerated extracts of omum showed significant antitussive effect measured by reduction of cough number (Boskabady *et al.*, 2005). Choudhury *et al.* (1998) showed the fruits of ajwain to have been used as an expectorant.

Analgesic and Antispasmodic Effect

Ajwain is mentioned to have some therapeutic effects on headache and joint pains in Iranian traditional literature. Using a tail-flick analgesiometer device, Dashti-Rahmatabadi *et al.* (2007) proved the claims of Iranian traditional medicine showing that Carum copticum extract possesses a definite analgesic effect. However, further investigations are required to evaluate the efficacy and safety of this herbal medication in man.

Ajwain has also been used as an antispasmodic agent, providing relief from stomach spasms and stomach ache. The major phenolic compound thymol, in ajwain has been found to be mainly responsible for the same (Javed *et al.*, 2012). Chaturbeeja churna (powder), made of ajwain, fenugreek. *Nigella sativa* (kalonji) and *Lepidium sativum*, a common ayurvedic prescription for dysmenorrhoea, was found to relieve stomach spasms in 25 patients. The antispasmodic effect of this churna was mainly due to presence of ajwain, which has high concentration of thymol. The effect is mediated through calcium channel blockade, which relieves the spasms and pain by its direct action on the myometrium (Dhiman and Chaudhary, 2012).

Thus it was indicated that the presence of calcium antagonist(s) in ajwain seeds provides sound mechanistic basis for some of their folkloric uses.

Gastroprotective Effect

Thymol of AEO is used in the treatment of gastro-intestinal ailments and bronchial problems. The ajwain fruit possesses gastric stimulant, and carminative properties. It is also an important remedial agent for flatulence, atonic dyspepsia and diarrhea (Bentely and Trimen, 1999).

Vasudevan *et al.* (2000) observed that the aqueous extract (10 per cent w/v) of ajwain had lower impact on gastric acidity in comparison with other spices (Red pepper, Fennel, Cardamom, Black pepper, Cumin and Coriander). Moreover, the fruit showed anti-ulcer activity in different ulcer models. Animals pre-treated with ethanolic extract showed significant decrease in ulcer index and higher percentage of ulcer protection in all models (Ramaswamy *et al.*, 2010).

Ajwain also cures abdominal tumours, abdominal pains and piles (Krishnamoorthy and Madalageri, 1999).

Natural Contraceptive and Galactogogue

A high risk of potential human fetotoxicity of *T. ammi (ajwain)*, based on teratogenicity was observed in rat fetuses by Nath *et al.* (1997). Paul and Kang (2011) are the first scientists to conduct series of experiments to determine the spermicidal and contraceptive efficacy of essential oil of ajwain on human sperm by *in vitro* viability and membrane integrity. The minimum effective dose of essential oil of ajwain that induced instant immobilization of human spermatozoa *in vitro* was 125 µg/ml and the effect was irreversible. A significant decrease inviability was also seen as assessed by eosin-nigrosin and fluorescence dual staining. Moreover, the treated sperm showed a significant loss of functional mitochondria and antioxidant enzyme, catalase (EC 1.11.1.6, CAT), when compared to control. The cholesterol:phospholipid ratio increased in treated sperm, which is an indicator of loss of binding ability of human spermatozoa to the zona pellucida. The scanning electron microscopic studies demonstrated the loss of membrane integrity in essential oil-treated human spermatozoa, which showed vacuolation, swelling of acrosomal cap, detachment of head portion and tail coiling. Thus, Paul and Kang (2012) concluded that ajwain could be useful in developing medicinal preparations as a male as well as vaginal contraceptive. The National Dairy Research Institute in India estimated the estrogenic content of *T. ammi* that is traditionally used to increase milk yield in dairy cattle as well as in humans. The total phytoestrogen content of dry *T. ammi* seed was 473 ppm (Kaur, 1998).

Antiurolithiatic Effect

Many medicinal plants have been employed since ages to treat urinary stones, though the rationale behind their use is not well established. Till date various plant extracts have been studied to reduce the incidence of urolithiasis but the identification of naturally occurring calcium oxalate (CaOx) inhibitory biomolecules from plants was hampered in past by limitation in analytical techniques. Fortunately, Kaur *et al.* (2009 a) isolated a novel calcium oxalate (CaOx) crystal growth inhibitor (an anti calcifying protein, having molecular weight 107 kDa and isolectric point 6.2) and purified by three step purification scheme (ammonium sulphate fractionation, anion exchange chromatography and molecular sieve chromatography) from the seeds of ajwain. The anti lithiatic potential of ajwain anticalcifying protein was confirmed by its ability to (a) maintain renal functioning and reduce renal injury; and (b) decrease crystal retention in renal tissues by preventing calcium oxalate deposition. This forms the basis for the development of anti lithiatic drug interventions through ajwain against urolithiasis (Kaur *et al.*, 2009 b).

Detoxificant

The seed extract of ajwain showed more than 91 per cent degradation of aflatoxin G1 (AFG1) in 24 hrs and 78 per cent in 6 hrs. Significant degradation of other aflatoxins AFB1, AFB2 and AFG2 was also observed by the dialyzed seeds. But the activity significantly reduced on boiling the extract (Velazhahan *et al.*, 2010).

Conclusions

The multiple benefits of ajwain have been scientifically well established with analytical explanation of the possible mechanisms involved. The antifertility property of ajwain is valuable in the present day context of overpopulation and hence commercial use of this property is worth exploring.

References

Aggarwal, H, Kotwal N (2009). Foods used as Ethno-medicine in Jammu. Ethnomed. 3 (1): 65–68.

Anilakumar KR, Saritha V, Khanum F, Bawa AS (2009). Ameliorative effect of ajwain extract on hexachlorocyclohexane-induced lipid peroxidation in rat liver. Food Chem. Toxicol. 47 (2): 279–82.

Bairwa R, Sodha RS, Rajawat BS (2012). *Trachyspermum ammi*, Pharmacogn. Rev. 6 (11): 56–60.

Bajrai, AA (2010). Prevalence of crude drugs used in Arab folk medicine available in Makkah Al-Mukarramah Area. International Journal of Medicine and Medical Sciences. 2 (9): 256–62.

Bentely R, Trimen H (1999). Medicinal Plants. Asiatic Publishing House. New Delhi. pp. 107–15.

Boskabady MH, Jandaghi P, Kiani S, Hasanzadeh L (2005). Antitussive effect of *Carum copticum* in guinea pigs. J. Ethnopharmacol. 97: 79–82.

Caccioni DL, Guizzardi M, Biondi DM (2000). Relationships between volatile components of citrus fruit essential oil and antimicrobial action on *Penicillium digitatum* and *Penicillium italicum*. Int. J. Food Microbiol. 88: 170–75.

Choudhury S (1998). Composition of the seed oil of *Trachyspermum ammi* (L.) Sprague from northeast India. J. Essent. Oil Res. 10: 588–90.

Choudhury S, Riyazuddin A, Kanjilal PB, Leclercq PA (1998). Composition of the seed oil of *Trachyspermum ammi* (L.) Sprague from northeast India. J. Essent. Oil Res. 10: 588–90.

Dashti-Rahmatabadi MH, Hejazian SH, Morshedi A, Rafati A (2007). The analgesic effect of *Carum copticum* extract and morphine on phasic pain in mice. J. Ethnopharmacol. 109 (2): 226–28.

Devasankaraiah G, Hanin I, Haranath PS, Ramanamurthy PS (1974). Cholinomimetic effects of aqueous extracts from *Carum copticum* seeds. Br. J. Pharmacol. 52 (4): 613–14.

Dhiman K, Chaudhary K (2012). Chaturbeeja in primary dysmenorrhoea: an observational study. Journal of Pharmaceutical and Scientific Innovation. 1 (3): 27 -31.

Dwivedi SN, Dwivedi S, Patel PC (2006). Medicinal plants used by the tribal and rural people of Satna district, Madhya Pradesh, for treatment of gastro-intestinal diseases and disorders. Explorer research article.Vol. 5 (1).

Garg SN, Kumar S (1998).

A new glucoside from *Trachyspermumammi*. Fitoterapia. 6: 511–12.

Gilani AH, Jabeen Q, Ghayur MN, Janbaz KH, Akhtar MS (2005). Studies on the anti-hypertensive, antispasmodic, broncho-dilator and hepato-protective activities of the Carum copticum seed extract. J. Ethnopharmacol. 98 (1-2): 127–35.

Gopalan C, Rama Sastri BV, Balasubramanian SC. (Revised and Updated by) Narasinga Rao BS, Deosthale, YG, Pant KC (2000). NIN, ICMR, Hyderabad, India.

Gupta M, Kapoor AC, Khetarpaul N (2003). Development, acceptability and nutrient composition of traditional supplementary foods consumed by lactating women in India. Nutr. Health. 17 (2): 147–55.

Hawrelak JA, Cattley T, Myers SP. (2009). Essential oils in the treatment of intestinal dysbiosis: A preliminary *in vitro* study. Altern. Med. Rev. 14 (4): 380–84.

Hussain S Z, Malik RN (2008). Ethnobotanical properties and uses of medicinal plants of Morgah bio-diversity park, Rawalpindi. Pak. J. Bot. 40 (5): 1897–911.

Ishikawah T, Sega Y, Kitajima J (2001). Water-soluble constituents of ajwain. Chem. Pharm. Bull. 49: 840–44.

Jabbar A, Iqbal Z, Khan MN (2006). *In vitro* anthelmintic activity of *Trachyspermum ammi* seeds. Pharmacogn. Mag. 2: 126–29.

Javed I, Iqbal Z, Rahman ZU, Khan FH, Muhammad F, Aslam B and Ali L (2006). Comparative Aantihyperlipidemic Efficacy of *Trachspermum ammi* Extracts in Albino Rabbits. Pakistan. Vet. J. 26 (1): 23–29.

Javed IM, Akhtar T, Khaliq MZ, Khan G, Muhammad M (2002). Antihyperlipidaemic effect of *Trachyspermum ammi* (Ajwain) in rabbits. In: Faisalabad: Proc 33rd All Pakistan Science Conference University of Agriculture. 80–81.

Javed S, Ahmad AS, Haider MS, Umeera A, Ahmad, R, Mushtaq S (2012). Nutritional, phytochemical potential and pharmacological evaluation of *Nigella sativa* and *Trachyspermum ammi*. Journal of Medicinal Plants Research. 6 (5): 768–75.

Kaur H (1998). Estrogenic activity of some herbal galactogogue constituents. Indian J. Anim. Nutr. 15: 232–34.

Kaur GJ, Arora DS (2009). Antibacterial and phytochemical screening of *Anethum graveolens, Foeniculum vulgare* and *Trachyspermum ammi*. BMC Complement. Altern. Med. 9: 30.

Kaur T, Bijarnia RK, Singla SK, Tandon C (2009 a). Purification and characterization of an anticalcifying protein from the seeds of *Trachyspermum ammi* (L.). Protein Pept. Lett. 16 (2): 173–81.

Kaur T, Bijarnia RK, Singla SK, Tandon C (2009 b). *In vivo* efficacy of *Trachyspermum ammi* anticalcifying protein in urolithiatic rat model. J. Ethnopharmacol. 126 (3): 459–62.

Khan R, Zakir M, Afaq SH, Latif A, Khan AU (2010 a). Activity of solvent extracts of *Prosopis spicigera, Zingiber officinale* and *Trachyspermum ammi* against multidrug resistant bacterial and fungal strains. J. Infect. Dev. Ctries. 4 (5): 292–300.

Khan R, Zakir M, Khanam Z, Shakil S, Khan AU (2010 b). Novel compound from *Trachyspermum ammi* (Ajowan caraway) seeds with antibiofilm and antiadherence activities against Streptococcus mutans: a potential chemotherapeutic agent against dental caries. J. Appl. Microbiol. 109 (6): 2151–59.

Kostyukovsky M, Rafaeli A, Gileadi C, Demchenko N, Shaaya E (2002). Activation of octopaminergic receptors by essential oil constituents isolated from aromatic plants: Possible mode of action against insect pests. Pest. Manage. Sci. 58: 1101–106.

Krishnamoorthy V, Madalageri MB (1999). Bishop weeds (*Trachyspermum ammi*): An essential crop for north Karnatka. J. Med. Aromat. Plant. Sci. 21: 996–98.

Kumari KS, Prameela M (1992). Effect of incorporating *Carum copticum* seeds in a high fat diet for albino rats. Med. Sci. Res. 20: 219–20.

Kwon Park Il, Junheon K, Sang-Gil L (2007). Nematicidal Activity of Plant Essential Oils and Components From Ajwain (*Trachyspermum ammi*), Allspice (*Pimenta dioica*) and Litsea (*Litsea cubeba*) Essential Oils Against Pine Wood Nematode (*Bursaphelenchus xylophilus*) J. Nematol. 39: 275–79.

Mathew N, Misra-Bhattacharya S, Perumal V, Muthuswamy K (2008). Antifilarial lead molecules isolated from *Trachyspermum ammi*. Molecules. 13 (9): 2156–68.

Mayaud L, Carricajo A, Zhiri A, Aubert G (2008). Comparison of bacteriostatic and bactericidal activity of 13 essential oils against strains with varying sensitivity to antibiotics. Lett. Appl. Microbiol. 47: 167-173.

Nagalakshmi S, Shankaracharya NB, Naik JP, Rao LJM (2000). Studies on chemical and technological aspects of ajowan (*Trachyspermum ammi* syn. *Carum copticum*) J. Food Sci. Technol. 37: 277–81.

Nath D, Sethi N, Srivastav S, Jain AK, Srivastava R (1997). Survey on indigenous medicinal plants used for abortion in some districts of Uttar Pradesh. Fitoterapia. 68: 223–25.

Paul S, Kang SC (2011). *In vitro* determination of the contraceptive spermicidal activity of essential oil of *Trachyspermum ammi* (L.) Sprague ex Turrill fruits. N. Biotechnol. 28 (6): 684–90.

Paul S, Kang SC (2012). Studies on the viability and membrane integrity of human spermatozoa treated with essential oil of *Trachyspermum ammi* (L.) Sprague ex Turrill fruit. Andrologia. 44. Suppl. 1: 117–25.

Pruthi JS (1992). Spices and Condiments. 4th ed. National Book Trust. New Delhi.

Ramaswamy S, Sengottuvelu S, Sherief S Haja, Jaikumar S, Saravanan R, Prasadkumar C *et al.* (2010). Gastro-protective Activity Of Ethanolic Extract of *Trachyspermum ammi* Fruit. Int. J. Pharm. Biosci. 1: 1–15.

Rasooli I, Fakoor MH, Yadegarinia D, Gachkar L, Allameh A, Rezaei MB (2008). Antimycotoxigenic characteristics of *Rosmarinus officinalis* and *Trachyspermum copticum* L. essential oils. Int. J. Food Microbiol. 122 (1-2): 135–39.

Saxena AP, Vyas KM (1986). Antimicrobial activity of seeds of some ethnomedicinal plants. J. Econ. Taxonomic. Bot. 8: 291–300.

Sidhu K, Kaur J, Kaur G, Pannu K (2007). Prevention and cure of digestive disorders through the use of medicinal plants. Journal of Hum.Ecol, 21 (2): 113–16.

Singh B, Kale RK (2010). Chemomodulatory effect of Trachyspermum ammi on murine skin and forestomach papillomagenesis. Nutr. Cancer. 62 (1): 74–84.

Singh G, Maurya S, Catalan C, De Lampasona MP. (2004) Chemical constituents, antifungal and antioxidative effects of ajwain essential oil and its acetone extract. J. Agric. Food Chem. 52 (11): 3292–96.

Singh I, Singh VP (2000). Antifungal properties of aqueous and organic extracts of seed plants against *Aspergillus flavus* and *A. niger*. Phytomorphology. 20: 151–57.

Singh DB, Singh SP, Gupta RC (1979). Antifungal effect of volatiles from seeds of some Umbelliferae. Trans. Br. Mycol. Soc. 73: 349–50.

Singh VK, Singh S, Singh DK (2003). Pharmacological effects of spices. In Recent Progress in Medicinal Plants. Phytochemistry Pharmacology. Vol. 2. Stadium Press. Houston, Texas, USA. pp. 321–53.

Srivastava KC (1988). Extract of a spice–omum (*Trachyspermum ammi*)-shows antiaggregatory effects and alters arachidonic acid metabolism in human platelets. Prostaglandins Leukot. Essent. Fatty Acids. 33 (1): 1–6.

Tambekar DH, Dahikar SB (2011). Antibacterial activity of some Indian ayurvedic preparations against enteric bacterial pathogens. Journal of Advanced Pharmaceutical Technology and Research. 2 (1): 24–29.

Tamurab T, Iwamoto H (2004). Thymol: A classical small molecule compound that has a dual effect (potentiating and inhibitory) on myosin. Biochem. Biophys. Res. Commun. 18: 786–91.

Thangam C, Dhananjayan R (2003). Anti-inflammatory Potential of the Seeds of *Carum copticum* Linn. Indian J. Pharmacol. 35: 388–91.

Vasudevan K, Vembar S, Veeraraghavan K, Haranath PS (2000). Influence of intragastric perfusion of aqueous spice extracts on acid secretion in anaesthetized albino rats. Indian J. Gastroenterol. 19 (2): 53–56.

Velazhahan R, Vijayanandraj S, Vijayasamundeeswari A, Paranidharan V, Samiyappan R, Iwamoto T, *et al.* (2010). Detoxification of aflatoxins by seed extracts of the medicinal plant, *Trachyspermum ammi* (L.) Sprague ex Turrill Structural analysis and biological toxicity of degradation product of aflatoxin G1. Food Control. 21: 719–25.

Wadhwa S, Bairagi M, Bhatt G, Panday M, Porwal A (2010). Antimicrobial activity of essential oils of *Trachyspermum ammi*. International Journal of Pharmaceutical and Biological Archives. 1 (2): 131–33.

Zahin M, Ahmad I, Aqil F (2010). Antioxidant and antimutagenic activity of *Carum copticum* fruit extracts. Toxicol. *In vitro*. 24 (4): 1243–49.

Chapter 2

Asafoetida

(*Ferula assafoetida*)

Asafoetida is also known as asant, food of the gods, giant fennel, Jowani badian, hing and tingis. In India it is known as Kaayam in Malayalam, Hing in Marathi, Gujarati, Hindi, Urdu, Ingua Telugu, and Perungayam in Tamil. Its overwhelming odor has given rise to its unusual names, "devil's dung" or 'stinking gum'. It was familiar in the early Mediterranean, having come by land across Iran. Though it is generally forgotten now in Europe, it emerged into Europe from a conquering expedition of Alexander the Great.

Asafoetida is the dried latex (gum oleoresin) exuded from the living underground rhizome or tap root of several species of Ferula (three of which grow in India). It is believed to be native to Iran. In India it is grown in Kashmir and in some parts of Punjab. The major supply of asafoetida to India is from Afghanistan and Iran. The species are distributed from the Mediterranean region to Central Asia. The Indian companies Laljee Godhoo and Laxmi Hing are the world's largest producers of compounded asafoetida.

It is a perennial plant growing to two metres tall, with stout, hollow, somewhat succulent stems 5-8 cm in diameter at the base of the plant. The leaves are 30–40 cm long, tripinnate or even more finely divided, with a stout basal sheath clasping the stem. The flowers are yellow, produced in large compound umbels.

Asafoetida is acrid and bitter in taste and emits a strong pungent odor due to the presence of sulphur compounds therein. Its odour and flavour become much milder and more pleasant on heating in oil or ghee, acquiring a taste and aroma reminiscent of sautéed onion and garlic. Since pure asafoetida is not preferred due to its strong flavour, it is mixed with starch and gum and sold as compounded asafoetida mostly in bricket form. It is also available in free flowing powder form. In India, it is used especially by Hindus and Jains in many vegetarian and lentil dishes not only to add flavour and aroma but also to reduce flatulence.

Varieties

There are two main varieties of asafoetida: 1. Hing Kabuli Safaid (Milky white Asafoetida) and 2. Hing Lal (Red Asafoetida). The white or pale variety is water soluble, while the dark variety is oil soluble.

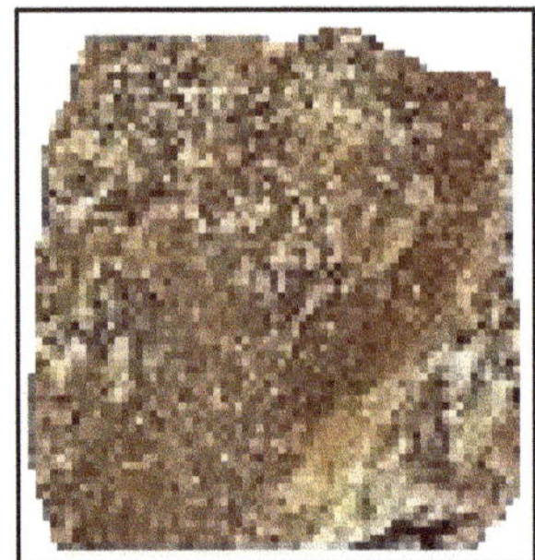

Hing Lal (Red Asafoetida)

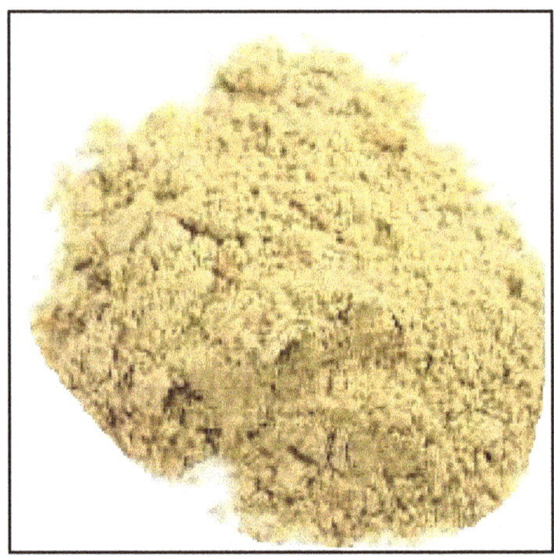

Kabuli Safaid (Milky white Asafoetida)

Chemical Composition

A wide range of chemical compounds including sugars, sesquiterpene coumarins and polysulfides have been isolated from hing plant (Iranshahy, 2011). Asafoetida contains Resin (40 – 65 per cent) chiefly asoresinotennol, free or combined with ferulic acid, Gum (25 per cent), Volatile oil (10–17 per cent) and ash (1.5-10 per cent). The resin portion is known to contain umbelliferone and four unidentified compounds (Singhal and Kulkarni, 1997). They are ferulic acid esters (60 per cent), free ferulic acid (1.3 per cent), coumarin derivatives – umbelliferone, foetidin and kamolonol and farnesiferoles A, B and C. One new sesquiterpene, asimafoetida- 1 was identified by Ghosh *et al.* (2009) the structure of which has been established from extensive 2D NMR spectral studies as 7'- [7–(1R,3S)–5- Hydroxy–6, 6 – dimethyl–2- methylene–cyclohexyl]–9-methyl–9- pentenyl]oxy]–2H – 1–benzo pyran – 2–one. Yet another new sesquiterpenoid coumarin, Saradaferin -1 named as [Decahydro–(3-alpha – hydroxyl–4,4,10 – trimethyl – 8 – methylene – 9–naphthenyl) -alpha- Hydroxy methyl] ether of umbelliferone was isolated from asafoetida resin by Bandyopadhyay *et al.* (2006). From the chloroform extract of the roots of asafoetida, two sesquiterpene coumarins designated assafoetidnol A and assafoetidnol B were isolated, in addition to six known compounds, gummosin, polyanthin, badrakemin, neveskone, samarcandin and galbanic acid (Abd El-Razek *et al.*, 2001).

The ethyl acetate-soluble fraction from a methanol extract of asafoetida has afforded six new sulfide derivatives, (1) (E)-3-methylsulfinyl-2-propenyl sec-butyl disulfide (foetisulfide A) (2) (Z)-3-methylsulfinyloxy-2-propenyl sec-butyl disulfide (foetisulfide B), (3) (E)-3-methylsulfinyloxy-2-propenyl sec-butyl disulfide (foetisulfide C), (4) bis(3-methylthio-2E-propenyl) disulfide (foetisulfide D), (5) 3,4,5-trimethyl-2-thiophenecarboxylic acid (foetithiophene A), (6) 3,4,5-trimethyl-2-(methylsulfinyloxymethyl) thiophene (foetithiophene B) along with other compounds (Duan *et al.*, 2002).

A new sesquiterpene ester, tunetanin A (1), a new sesquiterpene coumarin, tunetacoumarin A (2), together with eight known compounds, *i.e.*, coladin (3), coladonin (4), isosmarcandin (5), 13-hydroxyfeselol (6), umbelliprenin (7) propiophenone (8), beta-sitosterol (9), and stigmasterol (10), were isolated from the roots of Ferula tunetana (Jabrane *et al.*, 2010).

Volatile oil has sulfur-containing compounds: disulfides, symmetric tri- and tetrasulfides. Glucuronic acid, galactose, arabinose and rhamnose have also been isolated from the gum (Eigner and Scxhloz, 1999).

Traditional Therapeutic Usage

Ferula asafoetida is a well known phyto-medicine used in different parts of the world for various purposes. Not only is it used as a culinary spice but also traditionally used to treat various diseases, including asthma, gastrointestinal disorders (flatulence, abdominal pains and constipation), infections etc. The oleo-gum-resin of asafoetida has been known to possess antifungal, antidiabetic, anti-inflammatory, antimutagenic and antiviral activities (Iranshahy, 2011). Not only is asafoetida used as a phyto-medicine in India, its use has also been reported in western countries as a home remedy for various conditions. Residents of western countries such as Trinidad and Tobago, where the knowledge of use of natural foods as medicine was obtained from Chinese immigrants, reported the use of asafoetida as a carminative (Lans, 2007).

Asafoetida is said to be helpful in asthma and bronchitis. It also helps in relieving toothache, in treating migraines and tension headaches when mixed with water. It was one of the most commonly prescribed herbs for the treatment of hysteria and for many symptoms associated with mood swings and depression. A folk traditional remedy for children's colds is to make a paste and hang in a bag around the afflicted child's neck. It is an effective remedy for impotency. It is believed to be efficient in preventing snake bites and repelling insects when mixed with garlic.

Interestingly, in Jamaica, asafoetida is traditionally applied to a baby's anterior fontanel (Jamaican patois "mole") in order to prevent spirits (Jamaican patois "duppies") from entering the baby through the fontanel. In the African-American Hoodoo tradition, Asafoetida is used in magic spells as it is believed to have the power to curse.

In Thailand and India, it is used to aid digestion and is smeared on the abdomen in an alcohol or water tincture known as maha hing. In the Jammu region of India, Asafoetida is used as a medicine for flatulence and constipation by 60 per cent of locals (Aggarwal and Kotwal, 2009; Dwivedi *et al.*, 2006). The use of Asafoetida in different villages of Keshavraipatan tehsil in Bundi district, Rajasthan for abdominal pain was reported to yield positive results as evident from the reduction or total cure of abdominal pain (Shekhawat and Batra, 2006).

In Unani, Ayurveda and Arab traditional medicine asafoetida is used for various ailments, including spasms, flatulence, constipation, flatulent colic and as carminative (Leung 1980; Newall *et al.*, 1996). Asafoetida oleo-gum-resin has been reported to be antiepileptic in classical Unani, as well as ethno-botanical literature (Abdin *et al.*, 2006). In Pakistan it is used as antibiotic and to keep small children healthy by protecting them from diseases. In Ayurveda, asafoetida is considered to be one of the best spices for balancing the vata dosha. (Amadea and Desai, 1991). It is claimed to be a nerve stimulant. It is also claimed to have antispasmodic, hypotensive (Fatehi *et al.*, 2004)), anticancer (Mallikarjuna *et al.*, 2003) and antidiabetic properties (Abu-Zaiton, 2010).

A survey conducted in southern parts of India reported the use of asafoetida as a home remedy for treating dyspepsia, flatulence, whooping cough and bronchitis among children. It was also used as an anthelmentic. The information was gathered from local people, personal diaries of foresters, indigenous doctors, plant collectors, tribes and herbal vendors of Puducherry and nearby areas of Tamilnadu (Dixit, 2011).

Some of the medicinal properties/applications of asafoetida have been thoroughly studied and confirmed as listed below.

Asafoetida as an Antioxidant

Animal studies have shown that asafoetida possesses antioxidant ((Mallikarjuna *et al.*, 2003) and cholesterol lowering properties (Srinivasan and Srinivasan, 1995). Acetyl choline esterase (AChE) inhibitors and memantine have shown clinical efficacy in improving cognitive function in mild to moderate AD (Upadhyaya *et al.*, 2010).

Reports reveal that asafoetida has acetyl-cholinesterase inhibiting property as evidenced by *in vitro* assay and *in vivo* action on snail nervous system (Kumar *et al.*, 2009). It exhibited a consistent enzyme inhibition activity when measured on two separate occasions. This can be taken as an indirect evidence of its ability to cross blood brain barrier effectively (Vijayalakshmi *et al.*, 2012). It consistently increased total protein thiols (antioxidants) in serum at 400 mg dose. This finding is in agreement with earlier reports which demonstrated asafoetida's antioxidant potential and inhibition of lipid peroxidation in rats (Mallikarjuna *et al.*, 2003). The protective effect of asafoetida extract may be partly attributed to its antioxidant property by virtue of which brain cells are subjected to less oxidative stress resulting in less brain damage and improved neuronal function, thereby enhancing memory.

Among the flower, stem and leaf extracts of asafoetida as antioxidant and antihemolytic agents, the leaf aqueous-ethanol extract showed the highest activity in DPPH radical scavenging activity. All extracts showed weak nitric oxide scavenging activity. The stem extract had better activity in nitric oxide scavenging model than the other extracts. These biological effects may be attributed to the presence of phenols and flavonoids in the extract. (Nabavi *et al.*, 2011).

Antimicrobial

Asafoetida was used in 1918 to fight the Spanish influenza pandemic. In 2009, scientists at the Kaohsiung Medical University in Taiwan reported that the roots of asafoetida produce natural antiviral drug compounds that kill the swine flu virus, H1N1. In an article published in the American Chemical Society's Journal of Natural Products, the researchers said the compounds may serve as promising lead components for new drug development against this type of flu (Lee *et al.*, 2009).

Asafoetida has a broad range of uses in traditional medicine as an antimicrobial agent with well documented uses for treating chronic bronchitis and whooping cough, as well as reducing flatulence (Srinivasan, 2005).

Asafoetida decreased counts and viability of all tested isolates of blastocystis sp. subtype 3 which was confirmed by microscopy. The degree of the inhibitory effect was dependent on the concentration, form, as well as the time of incubation with asafoetida extracts. The lowest concentrations of 16 and 40 mg/ml, of asafoetida powder and oil respectively caused 100 per cent inhibition of blastocystis growth and 100 per cent inhibition of multiplication (El Deeb *et al.*, 2012).

Asafoetida had a potent antiparasitic effect on *T. vaginalis* compared to metronidazole, thus, worth further investigation on its applicability in treatment of parasitic infections (Ramadan and Khadrawy, 2003). Ramadan *et al.* (2004) confirmed a highly significant antiparasitic effect of asafoetida with regard to the mean worm burden and tissue egg count in mice experimentally infected with *Schistosoma mansoni* (intestinal parasite). Both the oil and the powder form of asafoetida were effective as compared to the control group.

Antidiabetic

Asafoetida induced significant reduction in blood glucose concentration. A significant rise in insulin secretion was seen in diabetic animals treated with asafoetida extract in comparison with control diabetic animals. Thus, Abu-Zaiton (2010) confirmed that treatment with the extract exerts therapeutic protective effect in diabetes by preserving pancreatic beta-cells integrity and activity, which supports traditional usage of asafoetida to prevent diabetic complications.

Anticarcinogenic

Using human umbilical vein endothelial cell (HUVEC) model, galbanic acid isolated from asafoetida was found to exert anticancer activity in association with antiangiogenic and anti-proliferative actions (Kim *et al.*, 2011). The 50 per cent inhibitory concentration (IC-50) of coumarin-derived sesquiterpene galbanic acid against protein farnesyltransferase in an enzyme-based assay was calculated as 2.5 μM. This compound also demonstrated potent inhibition of the proliferation of oncogenic RAS-transformed NIH3T3/Hras-F in a dose-dependent manner (Cha *et al.*, 2011). Lee *et al.* (2009) found some compounds from the chloroform fraction of asafoetida extract to show excellent potency against influenza A virus (H(1)N(1) and some others to exhibit the best potency against the HepG2, Hep3B, and MCF-7 cancer cell lines. Orally administered asafoetida, however, showed a weak sister-chromatid exchanges-inducing effect in spermatogonia of mice (Abraham and Kesavan, 1984).

Acetone extract from asafoetida afforded two drimane sesquiterpene dienones (fetidones A and B) and several known sesquiterpene coumarin ethers, one of which (8-acetoxy-5-hydroxyumbelliprenin, 2a) showed potent and specific NF-kappa B-inhibiting properties. This, coupled with a negligible cytotoxicity, qualifies 8-acetoxy-5-hydroxyumbelliprenin, 2a as a new anti-inflammatory chemotype, and its occurrence in asafoetida might rationalize the use of this gum resin to alleviate and prevent colon inflammatory disturbances (Appendino *et al.*, 2006). Asafoetida treatment resulted in a significant reduction in the levels of cytochrome P450 and b5 and in the multiplicity ($p < 0.001$) and size of palpable mammary tumours ($p < 0.005$-0.001), and a delay in mean latency period of tumour appearance ($p < 0.005$). From these observations Mallikarjuna *et al.* (2003) indicated the chemopreventive potential of asafoetida against N-methyl-N-nitrosourea-induced mammary carcinogenesis in Sprague-Dawley rats. Saleem *et al.* (2001) concluded from their study, that asafoetida is a potent antioxidant and can afford protection against free radical mediated diseases such as carcinogenesis, as the pretreament of animals with asafoetida recovered the antioxidant level and reversed the induced ODC activity and DNA synthesis significantly.

Antispasmodic

The role of asafoetida in treating abdominal pain and spasms could be attributed to its effects on variety of muscarinic, adrenergic and histamine receptor activities or with mobilization of calcium ions required for smooth muscle contraction. The asafoetida gum extract was found to cause relaxation of the precontracted ileum in a concentration dependent manner, thus exhibiting its antispasmodic potential (Fatehi *et al.*, 2004) and supporting its age-old use in Unani and Ayurvedic medicines. It is prescribed in Unani medicine for relieving abdominal spasms in dysmennorhoea (Arif *et al.*, 2012) and is an essential component of Shankha-vati, a classical ayurvedic formulation for gastro-intestinal disorders such as Shula, Gulma, Udara, Anhana, Krimi and is well known for pacifying Vata and Kapha (Kodlady and Patgiri, 2012).

Hypotensive

Asafoetida gum extract (0.3-2.2 mg/100 g body weight) significantly reduced the mean arterial blood pressure in anaesthetized rats. Fatehi *et al.* (2004) concluded that the relaxant compounds in asafoetida gum extract might interfere with a variety of muscarinic, adrenergic and histaminic receptor activities or with the mobilization of calcium ions required for smooth muscle contraction non-specifically.

Contraceptive

Asafoetida has also been reported to have contraceptive/abortifacient activity (Riddle 1992) and is related to (and considered an inferior substitute for) the ancient Ferulaspecies Silphium. Treatment of rats from days 1 to 7 of pregnancy with the extract resulted in pregnancy failure in about 65-85 per cent of the animals. Asafoetida appeared to interrupt the Hexosemonophosphate metabolic pathway more significantly. Keshri *et al.* (2004) thus concluded that plants lacking phyto-estrogens may intercept pregnancy by their ability to disrupt energy metabolism in rat uterus during implantation, especially the oxidative pathway.

Memory Booster

Certain plant products and diet rich in antioxidants are said to be neuroprotective and hence may have a role in improving cognition in aging and neurodegenerative diseases (Balenahalli *et al.*, 2010; Joseph *et al.*, 2009). Oral administration of two doses (200 mg/kg and 400 mg/kg) of asafoetida aqueous extract with rivastigmine as positive control produced significant improvement in memory score *i.e.* step through latency at 400 mg/kg dose in passive avoidance model ($P < 0.05$) and dose-dependent improvement of transfer latency in elevated plus maze model ($P < 0.001$). Dose-dependent inhibition of brain cholinesterase ($P < 0.001$) and significant improvement in antioxidant levels ($P < 0.05$) were also noted. Vijayalakshmi *et al.* (2012) attributed this memory enhancing potential of asafoetida to inhibition of acetyl cholinesterase and antioxidant properties. Hence, it can be employed as an adjuvant to existing antidementia therapies.

Conclusions

Apart from the fact that many studies have been conducted on the therapeutic benefits of asafoetida, there is paucity of research on the growth of gut microflora and flatulence that would confirm few more traditional beliefs.

References

Abd El-Razek MH, Ohta S, Ahmed AA, Hirata T (2001). Sesquiterpene coumarins from the roots of Ferula assa-foetida. Phytochemistry. 58 (8): 1289-95.

Abdin, MZ Abdin, Abrol YP (2006). Traditional Systems of Medicine. Published by Alpha Science Int'l Ltd. ISBN 81-7319-707-5.

Abraham SK, Kesavan PC (1984). Genotoxicity of garlic, turmeric and asafoetida in mice. Mutat. Res. 136 (1): 85-88.

Abu-Zaiton AS (2010). Antidiabetic activity of Ferula assafoetida extract in normal and alloxan-induced diabetic rats. Pak. J. Biol. Sci. 13 (2): 97–100.

Aggarwal H and Kotwal N (2009). Foods Used as Ethno-medicine in Jammu. Ethno-Med. 3 (1): 65–68.

Amadea M and Desai U (1991). The Ayurvedic Cookbook by Lotus Light, p. 74.

Appendino G, Maxia L, Bascope M, Houghton PJ, Sanchez-Duffhues G, Muñoz E, Sterner O (2006). A meroterpenoid NF-kappaB inhibitor and drimane sesquiterpenoids fromAsafoetida. J. Nat. Prod. 69 (7): 1101–1104.

Arif Zaidi SM, Khatoon K, Aslam KM (2012). Role of herbal remedies in Ussuruttams (Dysmenorrhoea). J. Acad.Indus.Res. 1 (3).

Balenahalli NR, Sathyanarayana Rao TS, Annamalai P, Kumar S, Jagannatha Rao KS (2010). Neuronutrition and Alzheimer's disease. J. Alzheimers Dis. 19: 1123–39.

Bandyopadhyay D, Basak B, Chatterjee A, Lai TK, Banerji A, Banerji J, Neuman A, Prangé T (2006). Saradaferin, a new sesquiterpenoid coumarin from Ferula assafoetida. Nat. Prod. Res. 20 (10): 961–65.

Cha MR, Choi YH, Choi CW, Kim YS, Kim YK, Ryu SY, Kim YH, Choi SU (2011). Galbanic acid, a cytotoxic sesquiterpene from the gum resin of *Ferula asafoetida*, blocks protein farnesyltransferase. Planta. Med. 77 (1): 52–54.

Dixit AK (2011). Some herbal remedies for common ailments of children in South India. J. Biosci. Tech. 2 (5): 379–84.

Duan H, Takaishi Y, Tori M, Takaoka S, Honda G, Ito M, Takeda Y, Kodzhimatov OK, Kodzhimatov K, Ashurmetov O (2002). Polysulfide derivatives from *Ferula foetida*. J. Nat. Prod. 65 (11): 1667–69.

Dwivedi SN, Sangeeta Dwivedi, Patel PC, 2006, Medicinal plants used by the tribal and rural people of Satna district, Madhya Pradesh.Explorer research article. 5 (1).

Eigner D, Scholz D (1999). *Ferula assafoetida* and *Curcuma longa* in traditional medical treatment and diet in Nepal. J. Ethnopharmacol. 67: 1–6.

El Deeb HK, Al Khadrawy FM, El-Hameid AK (2012). Inhibitory effect of *Ferula asafoetida* L. Umbelliferae) on *Blastocystis* sp. subtype 3 growth *in vitro*. Parasitol. Res.. [Epub ahead of print].

Fatehi M, Farifteh F, Fatehi-Hassanabad Z (2004). Antispasmodic and hypotensive effects of Ferula F. Foetida gum extract. J. Ethnopharmacol. 91: 321–24.

Ghosh A, Banerji A, Mandal S, Banerji J (2009). A new sesquiterpenoid coumarin from Ferula assafoetida. Nat. Prod. Commun. 4 (8): 1023–24.

Iranshahy M (2011). Traditional uses, phytochemistry and pharmacology of asafoetida (Ferula assa-foetida oleo-gum-resin)-a review. J. Ethnopharmacol. 134 (1): 1–10.

Jabrane A, Ben Jannet H, Mighri Z, Mirjolet JF, Duchamp O, Harzallah-Skhiri F, Lacaille-Dubois MA (2010). Two new sesquiterpene derivatives from the Tunisian endemic Ferula tunetana Pom. Chem. Biodivers. 7 (2): 392–99.

Joseph JA, Shukitt-Hale B, Willis LM (2009). Grape juice berries, and walnuts affect brain aging and behavior. J. Nutr. 139: 1813S–17.

Keshri G, Bajpai M, Lakshmi V, Setty BS, Gupta G (2004). Role of energy metabolism in the pregnancy interceptive action of *Ferula assafoetida* and *Melia azedarach* extracts in rat. Contraception. 70 (5): 429–32.

Kim KH, Lee HJ, Jeong SJ, Lee HJ, Lee EO, Kim HS, Zhang Y, Ryu SY, Lee MH, Lü J, Kim SH (2011). Galbanic acid isolated from *Ferula assafoetida* exerts *in vivo* anti-tumour activity in association with anti-angiogenesis and anti-proliferation. Pharm. Res. 28 (3): 597–609.

Kodlady N, Patgiri, BJ (2012). Varieties in Shankha vati- an ayurvedic classical formulation for gastro-intestinal disorders, Ann Ayurvedic Medicine 1 (3).

Lans C (2007). Comparison of plants used for skin and stomach problems in Trinidad and Tobago with Asian ethnomedicine. Journal of Ethnobiology and Ethnomedicine. 3: 3.

Lee CL, Chia-Lin Lee, Lien-Chai Chiang, Li-Hung Cheng, Chih-Chuang Liaw, Mohamed H. Abd El-Razek, Fang-Rong Chang, Yang-Chang Wu (2009). Influenza A (H1N1) Antiviral and Cytotoxic Agents from *Ferula assafoetida*. Journal of Natural Products. 72 (9): 1568–72.

Leung AY (1980). Encyclopedia of common natural ingredients used in food, drugs and cosmetics. John Wiley and Sons. 409.

Mallikarjuna GU, Dhanalakshmi S, Raisuddin S, Rao A (2003). Chemomodulatory influence of *Ferula foetida* on mammary epithelial differentiation, hepatic drug metabolizing enzymes, antioxidant profiles and *N*-methyl-*N*-nitrosourea-induced mammary carcinogenesis in rats. Breast Cancer Res. Treat. 81: 1–10.

Nabavi SM, Ebrahimzadeh MA, Nabavi SF, Eslami B, Dehpour AA (2011). Antioxidant and antihaemolytic activities of *Ferula foetida* regel (Umbelliferae). Eur. Rev. Med. Pharmacol. Sci. 15 (2): 157–64.

Newall CA, Anderson LA, Phillipson JD (1996). Herbal Medicines–A guide for healthcare professionals. Pharmaceutical Press, London. pp. 1–296.

Ramadan NI, Abdel-Aaty HE, Abdel-Hameed DM, El Deeb HK, Samir NA, Mansy SS, Al Khadrawy FM (2004). Effect of *Ferula assafoetida* on experimental murine *Schistosoma mansoni* infection. J. Egypt. Soc. Parasitol. 34 (3 Suppl): 1077–94.

Ramadan NI, Al-Khadrawy FM (2003). The *in vitro* effect of Asafoetida on *Trichomonas vaginalis*. J. Egypt. Soc. Parasitol. 33 (2): 615–30.

Riddle, JM (1992). Contraception and abortion from the ancient world to the enaissance. Harvard University Press p. 28.

Saleem M, Alam A, Sultana S (2001). Asafoetida inhibits early events of carcinogenesis: a chemo-preventive study. Life Sci. 68 (16): 1913–21.

Shekhawat D, Batra B (2006). Household remedies of Keshavraipatan tehsil in Bundi district, Rajasthan. Indian Journal of Traditional Knowledge. 5 (3): 362–67.

Singhal RS and Kulkarni PR (1997). Handbook of Indices of Food Quality and Authenticity, Woodhead Publishing, Food industry and trade. ISBN 1-85573-299–98.

Srinivasan K (2005). Role of Spices Beyond Food Flavouring: Nutraceuticals with Multiple Health Effects. Food Reviews International. 21 (2): 167–88.

Srinivasan MR, Srinivasan K (1995). Hypo-cholesterolemic efficacy of garlic smelling flower *Adenocalymma alliaceum* Miers.in experimental rats. Indian J. Exp. Biol. 33: 64–66.

Upadhyaya P, Seth V, Ahmad M (2010). Therapy of Alzheimer's disease: An update. Afr. J. Pharm. Pharmacol. 4: 408–21.

Vijayalakshmi, Adiga S, Bhat P, Chaturvedi A, Bairy KL, Kamath S (2012). Evaluation of the effect of *Ferula asafoetida* Linn. gum extract on learning and memory in Wistar rats. Indian J. Pharmacol. 44 (1): 82–87.

Chapter 3

Cinnamon

(*Cinnamomon zeylanicun*)

Cinnamon has been known from time immemorial. The Hebrew Bible makes specific mention of the spice many times. Though its source was kept mysterious in the Mediterranean world for centuries by the middlemen who handled the spice trade to protect their monopoly as suppliers, cinnamon is native to Sri Lanka (Encyclopaedia Britannica. 2008). Asian cultures considered cinnamon a key to long life. Cinnamon has been used as a spice for centuries. It is an ancient herbal medicine mentioned in Chinese texts as long as 4,000 years ago. It belongs to the family of Lauraceae. The name cinnamon comes from Greek kinnámômon, from Phoenician and akin to Hebrew qinnâmôn, which means sweet wood. Most people are familiar with the sweet but pungent taste of the oil, powder, or sticks of bark from the cinnamon tree. Cinnamon trees grow in a number of tropical areas, including parts of India, China, Madagascar, Brazil, and the Caribbean.

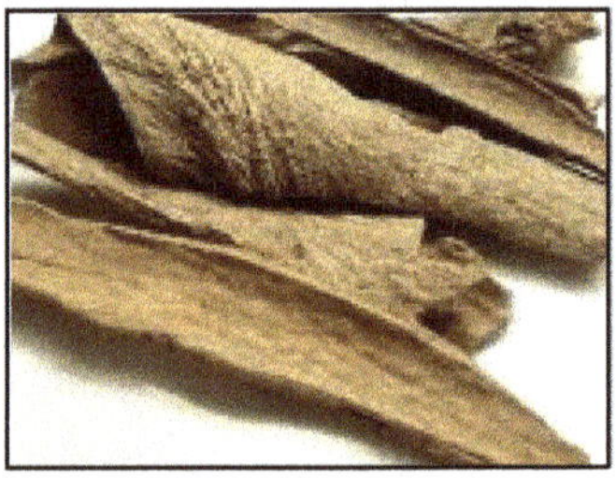

Cinnamon Bark

According to the International Herald Tribune, in 2006 Sri Lanka produced 90 per cent of the world's cinnamon, followed by China, India, and Vietnam. According to the FAO, Indonesia produces 40 per cent of the world's *Cassia* genus of cinnamon. The physical characteristics of cinnamon vary with the variety. *e.g. Ceylon cinnamon*, has a finer, less dense and more crumbly texture, and is less stronger than *C. aromaticum* (cassia-Chinese cinnamon) whereas Cassia is generally a medium to light reddish brown, hard and woody in texture and thicker (2–3 mm).

Sri Lankan cinnamon and cinnamon from the Seychelles Island are considered to be the best. In India, cinnamon is grown on the West coasts. It is also called Darchini in Hindi, Lavangpattai in Kannada, Darushila in Sanskrit and Sanna-lavangapattai in Tamil. In 1767 Lord Brown of East India Company established Anjarakkandy Cinnamon Estate near Anjarakkandy in Cannanore (now Kannur) district of Kerala, and this estate became Asia's largest cinnamon estate.

Different Varieties of Cinnamon

- ☆ *C. verum* (Sri Lanka cinnamon or Ceylon cinnamon).
- ☆ *C. burmannii* (Korintje or Indonesian cinnamon).
- ☆ *C. loureiroi* (Saigon cinnamon or Vietnamese cinnamon).
- ☆ *C. aromaticum* (Cassia or Chinese cinnamon).

Processing of Cinnamon

The outer bark of the branches of the tree, *i.e.*, the woody portion is discarded. Then by beating the branch evenly with a hammer the thin inner bark (0.5 mm/0.020 in) is loosened and dried or powdered. Thus Cinnamon, the brown bark of the cinnamon tree, is available in its dried tubular form known as a quill or as ground powder.

The barks, when whole, are easily distinguished, and their microscopic characteristics are also quite distinct. Ceylon Cinnamon sticks (or quills) have many thin layers and can easily be made into powder using a coffee or spice grinder, whereas cassia sticks are much harder. Indonesian cinnamon is often sold in neat quills made up of one thick layer. Saigon cinnamon and Chinese cinnamon are always sold as broken pieces of thick bark, as the bark is not supple enough to be rolled into quills. The powdered bark is harder to distinguish, but if it is treated with tincture of iodine (a test for starch), little effect is visible with pure Ceylon cinnamon, but when Chinese cinnamon is present, a deep-blue tint is produced (Pereira, 1854) exhibiting a difference in their composition.

Nutritional/Chemical Composition

Cinnamon is highly valued for its essential oil which is obtained from various parts of the cinnamon tree. The green leaves of cinnamon yield 1 per cent essential oil on steam distillation. The leaf oil is yellow to yellowish brown in colour with a slight camphoraceous odor resembles that of clove oil. The root bark of cinnamon yields 3 per cent oil, which differs from both stem bark and leaf oils. The seeds of cinnamon contain 33 per cent fixed oil, formerly used for making candles. Medicinal oil also called 'cinnamon suet', can be obtained from its fruits by heating to boil crushed ripe fruits suspended in water. The oleaginous matter rises to the surface and solidifies on cooling.

Various terpenoids found in the volatile oil are believed to account for cinnamon's medicinal effects. Important among these compounds are eugenol and cinnamaldehyde. Cinnamon oil, an aromatic essential oil that makes up to 0.5 per cent–1 per cent of its composition is responsible for its aroma. The pungent taste and

Nutritional Composition of Cinnamon

Nutrient	*Amount*	*Nutrient*	*Amount*
Calcium (mg)	1002	Iron (mg)	8.32
Magnesium (mg)	60	Phosphorus (mg)	64
Potassium (mg)	431	Sodium (mg)	10
Zinc (mg)	1.83	Nutrient	Amount
Energy (kcals)	247	Carbohydrate (gm)	80.59
Protein gm	3.99	Fat (gm)	1.24
Thiamin (mg)	0.022	Riboflavin (mg)	0.041
Niacin (mg)	1.332	Vitamin A (IU)	295
Vitamin K (μg)	31.2	Folate (μg)	6
Vitamin B6 (mg)	0.158		

USDA (2012).

scent come from cinnamic aldehyde or cinnamaldehyde (about 60 per cent of the bark oil). The colour gets darkened by the absorption of oxygen and develops resinous compounds. Other chemical components of the essential oil include ethyl cinnamate, eugenol (found mostly in the leaves), beta-caryophyllene, linalool, and methyl chavicol. Cinnamon contains a moderately toxic component called coumarin. This is present in much lower amount in Cinnamomum burmannii due to its low essential oil content. Ceylon cinnamon is said to have negligible amounts of coumarin (Blumenthal *et al.*, 1998).

Culinary Uses of Cinnamon

Cinnamon has a broad range of historical uses in different cultures. Cinnamon powder has long been an important spice in Persian cuisine, used in a variety of thick soups, drinks, and sweets. It is often mixed with rose water or other spices to make a cinnamon-based curry powder for stews or just sprinkled on sweet treats. It is used in the preparation of chocolate, especially in Mexico, which is the main importer of true cinnamon. It is also used in the preparation of some kinds of desserts, such as apple pie, donuts, buns, spicy candies, tea, hot cocoa, and liqueurs. True cinnamon, rather than cassia, is more suitable for use in sweet dishes. In the Middle East, it is often used in savory dishes of chicken and lamb. In the United States, cinnamon and sugar are often used to flavour cereals, bread-based dishes, and fruits, especially apples, cakes, sweets and curry powder. A cinnamon-sugar mixture is even sold separately for such purposes. Cinnamon can also be used in pickling and pharmaceutical preparations. Cinnamon oil is used for flavouring sweets, confectionery and pharmaceutical preparations. Cinnamon buds are as good for flavouring and spicing as the bark itself.

Traditional Therapeutic Uses/Folkloric Beliefs of Cinnamon

The combination of Honey and Cinnamon is considered a very effective medicine for most kinds of diseases. Honey and cinnamon revitalize the clogged arteries and veins by unclogging. It is believed that arthritis gets cured by consuming two spoons of honey and one small teaspoon of cinnamon powder in one cup of hot water daily morning and night. Two tablespoons of cinnamon powder and one teaspoon of honey, in a glass of lukewarm water seems to cure bladder Infections.

Cinnamon is often used to cure common cold. Coarsely powdered and boiled cinnamon in a glass of water with a pinch of pepper powder and honey can be beneficially used as medicine in cases of influenza, sore throat, and malaria. Cinnamon oil, mixed with honey, gives relief from cold. As a part of home remedy its decoction is used to combat cough.

Cinnamon is aromatic, astringent, stimulant and carminative. It prevents nausea and vomiting and also stimulates digestion. A tablespoon of cinnamon water consumed half an hour after meals relieves flatulence and indigestion.

A pinch of cinnamon powder mixed with honey prevents nervous tension, improves complexion and memory if taken regularly every night. Cinnamon can be used for natural birth-control. It has the remarkable effect of checking the early release of ova after child-birth. Cinnamon if taken every night for a month after delivery is believed to delay menstruation and thus early conception by more than 15 to 20 months. It indirectly helps in the secretion of breast milk.

Cinnamon leaves are used in the form of powder or decoction to increase secretion and discharge of urine. Cinnamon is often used as a good mouth freshener. Applying a paste of finely powdered cinnamon mixed in water on the temples and forehead readily cures headache caused by exposure to cold air. Paste of cinnamon powder prepared with a few drops of fresh lime juice can be applied over pimples and blackheads with beneficial results. Cinnamon is highly beneficial in the treatment of several other ailments, including spasmodic afflictions, asthma, paralysis, excessive menstruation, uterus disorders and gonorrhea. It is sometimes used as a prophylactic agent, to control German measles. Scientific evidence for some of the therapeutic benefits of cinnamon is discussed below.

Antimicrobial Agent

The essential oil of cinnamon has antimicrobial properties (Lopez *et al.*, 2005). Preliminary human studies confirmed this effect in a clinical trial with AIDS patients suffering from oral candida (thrush) infections that improved with topical application of cinnamon oil (Quale *et al.*, 1996). *Cinnamomum cassia* bark extract was very effective against HIV-1 and HIV-2 (Premanathan *et al.*, 2000).

Antibacterial actions have also been demonstrated for cinnamon (Azumi *et al.*, 1997). Meades *et al.* (2010) studied cinnamon oil, its major component, TRANS-cinnamaldehyde, and an analogue, 4-hydroxy-3-methoxy-TRANS- cinnamaldehyde against bacterial acetyl-CoA carboxylase in an attempt to elucidate the mechanism of action. They found inhibition of the carboxyltransferase component of *E. coli*, acetyl-CoA carboxylase but no effect on the activity of the biotin carboxylase component. The inhibition patterns indicated that these products bound to the biotin binding site of carboxyltransferase with Trans-cinnamaldehyde. Thus, Meades *et al.* (2010) confirmed the antibacterial activity of Cinnamon.

Diabetes and CVD

Cinnamon has a long history as an antidiabetic spice. The cinnamon extract seems to have a moderate effect in reducing fasting plasma glucose (FBG) concentrations in diabetic patients with poor glycaemic control (Mang *et al.*, 2006). The beneficial effects of cinnamon on blood glucose control appear to be in part due to doubly-linked polyphenol type-A compounds (Anderson *et al.*, 2004). Over the past two decades, *in vitro* and *in vivo* data have been accumulating which support the role of cinnamon on glycemic control. For example, Jarvill-Taylor *et al.* (2001) reported that cinnamon stimulated glucose uptake, glycogen synthesis, and activated glycogen synthase in 3T3-L1 adipocytes. In rats, cinnamon enhanced glucose uptake by enhancing insulin-stimulated tyrosine phosphorylation of insulin receptor-β, insulin receptor substrate-1, and phosphatidyl inositol 3-kinase in a dose-dependent fashion (Qin *et al.*, 2003; 2004). Solomon and Blannin (2009) observed that while cinnamon improved glycemic control and insulin sensitivity, the effects were also quickly reversed.

Cinnamon has been reported to have remarkable pharmacological effects in the treatment of type 2 diabetes mellitus (DM) and insulin resistance (Verspohol *et al.*, 2005). Early *in vitro* studies showed that cinnamon can augment the action of insulin (Berrio *et al.*, 1992). But later, the same effect has also been proved in human trials. Recent advancement in phytochemistry has shown that cinnamtannin B1 isolated from *C. verum* is therapeutically effective in type 2 diabetes. Procyanidin oligomers in cinnamon are thought to be responsible for the biological activity in the treatment of diabetes mellitus (DM). Lu *et al.* (2010) found that administration of the cinnamon extracts significantly increased the consumption of extracellular glucose in insulin-resistant and normal HepG2 cells compared with the control group. These results suggest that both A- and B-type procyanidin oligomers in different Cinnamon species have hypoglycaemic activities and may improve insulin sensitivity in type 2 DM.

According to Sheng *et al.* (2008) cinnamon in its water extract form can act as a dual activator of Peroxisome proliferator-activated receptors (PPAR) gamma and alpha, and may be an alternative to PPAR gamma activator in managing obesity-related diabetes and hyper lipidemia. Kim and Choung (2010) confirmed that cinnamon extract significantly increases insulin sensitivity, reduces serum, and hepatic lipids, and improves hyperglycemia and hyperlipidemia possibly by regulating the PPAR-mediated glucose and lipid metabolism as the fasting and postprandial blood glucose levels in the cinnamon treated group were significantly lower than those in the control group; and the serum lipids and hepatic lipids were also improved.

Khan *et al.* (2003) demonstrated that intake of 1, 3, or 6 g of cinnamon per day reduces serum glucose, triglyceride, LDL cholesterol, and total cholesterol in people with type 2 diabetes and suggested that the inclusion of cinnamon in the diet of people with type 2 diabetes will reduce risk factors associated with diabetes and cardiovascular diseases. Mang *et al.* (2006) reported significantly higher reduction in fasting plasma glucose level without any adverse effects in the cinnamon treated diabetics (10.3 per cent) than in the placebo group (3.4 per cent). The decrease in plasma glucose correlated significantly with the baseline concentrations, indicating that subjects with a higher initial plasma glucose level may benefit more from cinnamon intake. However, no significant intra group or intergroup differences were observed regarding in HbA1c on cinnamon intervention.

Ziegenfuss *et al.* (2006) proved the efficacy of Cinnulin PF(R) supplementation on reducing FBG and systolic blood pressure (SBP), and improving body composition in men and women with the metabolic syndrome and suggested that this naturally-occurring spice can reduce risk factors associated with diabetes and cardiovascular diseases. But Kirkhaum *et al.* (2009) while proving the anti postprandial hyperglycaemic properties of cinnamon, felt that further research is required to confirm a possible correlation between baseline FBG and its reduction post supplementation and also to assess the potential of cinnamon to reduce pathogenic diabetic complications.

Dugoua *et al.* (2007) did not observe any beneficial effect of *Cassia cinnamon*, on glycosylated hemoglobin (HbA1c). But Saraswat *et al.* (2009) indicated the potential of certain dietary components to prevent and/or inhibit protein glycation. Supporting this, a daily intake of 2 g of cinnamon for 12 weeks resulted in decrease in glycated hemoglobin by 0.36 per cent, while the placebo group showed an increase of 0.12 per cent (P =.002). Changes in systolic (-4 mm Hg vs +1 mm Hg, P <.001) and diastolic (-4 mm Hg vs -1 mm Hg, P <.001) blood pressure also favoured the cinnamon group along with non significant differences in body weight (-2.9 per cent vs -0.5 per cent, P = 0.183) and waist circumference (-2.4 cm vs -0.6 cm, P =.354) as reported by Akilen *et al.* (2010). *In vitro* studies have demonstrated the mechanism of action of cinnamon on blood glucose which involve action of cinnamon as insulin mimetic, potentiation of insulin activity and/or stimulation of cellular glucose metabolism. Further, animal studies also have demonstrated strong hypoglycaemic properties of cinnamon. Thus, the use of cinnamon as an adjunct to the treatment of type 2 diabetes mellitus is the most promising area, but further research is needed before definite recommendations can be made (Gruenwald *et al.*, 2010).

Cinnamon in Metabolic Syndrome

In addition to the positive effects of cinnamon on glucose regulation, there are data which support the beneficial effects of cinnamon on blood pressure (Preuss *et al.*, 2006) and hyperlipidemias (Khan *et al.*, 2003). Compounds that improve insulin sensitivity include Chromium and polyphenols found in cinnamon. The beneficial effects and the responses are related to the duration of the study, form of Cr or cinnamon used and the extent of obesity and glucose intolerance of the subjects (Anderson, 2008). Qin *et al.* (2010) reviewed the available *in vitro* and *in vivo* studies on the clinical benefits of cinnamon. Human studies involving control subjects and subjects with metabolic syndrome, type 2 diabetes mellitus, and polycystic ovary syndrome all showed beneficial effects of whole cinnamon and/or aqueous extracts of cinnamon on glucose, insulin, insulin sensitivity, lipids, antioxidant status, blood pressure, lean body mass, and gastric emptying. However, not all studies have shown positive effects of cinnamon. The type and amount of cinnamon as well as the type of subjects and drugs consumed by the subjects are likely to affect the response to cinnamon. Thus, the components of cinnamon may be important in the alleviation and prevention of the signs and symptoms of metabolic syndrome, type 2 diabetes, and cardiovascular and related diseases.

Cinnamon as an Antioxidant

The role of cinnamon in oxidative stress has been well investigated and confirmed (Shan *et al.*, 2005; Blomhoff 2004: Mancini-Filho *et al.*, 1998; Chrysohoou *et al.*, 2006). Chrysohoou *et al.* (2006) recently reported an inverse relationship between body fat and antioxidant capacity, even after controlling for smoking, physical activity patterns, dietary habits, blood pressure, glucose levels, and lipid concentrations. Regular consumption of tea made from the bark of Sri Lanka cinnamon was reported to be beneficial in people with oxidative stress related illness in humans, as this part of the plant contains significant antioxidant potential.

Peng *et al.* (2008) reported for the first time that pro-anthocyanidins can effectively scavenge reactive carbonyl species and thus inhibit the formation of AGEs. As pro-anthocyanidins behave in a similar fashion as aminoguanidine, (the first AGE inhibitor explored in clinical trials), they show great potential to be developed as agents to alleviate diabetic complications.

Cancer

Colourectal cancer is a major cause of tumour-related morbidity and mortality worldwide. Pharmacological experiments suggest that the cinnamon-derived dietary factor cinnamic aldehyde (cinnamaldehyde) activates the nuclear factor-2-dependent antioxidant response in human epithelial colon cells and may therefore represent an experimental chemo-preventive dietary factor targeting colourectal carcinogenesis (Wondrak *et al.*, 2010). *In vitro* studies also showed that components of cinnamon control angiogenesis associated with the proliferation of cancer cells (Qin *et al.*, 2010).

Cinnamon extract inhibited vascular endothelial growth factor-induced endothelial cell proliferation, migration, and tube formation *in vitro*, sprouts formation from aortic ring *ex vivo*, and tumour-induced blood vessel formation *in vivo* (Lu *et al.* (2010). Thus, they reported that cinnamon could potentially be useful in cancer prevention and/or treatment.

Other Uses

The diterpenes in the volatile oil of cinnamon have shown antiallergic activity (Nagai *et al.*, 1982) as well. In addition, water extracts may help reduce ulcers (Akira *et al.*, 1986). Cinnamon has been shown to improve diarrhoea, rheumatism, and certain menstrual disorders *in vitro*, animal, and/or human studies (Leung and Foster, 1996).

Cinnamon bark is used extensively as an antimicrobial material and thus can be used as preservative. Both cinnamaldehyde and cinnamon oil vapours are potent antifungal compounds (Singh *et al.*, 1995).

Toxic Element

European health agencies have recently warned against consuming large amounts of cassia due to the presence of a moderately toxic component called coumarin which is known to cause liver and kidney damage in high concentrations. Therefore, only small amounts should be used initially in people who have not previously had contact with cinnamon, and anyone with a known allergy should avoid it. Chronic use of the concentrated oil may cause inflammation in the mouth. According to the German Commission E monograph, cinnamon is not recommended for use by pregnant women (Blumenthal *et al.*, 1998).

Safety Levels

Coumarin is a secondary phytochemical with hepatotoxic and carcinogenic properties. For the carcinogenic effect, a genotoxic mechanism was considered possible, but was discounted by the European Food Safety Authority in 2004 based on new evidence. This allowed the derivation of a tolerable daily intake (TDI) for the first time, and a value of 0.1 mg/kg body weight was arrived at based on animal hepatotoxicity data. The cause of the high susceptibility is currently unknown. The human data confirmed the TDI of the European Food Safety Authority. Nutritional exposure may be considerably, and is mainly due to use of cassia cinnamon, which is a popular spice especially, used for cookies and sweet dishes (Abraham *et al.*, 2011). Heavy consumers of *Cassia cinnamon* may reach a daily coumarin intake corresponding to the TDI. But the German Commission E monograph suggests half to 3/4 teaspoon (2–4 grams) of the powder per day (Blumenthal *et al.*, 1998) as a safe dose.

Conclusion

The use of cinnamon as an adjunct to the treatment of type 2 diabetes mellitus and CVD is the most promising area. But, scientific research is awaited on the anti-inflammatory properties and its effect on arthritis.

References

Abraham K, Wöhrlin F, Lindtner O, Heinemeyer G, Lampen A. (2010). Toxicology and risk assessment of coumarin: focus on human data. Mol. Nutr. Food Res. 54 (2): 228–39.

Anderson RA (2008). Chromium and polyphenols from cinnamon improve insulin sensitivity. Proc Nutr Soc. 67 (1): 48–53.

Anderson RA, Broadhurst CL, Polansky MM *et al.* (2004). Isolation and characterization of polyphenol type-A polymers from cinnamon with insulin-like biological activity. Agric. Food Chem. 52: 65–70.

Akilen R, Tsiami A, Devendra D, Robinson N (2010). Glycated Haemoglobin and Blood Pressure-Lowering Effect of Cinnamon in Multi-Ethnic Type 2 Diabetic Patients in the UK: A Randomized, Placebo-Controlled, Double-Blind Clinical Trial. *Diab Med.* 27: 1159-1167.

Azumi S, Tanimura A, Tanamoto K (1997) A novel inhibitor of bacterial endotoxin derived from cinnamon bark. *Biochem Biophys Res Commun* 234: 506–10.

Blomhoff R. (2004). Antioxidants and oxidative stress (Review) Tidsskr Nor Laegeforen. 124: 1643–45.

Blumenthal M, Busse WR, Goldberg A, *et al.* (eds). (1998). *The Complete Commission E Monographs: Therapeutic Guide to Herbal Medicines.* Boston, MA: Integrative Medicine Communications, 110–111.

Chrysohoou C, Panagiotakos DB, Pitsavos C, *et al.* (2006). The implication of obesity on total antioxidant capacity in apparently healthy men and women: The ATTICA study. Nutr Metab Cardiovasc. Dis.

Dugoua JJ, Seely D, Perri D, Cooley K, Forelli T, Mills E, Koren G (2007). From type 2 diabetes to antioxidant activity: a systematic review of the safety and efficacy of common and cassia cinnamon bark. Can. J. Physiol. Pharmacol. 85 (9): 837–47.

Encyclopaedia Britannica. (2008). Cinnamon. (species *Cinnamomum zeylanicum*).

Gruenwald J, Freder J, Armbruester N. (2010). Cinnamon and health. Crit Rev Food Sci Nutr. 50 (9): 822-34.

Jarvill-Taylor KJ, Anderson RA, Graves DJ. (2001). A hydroxychalcone derived from cinnamon functions as a mimetic for insulin in 3T3-L1 adipocytes. J. Am. Coll. Nutr. 20: 327–36.

Khan A, Safdar M, Ali Khan MM, Khattak KN, Anderson RA (2003). Cinnamon improves glucose and lipids of people with type 2 diabetes. Diabetes Care. 26 (12): 3215–18.

Kim SH, Choung SY (2010). Antihyperglycemic and antihyperlipidemic action of Cinnamomi Cassiae (Cinnamon bark) extract in C57BL/Ks db/db mice. Arch. Pharm. Res. 33 (2): 325–33.

Kirkham S, Akilen R, Sharma S, Tsiami A (2009). The potential of cinnamon to reduce blood glucose levels in patients with type 2 diabetes and insulin resistance. Diabetes Obes. Metab. (12):1100–113.

Leung AY, Foster S (1996). *Encyclopedia of Common Natural Ingredients Used in Foods, Drugs, and Cosmetics,* 2d ed. New York: John Wiley and Sons, 168–70.

López P, Sánchez C, Batlle R, Nerín C (2005). Solid- and vapor-phase antimicrobial activities of six essential oils: susceptibility of selected foodborne bacterial and fungal strains. J. Agric. Food Chem. 53 (17): 6939–46.

Lu Z, Jia Q, Wang R, Wu X, Wu Y, Huang C, Li Y (2010). Hypoglycaemic activities of A- and B-type procyanidin oligomer-rich extracts from different Cinnamon barks. Phytomedicine. 18.

Mancini-Filho J, Van-Koiij A, Mancini DA, Cozzolino FF, Torres RP (1998). Antioxidant activity of cinnamon (*Cinnamomum zeylanicum,* Breyne) extracts. Boll. Chim. Farm. 137 (11): 443–47.

Mang B, Wolters M, Schmitt B, Kelb K, Lichtinghagen R, Stichtenoth DO, Hahn A. (2006). Effects of a cinnamon extract on plasma glucose, HbA, and serum lipids in diabetes mellitus type 2. Eur. J. Clin. Invest. 36 (5): 340–44.

Meades G Jr, Henken RL, Waldrop GL, Rahman MM, Gilman SD, Kamatou GP, Viljoen AM, Gibbons S (2010). Constituents of cinnamon inhibit bacterial acetyl CoA carboxylase. Planta. Med. 76 (14): 1570–75.

Nagai H, Shimazawa T, Matsuura N, Koda A (1982). Immunopharmacological studies of the aqueous extract of *Cinnamomum cassia* (CCAq). I. Anti-allergic action. Jpn. J. Pharmacol. 32: 813–22.

Peng X, Cheng KW, Ma J, Chen B, Ho CT, Lo C, Chen F, Wang M (2008). Cinnamon bark proanthocyanidins as reactive carbonyl scavengers to prevent the formation of advanced glycation endproducts. J. Agric. Food Chem. 56 (6): 1907 – 1911.

Pereira J (1854). Elements of Materia Medica and Therapeutics. Vol. 2. p. 390.

Premanathan M, Rajendran S, Ramanathan T, Kathiresan K, Nakashima H, Yamamoto N (2000). A survey of some Indian medicinal plants for anti-human immunodeficiency virus (HIV) activity. The Indian journal of medical research. 112: 73–77.

Qin B, Nagasaki M, Ren M, *et al.* (2003). Cinnamon extract (traditional herb) potentiates *in vivo* insulin-regulated glucose utilization via enhancing insulin signaling in rats. Diabetes Res. Clin. Pract. 62: 139–48.

Qin B, Nagasaki M, Ren M, *et al.* (2004). Cinnamon extract prevents the insulin resistance induced by a high-fructose diet. Horm Metab Res. 36: 119–25.

Qin B, Panickar KS, Anderson RA (2010). Cinnamon: potential role in the prevention of insulin resistance, metabolic syndrome, and type 2 diabetes. J. Diabetes Sci. Technol. 4 (3): 685–93.

Quale JM, Landman D, Zaman MM, *et al.* (1996). *In vitro* activity of *Cinnamomum zeylanicum* against azole resistant and sensitive *Candida* species and a pilot study of cinnamon for oral candidiasis. *Am. J. Chin. Med.* 24: 103–109.

Saraswat M, Reddy PY, Muthenna P, Reddy GB (2009). Prevention of non-enzymic glycation of proteins by dietary agents: prospects for alleviating diabetic complications. Br J Nutr. 101 (11): 1714-21.

Shan B, Cai YZ, Sun M, Corke H (2005). Antioxidant capacity of 26 spice extracts and characterization of their phenolic constituents. J. Agric. Food Chem. 53 (20): 7749–59.

Sheng X, Zhang Y, Gong Z, Huang C, Zang YQ (2008). Improved Insulin Resistance and Lipid Metabolism by Cinnamon Extract through Activation of Peroxisome Proliferator-Activated Receptors. PPAR Res. 2008: 581348.

Sheng X, Zhang Y, Gong Z, Huang C, Zang YQ.(2008). Improved Insulin Resistance and Lipid Metabolism by Cinnamon Extract through Activation of Peroxisome Proliferator-Activated Receptors. PPAR Res.: 581348.

Singh HB, Srivastava M, Singh AB, Srivastava AK (1995). Cinnamon bark oil, a potent fungitoxicant against fungi causing respiratory tract mycoses. *Allergy*. 50: 995–99.

Solomon TP, Blannin AK (2009). Changes in glucose tolerance and insulin sensitivity following 2 weeks of daily cinnamon ingestion in healthy humans. Eur J Appl Physiol. 105 (6): 969–76.

Verspohl, Eugen J., Bauer, K; Neddermann, E (2005). Antidiabetic effect of *Cinnamomum cassia* and *Cinnamomum zeylanicum In vivo* and *In vitro*. Phytotherapy Research 19 (3): 203–206.

Wang JG, Anderson RA, Graham GM, Chu MC, Sauer MV, Guarnaccia MM, Lobo RA. (2007). The effect of cinnamon extract on insulin resistance parameters in polycystic ovary syndrome: a pilot study. Fertil. Steril. 88 (1): 240–43.

Wondrak GT, Villeneuve NF, Lamore SD, Bause AS, Jiang T, Zhang DD (2010). The Cinnamon-Derived Dietary Factor Cinnamic Aldehyde Activates the Nrf2-Dependent Antioxidant Response in Human Epithelial Colon Cells. Molecules 15 (5): 3338–55.

USDA (2012). National Nutrient Data base for standard reference, release 25.

Ziegenfuss TN, Hofheins JE, Mendel RW, Landis J, Anderson RA. (2006) Effects of a water-soluble cinnamon extract on body composition and features of the metabolic syndrome in pre-diabetic men and women. J. Int. Soc. Sports Nutr. 3 (2): 45–53.

Chapter 4

Cloves

(*Syzygium aromaticum*)

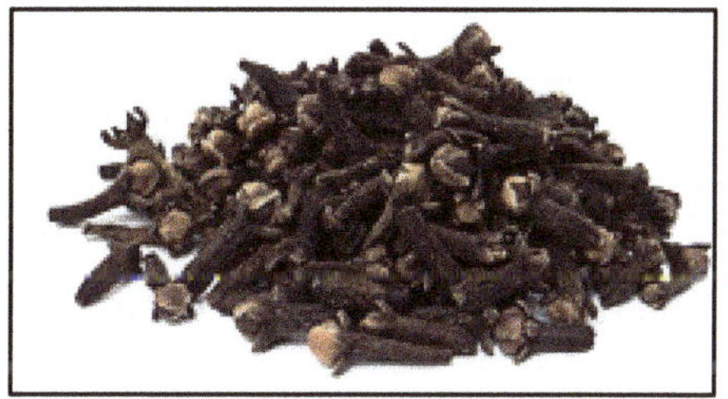

Cloves are one of the oldest spices in the world. The English name comes from Latin clavus 'nail' (also the origin of French clou and Spanish clavo, 'nail') as the buds vaguely resemble small irregular nails in shape. The synonyms are: *Caryophyllus aromaticus* L., *Eugenia aromatica* (L.) Baill, *Eugenia caryophyllata* Thunb. *Eugenia caryophyllus* (Spreng).

Cloves are the aromatic dried flower buds of a tree namely *Eugenia aromatica*, belonging to the family Myrtaceae. It is believed that the oldest clove tree in the world (350 and 400 years old), named "Afo," is found on Ternate. Cloves are native to the Maluku islands (historically called the Spice Islands), including Bacan, Makian, Moti, Ternate, and Tidore (in Indonesia) and used as a spice in cuisines all over the world. They are harvested primarily in Indonesia, India, Madagascar, Zanzibar, Pakistan, Tanzania,and Sri Lanka. During the 17th and 18th centuries, cloves were worth at least their weight in gold, due to the high cost of importing them in Britain.

Chemical Constituents

The oil extracted from various parts of the clove plant showed different chemical composition. The essential oil of clove buds was found to contain 36 different components, the most important being Eugenol (72-90 per cent) Chaieb *et al.* (2007a) which varied significantly between 15 clove samples cultivated in various countries

(Indonesia, Singapore, and China) (Yun *et al.*, 2010). Two new apigenin triglycosides, apigenin 6-C-[beta-D-xylopyranosyl-(1'''→2'')-beta-D-galactopyranoside]-7-O-beta-D-glucopyranoside and apigenin 6-C-[beta-D-xylopyranosyl–(1'''→2'')–beta-D-galactopyranoside]-7-O-beta-D-(6-O-p-coumaryl glucopyranoside) were isolated from the ethanol extract of the buds of cloves (Nassar, 2006) and eugenyl acetate 5.6 per cent, beta-caryophyllene 1.4 per cent and 2-heptanone 0.9 per cent in the clove bud oil (Chaieb *et al.*, 2007 a).

Gallic acid, caffeic acid, and syringic acid were present at levels of 1.58, 0.06, and 0.05 per cent (w/w), respectively, in *S. aromaticum* (Rastogi *et al.*, 2008). Liu *et al.* (2008) separated five compounds from the water extracts, identified as quercetin-3-O-glucuronide, quercetin-3-O-glucuronide 6''-methyl ester, quercetin-3-O-glucopyranoside, eugenyl-beta-rutinoside and myricetin.

The commercially rectified clove leaf essential oil contains a total of 23 constituents in including eugenol (76.8 per cent); beta-caryophyllene (17.4 per cent); alpha-humulene (2.1 per cent) and eugenyl acetate (1.2 per cent) as the main components (Jirovetz *et al.*, 2006). Eugeniin purified from *S. aromaticum* extract exhibited antiherpesvirus (HSV) activity in mice (Kurokawa *et al.*, 1998).

Nutritive Value of Cloves

Cloves are rich in iron, manganese, magnesium, phosphorus, sodium, calcium, potassium, and the vitamins C, K and A, besides dietary fiber.

Nutritional Value per 100 g

Nutrient	*Amount*	*Nutrient*	*Amount*
Energy (kcal)	25.2	Carbohydrates (g)	46.0
Dietary fiber (g)	9.5	Fat (g)	8.9
Protein (g)	5.2	Calcium (mg)	740.0
Iron (mg)	11.7	Magnesium (mg)	130.0
Phosphorus (mg)	100.0	Zinc (mg)	1.47
Thiamine (Vit. B1) (mg)	0.08	Riboflavin (Vit. B2) (mg)	0.13
B carotene (μg)	253.0		

Gopalan *et al.*, 2010.

Traditional Therapeutic Uses of Cloves

Due to their sweet aromatic flavour and powerful essential oil compounds, cloves have been used for hundreds of years as a nutritional spice for food and a remedy for a variety of health concerns. Thyme and cloves are routinely used as food additives in Omani food menus. Due to their strong aromatic flavour they mask the smell of poorly-kept foods and therefore used to preserve foods. In Mexican cuisine, cloves are best known as clavos de olor, and often used together with cumin and cinnamon.

Cloves are natural antiviral, antimicrobial, antiseptic, and antifungal agents. They also hold aphrodisiac and circulation-stimulating capacities. The oil of cloves has been used in a variety of health conditions including indigestion, generalized stress, parasitic infestations, cough, toothaches, headache, and blood impurities. In fact, the expert panel of German Commission recently approved the use of its essential oil as a topical antiseptic and anesthetic.

In West Africa, the Yorubas use water infusion of cloves called Ogun Jedi-jedi as a treatment for stomach upsets, vomiting and diarrhea. Cloves may be used internally as a tea and topically as oil for hypotonic muscles, including for multiple sclerosis. Use of clove as a memory booster is worth mentioning.

Eugenol, the chemical constituent of clove oil is responsible for its powerful analgesic, anesthetic, anti-inflammatory, and antibacterial effects, as well as its distinctive aromatic smell. The analgesic property of clove oil has been in use for treatment of various dental problems like tooth aches. They have a numbing effect on mouth. A cotton ball soaked in the clove oil is believed to work wonders on the aching tooth. Clove oil is also used to relieve pain from sore gums and to improve overall dental health. Thus nowadays it is a common ingredient in various dental creams, toothpastes, mouth wash, and throat sprays.

Cloves are also used to improve blood circulation and other ailments related to the heart, liver and stomach (stomach ulcers, loose stools, indigestion, nausea, gastric irritability and vomiting, flatulence and dyspepsia) since they stimulate the body's enzymes and boost digestion and help to fight against various diseases.

As Cloves and clove oil are antiseptic in nature they are expected to work as an effective remedy for some common problems such as cuts, fungal infections, burns, wounds, athlete's foot and bruises. Aroma therapists often use clove oil to treat the symptoms of rheumatism and arthritis. The aromatic clove oil, when inhaled, can relieve certain respiratory conditions like coughs, colds, asthma, bronchitis and sinusitis.

The scientific evidence for effect of cloves in various clinical conditions has been extensively studied and documented.

Oxidative Stress

Cloves contain a variety of flavonoids which contribute to its antioxidant and anti-inflammatory properties.

Eugenol which was the most abundant ingredient in plant extracts, showed the most potent antioxidative activity [ORAC(Oxygen radical absorbance capacity) value of 39,270 μmol TE (trolox equivalent)/g]. (Yoshimura *et al.*, 2011). Four eugenol-like molecules, daku-diisoeugenol, hydroxymethyleugenol, dihydroeugenol and 1,3-dioxanylphenol, synthesized using eugenol or isoeugenol of the essential oil of clove bud dried fruits from Eugenia caryophyllus had a more potent free radical scavenger activity than the reference compounds. Particularly, daku-diisoeugenol and 1,3-dioxanylphenol, were 3-fold more potent than vitamin E (Arenas *et al.*, 2011).

Petrovic *et al.* (2011) found that supplementation of the diet with clove flower buds powder combined with lemon balm extract or agrimony extract dissolved in drinking water has a potential to increase the antioxidant status but fails to influence either the growth performance or the selected lipid metabolism indices of broilers.

The clove bud essential oil showed the highest antioxidant activities among other sources. Mixtures containing clove bud essential oil also strongly inhibited oxidation of hexanal (Misharina and Samusenko, 2008). The clove extract-fed group had the smallest increase in body weight and height and the strongest antioxidant activity following a 5-week high cholesterol diet. Hydrophilic ingredients of cinnamon and clove showed potent activities to suppress the incidence of atherosclerosis and diabetes via strong antixidant potential, prevention of apoA-I glycation and LDL-phagocytosis, inhibition of cholesteryl ester transfer protein and hypolipidemic activity (Jin and Cho, 2011).

Between the two aroma extracts (Eucalyptus leaves and clove buds) tested, cloves exhibited the most potent antioxidant activities. The extracts inhibited malonaldehyde formation by 23 and 48 per cent, respectively, at the level of 400 μg/ml. Eugenol, thymol and benzyl alcohol inhibited malonaldehyde formation by 57, 43 and 32 per cent, respectively, at the level of 400 μg/ml (Lee and Shibamoto, 2001).

The antioxidant property of cloves due to their essential oil makes them suitable for food preservation. Even at lower concentrations, the scavenging activity of the essential oil against the 2,2-diphenyl-1-picryl hydracyl radical was reported to be higher than that of eugenol, butylated hydroxytoluene (BHT), butylated hydroxyanisole (BHA) and tert-butylated hydroxytoluene. This essential oil also showed a significant inhibitory effect against hydroxyl radicals and acted as an iron chelator. With respect to the lipid peroxidation, the inhibitory activity of clove oil determined using a linoleic acid emulsion system indicated a higher antioxidant activity than the standard BHT (Jirovetz *et al.*, 2006, Chaieb *et al.*, 2007b). Eugenol together with isoeugenol, thymol and carvacrol are attractive molecular models in pharmacological and biological studies related to Reactive Oxygen Species inhibition (Masteliæ *et al.*, 2008).

Inflammation

Leukotrienes are implicated in pathophysiology of allergic and inflammatory disorders like asthma, allergic rhinitis, arthritis, inflammatory bowel disease and psoriasis. 5-lipoxygenase (5-LO) is the key enzyme in biosynthetic pathway of leukotrienes. Raghavendra *et al.* (2006) reported that the inhibitory effect of eugenol, the active principle of clove on 5-LO was of a non-competitive nature. Further, eugenol significantly inhibit the formation of leukotriene C(4) in calcium ionophore A23187 and arachidonic acid stimulated Polymorphonuclear leukocytes cells.

Treatment of mice with water extract of clove was found to inhibit macrophages to produce proinflammatory cytokines both IL-1beta and IL-6. The essential oil of Clove also inhibited the production of these cytokines *in vitro* suggesting an anti-inflammatory action of this spice (Rodrigues *et al.*, 2009).

Bachiega *et al.* (2009) showed that clove administration to mice did not influence the Th1/Th2 cytokine balance. Later Bachiega *et al.* (2012) explained that the immunomodulatory/anti-inflammatory effects of cloves could be due to inhibition of LPS (Lipo Polysaccharide) action. A possible mechanism of action probably involved the suppression of the nuclear factor-ê pathway by eugenol. Further studies using different extract concentrations and different intake periods on cytokine expression and production will provide a better understanding of clove's immunomodulatory and anti-inflammatory actions.

Immunomodulation

Carrasco *et al.* (2009) established that the immunestimulatory activity found in mice treated with clove essential oil is due to improvement in humoral and cell-mediated immune response mechanisms. Clove essential oil increased the total white blood cell (WBC) count and enhanced the delayed-type hypersensitivity (DTH) response in mice. Moreover, it restored cellular and humoral immune responses in cyclophosphamide-immunosuppressed mice in a dose-dependent manner.

Clove oil administration produced a significant increase in the primary as well as secondary humoral immune response measured by the hemagglutination titre to sheep red blood cells. In addition, it also produced a significant decrease in foot pad thickness (measuring delayed type hypersensitivity) as compared to the control group thus suggesting that clove oil can modulate the immune response by augmenting humoral immunity and decreasing cell mediated immunity (Halder *et al.*, 2011).

Infections

The antimicrobial potential of cloves was established when its essential oil extracts killed many Gram positive and Gram negative organisms including some fungi (Gijzen *et al.*, 1991; Gislene *et al.*, 1999). The antimicrobial activity of clove is attributable to eugenol, oleic acid and lipids found in its essential oils (Hammer *et al.*, 1999). The biological activity of *Eugenia caryophyllata* has been proved on several microorganisms and parasites, including pathogenic bacteria, *Herpes simplex* and hepatitis C viruses and also against a large number of multiresistant *Staphylococcus epidermidis* isolated from dialysis biomaterials (Chaieb *et al.*, 2007 b).

Antibacterial

When the antibacterial activity of the clove oil and its major compounds, eugenol and β-caryophyllene were compared, the same was higher for clove oil than β-caryophyllene but was similar to eugenol against all tested oral bacteria suggesting that the clove oil and eugenol could be employed as a natural antibacterial agent against cariogenic and periodonto-pathogenic bacteria (Moon *et al.*, 2011). Eugenol from clove inactivated *Salmonella typhi* within 60 min exposure. The chemo-attractant property of eugenol combined with the observed high antibacterial activity at alkaline pH favours the fact that the compound can work more efficiently when given *in vivo*. Eugenol increased the permeability of the membrane and thus Devi *et al.* (2010) confirmed the disruptive action of eugenol on cytoplasmic membrane. A crude methonolic extract of clove exhibited preferential growth-inhibitory activity against Gram-negative anaerobic periodontal oral pathogens, including *Porphyromonas gingivalis* and *Prevotella intermedia*. Also the flavones, kaempferol and myricetin, isolated from cloves showed potent growth-inhibitory activity against the Periodontal pathogens *P. gingivalis* and *P. intermedia* (Cai and Wu, 1996). The water extract of clove oil showed inhibition of several organisms tested except *S. pyogenes*, *B. fragilis* and *C. albicans*, proving the fact that the anti bacterial effect of cloves is present in the oil fraction.

The oil was found to be extremely successful in the treatment of experimental murine vaginitis in model animals. There was a significant decrease in bacterial colonization after short-term feeding with clove oil compared with the controls ($p < 0.05$). Thus, dietary supplementation with clove oil protects against bacterial colonization of the lungs (Saini *et al.*, 2009).

Antifungal

Cloves displayed an important antifungal effect against the tested 53 human pathogenic yeasts using a disc paper diffusion method (Chaieb *et al.*, 2007b). The Essential oil of cloves and Eugenol showed inhibitory activity against all the tested *Candida*, *Aspergillus* and *dermatophytes* and American Type Culture Collection strains. Clove oil and eugenol also caused a considerable reduction in the quantity of ergosterol, a specific fungal cell membrane component. Clove oil was found to possess strong antifungal activity against opportunistic fungal pathogens such as *Candida albicans*, *Cryptococcus neoformans* and *Aspergillus fumigatus*, etc. Germ tube formation by *Candida albicans* was almost completely inhibited by oil and eugenol concentrations below the Minimum Inhibitory Concentration (MIC) values (Pinto *et al.*, 2009). Taguchi *et al.* (2005) demonstrated that oral intake of Clove suppressed the overgrowth of *C. albicans* in the alimentary tract including the oral cavity of Candida-infected mice. *C. albicans* was reported by several researchers (Hili *et al.*, 1997; Panizzi *et al.*, 1993; Piccaglia *et al.*, 1993) to be the most susceptible organism to thyme and Clove oil with concentration end-points of 0.1 per cent (1024) and 0.2 per cent (512) respectively.

On evaluating various formulations, topical administration of the liposomized clove oil was found to be most effective against treatment of vaginal candidiasis (Ahmad *et al.*, 2005).

Nzeako *et al.* (2006) showed that the country of origin/geographical location of cultivation has no effect on clove's antimicrobial activity as there was no significant difference between cloves obtained from Sri Lanka or Zanzibar. Eugenol was the most effective antifungal constituent of clove oil against the dermatophytes *T. mentagrophytes* and *M. canis* (Park *et al.*, 2007) and presented prominent antifungal action with MIC of 1 per cent and 4 per cent, respectively on fungal strains isolated from onychomycosis (Gayoso *et al.*, 2005). The activities of clove oil against the dermatophytes tested were highest (>60 per cent) at a concentration of 0.2 mg/ml. Clove oil also exhibited significant antifungal activity against *T. rubrum*, *E. floccosum*, and *M. gypseum*. Hyphal growth was completely inhibited in *T. mentagrophytes*, *T. rubrum*, and *M. gypseum* by treatment with clove oil at a concentration of 0.2 mg/ml.

Presence of anti-quorum sensing (QS) activity in clove oil and other essential oils has indicated new anti-infective activity. The identification of anti-QS phytoconstituents is needed to assess the mechanism of action against both *C. violaceum* and *P. aeruginosa* Because of its anti-QS activity clove bud essential oil might be important in reducing virulence and pathogenicity of drug-resistant bacteria *in vivo* (Khan *et al.*, 2009).

Antiparasitic

The Clove essential oil inhibited trophozoites adherence from the first hour of incubation and was able to kill almost 50 per cent of the parasite population in a time dependent manner. The eugenol inhibited *G. lamblia trophozoites* adherence only from the third hour and not induce cell lyses. On the basis of the above findings Machado *et al.* (2011) proposed that eugenol was responsible for the antigiardial activity of the S. aromaticum essential oil and both are potential for agents against giardiasis.

Treatment with essential oils (clove, basil and yarrow) and constituents (eugenol and linalool) demonstrated that they inhibit parasite growth, with clove essential being the most effective one (IC (50) =99.5 µg/ml for epimastigotes and 57.5 µg/ml for trypomastigotes). Ultrastructural alterations were observed mainly in the nucleus (Santoro *et al.*, 2007). In a filter paper diffusion bioassay with female *P. capitis*, the pediculicidal activity of the Eugenia bud and leaf oils was comparable to those of delta-phenothrin and pyrethrum on the basis of LT (50) values at 0.25 mg/cm. At 0.25 mg/cm, the compound most toxic to female *P. capitis* was eugenol followed by methyl salicylate. Acetyleugenol, beta-caryophyllene, alpha-humulene, isoeugenol, and methyleugenol were not effective. Eugenol at 0.25 mg/cm was as potent as delta-phenothrin and pyrethrum but was slightly less effective than the pyrethroids at 0.125 mg/cm (Yang *et al.*, 2003).

Atherosclerosis

Clove extract decreased serum cholesterol and TG levels by 68 per cent and 80 per cent respectively in hypercholesterolemic zebrafish model, as compared to the cinnamon extract (Jin and Cho, 2011). Hydrophilic ingredients of cinnamon and clove showed potent activities to suppress the incidence of atherosclerosis and diabetes via strong antioxidant potential, prevention of apoA-I glycation and LDL-phagocytosis, inhibition of cholesteryl ester transfer protein, and hypolipidemic activity.

Clove oil (OC) was found to be a potent inhibitor of platelet aggregation induced by arachidonic acid (AA), collagen and epinephrine; in this respect it was most effective against AA-induced aggregation. Inhibition of aggregation by OC seems to be mediated through a reduced formation of thromboxane as indicated by the following experimental evidence. (i) OC inhibited TxB2 formation in intact as well as lysed platelet preparations from added arachidonate, and (ii) it inhibited the formation of TxB2 from AA-labelled platelets after activation with Ca^{2+-} ionophore A23187 (Srivastava and Justesen (1987). Acetyl eugenol from clove oil was found to be a potent platelet inhibitor; arachidonate (AA)-induced aggregation at ca. 12 µM, a concentration needed to abolish the second phase of adrenaline-induced aggregation. Chemically synthesized acetyl eugenol showed similar effects on AA- and adrenaline-induced aggregation. A dose-dependent inhibition of collagen-induced aggregation was also observed. Acetyl eugenol did not inhibit either calcium ionophore A23187- or thrombin-induced aggregation. Inhibition of aggregation appeared to be mediated by a combination of two effects: reduced formation of thromboxane and increased generation of 12-lipoxygenase product (Srivastava and Malhotra (1991). Based on their IC50 values, it was found that both eugenol and acetyl eugenol were more potent than aspirin in inhibiting platelet aggregation induced by arachidonate, adrenaline and collagen. In arachidonate-induced aggregation eugenol was on a par with indomethacin. It was found that eugenol and acetyl eugenol when used in combination potentiated inhibition of platelet aggregation induced by arachidonate, adrenaline and collagen (Srivastava, 1993).

The *in vivo* experiments in rabbits showed that clove oil (50-100 mg/kg) offered 100 per cent protection against platelet-activating factor (11 mg/kg, i.v.) and 70 per cent protection against arachidonic acid (AA) (2.0 mg/kg, i.v.)-induced thrombosis and shock due to pulmonary platelet thrombosis. It also inhibited thromboxane-A2 and 12-HETE production by human platelets incubated with [C14] AA and thus acts as antithrombotic agent (Saeed *et al.*, 1994).

Cancer

Clove oil was found to be highly cytotoxic at concentrations as low as 0.03 per cent (v/v). Upto 73 per cent of this effect attributable to eugenol. Beta-caryophyllene did not exhibit any cytotoxic activity, indicating that other cytotoxic components may also exist within the parent oil (Prashar *et al.*, 2006).

Since the n-hexane extract of cloves demonstrated preferential growth-inhibitory activity against the causal cariogenic pathogens (S. mutans) in dental caries, Uju and Obioma (2011) suggested that clove extract be henceforth considered as a potential ingredient in toothpaste preparation.

The mechanism of the anticancer effect of eugenol isolated from cloves was first demonstrated by Yoo *et al.*, in 2005 and they observed that eugenol transduced the apoptotic signal via reactive oxygen species generation, thereby (a) inducing mitochondrial permeability transition, (b) reducing anti-apoptotic protein bcl-2 level, (c) inducing cytochrome c release to the cytosol, and (d) subsequent apoptotic cell death.

A methanol extract from clove showed a suppressive effect of the SOS-inducing activity on the mutagen 2-(2-furyl)-3-(5-nitro-2-furyl) acrylamide (furylfuramide) (Miyazawa and Hisama, 2001). A significant apoptogenic and antiproliferative properties and thereby the chemo-preventive potential of clove was demonstrated by Banerjee *et al.* (2006) in mice.

Banerjee and Das (2005) have shown that oral administration of aqueous infusions of clove at a dose of 100 microl per mouse per day not only delays the formation of papilloma but also reduces the incidence of papilloma as well as the cumulative number of papillomas per papilloma bearing mouse suggesting a promising role for cloves in restriction of the carcinogenesis process.

Dehydrodieugenol and trans-coniferyl aldehyde isolated from clove buds showed dramatic reductions in their mutagenic potential of 4-nitroquinolin 1-oxide (4NQO) and N-methyl-N'-nitro-N-nitrosoguanidine (MNNG), which do not require liver metabolizing enzymes, and aflatoxin B (1) (AfB (1)) and 3-amino-1,4-dimethyl-5H-pyrido[4,3-b]indole (Trp-P-1), which require liver metabolizing enzymes (Miyazawa and Hisama, 2003). The active compounds Erugenol and eugenol acetate isolated from the methanol extract of clove bud showed melanin inhibition of 60 per cent and 40 per cent in B_{16} melanoma cell with less cytotoxicity at the concentration of 100 and 200 µg/ml respectively (Arung *et al.*, 2011).

Diabetes

Clove extract acts like insulin in hepatocytes and hepatoma cells by reducing phosphoenolpyruvate carboxykinase (PEPCK) and glucose 6-phosphatase (G6Pase) gene expression. Much like insulin, clove-mediated repression is reversed by PI3K inhibitors and N-acetylcysteine (NAC). Prasad *et al.* (2005) thus demonstrate that cloves may have beneficial effects for the treatment of diabetes and indicate a potential role for compounds derived from clove as insulin-mimetic agents.

Studies indicate that the antihyperglycemic effects of clove-derived oleanolic acid (OA) are mediated in part through increased hepatic glycogen synthesis. Ngubane *et al.* (2011) found that OA administration restored these biochemical alterations (depleted glycogen levels and low activities of glycogenic enzymes in muscle and hepatic tissues in STZ-induced diabetic rats) to near normalcy.

In vitro evaluation showed the ethonolic extract had human peroxisome proliferator-activated receptor (PPAR)-daku ligand-binding activity in a GAL4-PPAR-daku chimera assay. Dehydro-dieugenol and dehydrodieugenol B fractions of the extract had potent PPAR-daku ligand-binding activities, whereas oleanolic acid, a major constituent in the extract, had moderate activity. Thus, clove is shown to be a potential functional food ingredient for the prevention of type 2 diabetes and that Dehydrodieugenol and dehydrodieugenol B fractions mainly contribute to its hypoglycaemic effects via PPAR-daku activation (Kuroda *et al.*, 2012).

Gastrointestinal Disorders

Gastrointestinal disorders constitute one of the most common diseases world-wide and the treatment of some of them has since constituted a great challenge to health workers. Clove has since been employed locally to treat constipation. Hot aqueous extract of clove increased the gut muscle propulsion similar to the standard drugs–carbachol and metoclopramide. In the ulcer models, the decoction reduced the ulcer number and ulcer area in the ethanol and HCl-ethanol models, with significant respective ulcer indices of 2.80 +/- 3.51 and 11.4 +/- 3.79 compared with controls. Agbaje (2008) confirmed the folkloric uses of cloves as an antiulcer and a purgative agent as well as its possible mechanism of action.

Eugenol of the essential oil of cloves stimulates the synthesis of mucus, an important gastroprotective factor. However, further pharmacological and toxicological investigations are required to enable its use for the treatment of gastric ulcer (Santin *et al.*, 2011).

Sexual Disorders

Spices are considered as sexual invigorators in the Unani System of Medicine. Cloves have been used as indigenous medicine for the treatment of male sexual disorders in Asian countries. Lower dose (15 mg) of the hexane extract of cloves increased the activities of Delta (5) 3 beta-HSD and 17 beta-HSD, and serum level of testosterone. The higher doses (30 and 60 mg) of extract inhibited these parameters and induced non-uniform degenerative changes in the seminiferous tubules associated with decrease in daily sperm production and depletion of 1C (round and elongated spermatids) population. Mishra *et al.* (2008) showed the biphasic action of hexane extract of Syzygium clove flower bud on testicular function, thereby advocating a cautious use of the flower bud as an aphrodisiac in indigenous systems of medicine in Asian countries.

Tajuddin *et al.* (2003; 2004) observed that 50 per cent ethanolic clove was found to stimulate the mounting behaviour of male mice, and also to significantly increase their mating performance. The drugs were devoid of any conspicuous general short term toxicity. The extract produced a significant and sustained increase in the sexual activity of normal male rats, without any conspicuous gastric ulceration and adverse effects. Thus, the resultant aphrodisiac effect of the extract lends support to the claims for its traditional usage in sexual disorders.

Other Benefits

Supplementation with hydro-alcoholic extract of dried clove buds significantly restored the serum alkaline phosphatase: 48.25 per cent, serum tartrate-resistant acid phosphatase: 33.51 per cent, calcium: 53.15 per cent, phosphate: 27.49 per cent, creatinine: 46.40 per cent in ovariectomised rats. Similar trend was seen with regard to bone density, bone mineral content, bone tensile strength and histological analysis. Based on these results, Karmarkar *et al.* (2012) proposed that hydro-alcoholic extract of dried clove buds has bone-preserving efficacy against hypogonadal osteoporosis.

Clove oil is an effective, local and natural anaesthetic. Many hatcheries use clove oil to immobilize fish for handling, sorting, tagging, artificial reproduction procedures and surgery and to suppress sensory systems during invasive procedures (Javahery *et al.*, 2012). Anaesthesia was associated with increased blood glucose, potassium, and sodium concentrations as well as Haematocrit and haemoglobin (Sladky *et al.*, 2001). The time required for anesthesia to take effect on Marine medaka (*Oryzias dancena*) decreased significantly as both anesthetic concentration and water temperature increased for both clove oil and lidocaine-HCl. As expected, both anesthetic exposure time and recovery time were significantly shorter for smaller fish than for larger fish (Park *et al.*, 2011).

The aqueous extract of cloves reduced the hydrolysis of acetylcholine by acetylcholine Esterase. This reducing effect was not due to the acidic nature of the extract and suggests that cloves contain some water soluble substance(s) with anti-choline esterase activity (Akinrimisi and Akinwande, 1975). Later, the same authors showed that all the extracts (water, saline and ethanol) of inhibited brain acetylcholinesterase activity. Inhibitory action of the saline extract was greater than that of other extracts. Therefore they (Akinrimisi and Akinwande, 1976) suggested that the active inhibitor is a complex glycoside containing phenol and uronic acid.

Food Preservation

The antimicrobial activity of clove oil has been explored in food preservation as well. Essential oil of clove dispersed (0.4 per cent v/v) in a concentrated sugar solution, had a marked germicidal effect against various bacteria and *Candida albicans. Staphylococcus aureus* (five strains), *Klebsiella pneumoniae, Pseudomonas aeruginosa, Clostridium perfringens, Escherichia coli* and *C. albicans* inoculated in laboratory broth were killed when supplemented with 63 per cent (v/w) of sugar, 0.4 per cent (v/w) of essential oil of clove. The concentrated sugar solution provided a good vehicle for obtaining an oil dispersion that is relatively stable for certain practical applications (Briozzo *et al.*, 1989).

Mycelial growth of the four test pathogens namely *P. vagabunda, P. expansum, B. cinerea* and *M. fructigena* was completely inhibited when treated with 150 microl l(-1) of volatile eugenol whether at 4 or 20 degrees C. Ethoxylate and Tween 80-eugenol formulations applied at room temperature were ineffective in reducing disease incidence. When heated to 50°C, both formulations induced phytotoxicity on apple surface and caused cuticle damages as revealed by scanning electronic microscopic observations. The application of heated lecithin-formulated eugenol could become a successful alternative to the traditional fungicides used in postharvest disease management of apple fruit (Amiri *et al.*, 2008).

Clove oil was found to be fungistatic and fungicidal against *Lasiodiplodia theobromae, C. musae* and *Fusarium proliferatum*, identified as causative agents responsible for crown rot in banana. The oil was fungistatic and fungicidal against the test pathogens within a range of 0.03-0.11 per cent (v/v). Ranasinghe *et al.* (2002) therefore suggest that clove essential oil could be used as alternative post-harvest treatments on banana. Banana treated with essential oil is chemically safe and acceptable to consumers. Benomyl (Benlate), which is currently used to manage fungal pathogens, can cause adverse health effects and could be replaced with volatile essential oils. Among selected oils–cinnamon, clove, ginger and holy basil, clove oil had the strongest inhibitory effect and exhibited a bactericidal mode of action against a fish pathogenic bacterium *Lactococcus garvieae*. Thus, Rattanachaikunsopon and Phumkhachorn (2009) indicated that clove oil has a protective effect on experimental *L. garvieae* infection in tilapia and the potential to replace antibiotics for controlling the disease.

Syzygium powder, at 3 per cent and in combination with Jute bags (JB)-packaging, effectively suppressed cross infection of healthy kernels (12 per cent moisture) by fungi from diseased kernels when both kernel types occurred in the same lot. Packaging with JB and Interlaced polypropylene bags with Syzygium powder gave 100 per cent protection against fungi up to 4 months, and insect infestation was also prevented (Awuah and Ellis, 2002).

Cava *et al.* (2007) indicated from their study the possibility of using the three essential oils (EO) (the cinnamon bark EO, cinnamon leaf EO and clove EO) in milk beverages as natural antimicrobials, especially because milk beverages flavoured with cinnamon and clove are consumed worldwide and have been increasing in popularity in recent years. But no antimicrobial effect of 1 per cent (w/w) clove powder on *L. monocytogenes* was observed in cheese after 1 or 2 weeks at the lower or higher temperature (Leuschner and Ielsh, 2003).

Synergistic Effect with Other Spices/Spice Products

Several researchers compared the antimicrobial activity of clove oil with other essential oils. Combinations of the two essential oils from clove and rosemary indicated their additive, synergistic or antagonistic effects against individual microorganisms and thus demonstrated clear bactericidal and fungicidal processes (Fu *et al.*, 2007). Cinnamon oil and clove oil strongly inhibited the growth of *E. coli* O157:H7 at neutral and acidic pH. A synergistic effect between the essential oils and the lower pH of the growth medium was evident by consistently lower MICs at pH 4.5. The addition of cinnamon and clove oils at 0.01 per cent vol/vol resulted in lower D-values of *E. coli* O157:H7 than those for cider alone, suggesting a synergistic effect and the potential efficacy of a mild heat treatment for apple cider (Knight and McKellar, 2007).

Mixtures of cinnamon and clove oils were tested for inhibitory activity against important spoilage microorganisms of intermediate moisture foods. A. flavus and Eurotium sp. proved to be the most resistant microorganisms out of four fungal species (*A. flavus, P. roqueforti, M.plumbeus* and *Eurotium* sp.). Cinnamon and clove oil added between 1000 and 4000 microL at a ratio of 1:1 were tested for minimum inhibitory volume (MIV) against molds and four yeasts species (*D. hansenii, P. membranaefaciens, Z. rouxii* and *C. lipolytica*). The gas phase above 1000 microL of the oil mixture inhibited growth of *C. lipolytica* and *P. membranaefaciens*; 2000 microL inhibited growth of *A. flavus, P. roqueforti, M. plumbeus, Eurotium* sp., *D. hansenii*, and *Z. rouxii*, while inhibition of A. flavus required the addition of 4000 microL. Higher ratios of cinnamon oil/clove oil were more effective for inhibiting the growth of *A. flavus* (Matan *et al.*, 2006). Chami *et al.* (2005) observed the antimicrobial activity of Oregano and Clove essential oils against yeast cells.

The antimicrobial activities of allspice, cinnamon, and clove bud oils in apple puree film-forming solutions formulated into edible films at 0.5 per cent to 3 per cent (w/w) concentrations showed that the same was more effective against *L. monocytogenes* than against the *S. enterica*. The antimicrobial activities against the 3 pathogens (*E. coli* O157:H7, *S. enterica*, and *L. monocytogenes*) were in the following order: cinnamon oil > clove bud oil > allspice oil (Du *et al.*, 2009).

Surfactant

The addition of clove oil–phospholipid mixtures caused a decrease in the mucus gel simulant (MGS: a polymeric gel consisting predominantly of gum tragacanth and simulating respiratory mucus), when compared with the effect of the phospholipid alone at low shear rates in case of dipalmitoyl phosphatidylcholine (PC), phosphatidylglycerol (PG) and PCPG. The combination of PC: PG with clove oil caused ratios of change in MGS viscosity < 1, *i.e.*, caused a decrease in the MGS viscosity. PC: PG with clove oil was capable of lowering MGS viscosity (Banerjee and Puniyani (2000).

As Dipalmitoyl phosphatidylcholine, the main component of lung surfactant is ineffective as a replacement surfactant due to its poor adsorption, Banerjee and Bellare (2001) found the presence of clove oil to cause a significant improvement in the adsorption and minimum surface tension of all the protein-free phospholipid suspensions.

Safety Concerns

Eugenol can be toxic in relatively small quantities–as low as 5 ml (Hartnoll *et al.*, 1993). Anesthesia induced with tricaine methanesulphonate or eugenol contributes to hypoxemia, hypercapnia, respiratory acidosis, and hyperglycemia in red pacu. Though similar to tricaine methanesulphonate, eugenol appears to be an effective immobilization compound; eugenol is characterized by more rapid induction, prolonged recovery, and a narrow margin of safety. Care must be taken when using high concentrations of eugenol for induction, because ventilatory failure may occur rapidly. In addition, analgesic properties of eugenol are unknown (Sladky *et al.*, 2001). Agbaje *et al.* (2009) from their study involving long term administration of clove aqueous extract revealed the toxicity of sub chronic administration of clove, and suggest that its prolonged usage must be avoided.

Conclusion

Among many affirmative health benefits studied experimentally, the most important quality of cloves and its essential oil is its antimicrobial benefit.

References

Agbaje EO (2008). Gastrointestinal effects of *Syzigium aromaticum* (L) Merr. and Perry (Myrtaceae) in animal models. Nig. Q. J. Hosp. Med. 18 (3): 137–41.

Agbaje EO, Adeneye AA, Daramola AO (2009). Biochemical and toxicological studies of aqueous extract of *Syzigium aromaticum* (L.) Merr. and Perry (Myrtaceae) in rodents. Afr. J. Tradit. Complement. Altern. Med. 6 (3): 241–54.

Ahmad N, Alam MK, Shehbaz A, Khan A, Mannan A, Hakim SR, Bisht D, Owais M (2005). Antimicrobial activity of clove oil and its potential in the treatment of vaginal candidiasis. J. Drug Target. 13 (10): 555–61.

Akinrimisi EO, Akinwande AI (1975). Effect of aqueous extract of *Eugenia caryophyllus* on brain acetylcholine esterase in rats. West Afr. J. Pharmacol. Drug Res. 2 (2): 127–31.

Akinrimisi EO, Akinwande AI (1976). Biochemical studies of acetylcholine esterase inhibitor present in *Eugenia caryophyllus*. West Afr. J. Pharmacol. Drug Res. 3 (2): 141–48.

Amiri A, Dugas R, Pichot AL, Bompeix G (2008). *In vitro* and *in vivo* [corrected] activity of eugenol oil (*Eugenia caryophylata*) against four important postharvest apple pathogens. Int. J. Food Microbiol. 126 (1-2): 13–19.

Arenas Merchán DR, Acevedo AM, Vargas Méndez LY, Kouznetsov VV (2011). Scavenger Activity Evaluation of the Clove Bud Essential Oil (*Eugenia *caryophyllus*) and Eugenol Derivatives Employing ABTS Decolourization. Sci. Pharm. 79 (4): 779–91.

Arung ET, Matsubara E, Kusuma IW, Sukaton E, Shimizu K, Kondo R (2011). Inhibitory components from the buds of clove (*Syzygium aromaticum*) on melanin formation in B16 melanoma cells. Fitoterapia. 82 (2): 198–202.

Awuah RT, Ellis WO (2002). Effects of some groundnut packaging methods and protection with Ocimum and syzygium powders on kernel infection by fungi. Mycopathologia. 154 (1): 29–36.

Bachiega TF, de Sousa JP, Bastos JK, Sforcin JM (2012). Clove and eugenol in noncytotoxic concentrations exert immunomodulatory/anti-inflammatory action on cytokine production by murine macrophages. J. Pharm. Pharmacol. 64 (4): 610–16.

Bachiega TF, Orsatti CL, Pagliarone AC, Missima F, Sousa JP, Bastos JK, Sforcin JM (2009). Th1/Th2 cytokine production by clove-treated mice. Nat. Prod. Res. 23 (16): 1552–58.

Banerjee R, Bellare JR (2001). Comparison of *in vitro* surface properties of clove oil-phospholipid suspensions with those of ALEC, Exosurf and Survanta. Pulm. Pharmacol. Ther. 14 (2): 85–91.

Banerjee S, Das S (2005). Anticarcinogenic effects of an aqueous infusion of cloves on skin carcinogenesis. Asian Pac. J. Cancer Prev. 6 (3): 304–308.

Banerjee S, Panda CK, Das S (2006). Clove (*Syzygium aromaticum* L.), a potential chemo-preventive agent for lung cancer. Carcinogenesis. 27 (8): 1645–54.

Banerjee R, Puniyani RR (2000). Effects of clove oil-phospholipid mixtures on rheology of gum tragacanth–possible application for surfactant action on mucus gel simulants. Biomed. Mater. Eng. 10 (3-4): 189–97.

Briozzo J, Núñez L, Chirife J, Herszage L, D'Aquino M (1989). Antimicrobial activity of clove oil dispersed in a concentrated sugar solution. J. Appl. Bacteriol. 66 (1): 69–75.

Cai L, Wu CD (1996). Compounds from *Syzygium aromaticum* possessing growth inhibitory activity against oral pathogens. J. Nat. Prod. 59 (10): 987–90.

Carrasco FR, Schmidt G, Romero AL, Sartoretto JL, Caparroz-Assef SM, Bersani-Amado CA, Cuman RK (2009). Immunomodulatory activity of *Zingiber officinale* Roscoe, *Salvia officinalis* L. and *Syzygium aromaticum* L. essential oils: evidence for humor- and cell-mediated responses. J. Pharm. Pharmacol. 61 (7): 961–67.

Cava R, Nowak E, Taboada A, Marin-Iniesta F (2007). Antimicrobial activity of clove and cinnamon essential oils against *Listeria monocytogenes* in pasteurized milk. J. Food Prot. 70 (12): 2757–63.

Chaieb K, Hajlaoui H, Zmantar T, Kahla-Nakbi AB, Rouabhia M, Mahdouani K, Bakhrouf A (2007a). The chemical composition and biological activity of clove essential oil, *Eugenia caryophyllata* (*Syzigium aromaticum* L. Myrtaceae): a short review. Phytother. Res. 21 (6): 501–506.

Chaieb K, Zmantar T, Ksouri R, Hajlaoui H, Mahdouani K, Abdelly C, Bakhrouf A (2007b). Antioxidant properties of the essential oil of *Eugenia caryophyllata* and its antifungal activity against a large number of clinical Candida species. Mycoses. 50 (5): 403–406.

Chami F, Chami N, Bennis S, Bouchikhi T, Remmal A (2005). Oregano and clove essential oils induce surface alteration of *Saccharomyces cerevisiae*. Phytother. Res. 19 (5): 405–408.

Devi KP, Nisha SA, Sakthivel R, Pandian SK (2010). Eugenol (an essential oil of clove) acts as an antibacterial agent against *Salmonella typhi* by disrupting the cellular membrane. J. Ethnopharmacol. 130 (1): 107–15.

Du WX, Olsen CW, Avena-Bustillos RJ, McHugh TH, Levin CE, Friedman M (2009). Effects of allspice, cinnamon, and clove bud essential oils in edible apple films on physical properties and antimicrobial activities. J. Food Sci. 74 (7): M 372–78.

Fu Y, Zu Y, Chen L, Shi X, Wang Z, Sun S, Efferth T (2007). Antimicrobial activity of clove and rosemary essential oils alone and in combination. Phytother. Res. 21 (10): 989–94.

Gayoso CW, Lima EO, Oliveira VT, Pereira FO, Souza EL, Lima IO, Navarro DF (2005). Sensitivity of fungi isolated from onychomycosis to *Eugenia cariophyllata* essential oil and eugenol. Fitoterapia. 76 (2): 247–49.

Gijzen M, Efraim L, Savage T, Croteau R (1991). Bioactive Volatile Compounds from Plants. In: Teranishi R, Buttery RG, Sugisawa H, editors. Conifer Monoterpenes: Biochemistry and Bark Beetle Chemistry Ecology. Ch. 2 ed. Washington DC: American Chemistry Society.

Gislene GF, Paulo C, Giuliana L (2000). Antibacterial Activity of Plant Extracts and Phytochemicals on Antibiotic Resistant Bacteria. Braz. J. Microbiol. 31: 314–25.

Halder S, Mehta AK, Mediratta PK, Sharma KK (2011). Essential oil of clove (*Eugenia caryophyllata*) augments the humoral immune response but decreases cell mediated immunity. Phytother. Res. 25 (8): 1254–56.

Hartnoll, G; Moore, D; Douek, D (1993). Near fatal ingestion of oil of cloves. Archives of Disease in Childhood. 69 (3): 392–93.

Hili P, Evans CS, Veness RG (1997). Antimicrobial Action of Essential Oils: The Effect of Dimethylsulphoxide on the Activity of Cinnamon Oil. Lett. Appl. Microbiol. 24: 269–75.

Javahery S, Nekoubin H, Moradlu AH (2012). Effect of anaesthesia with clove oil in fish (review). Fish. Physiol. Biochem. 2012 Jun 30. [Epub ahead of print].

Jin S, Cho KH (2011). Water extracts of cinnamon and clove exhibits potent inhibition of protein glycation and antiatherosclerotic activity *in vitro* and *in vivo* hypolipidemic activity in zebrafish. Food Chem. Toxicol. 49 (7): 1521–29.

Jirovetz L, Buchbauer G, Stoilova I, Stoyanova A, Krastanov A, Schmidt E (2006). Chemical composition and antioxidant properties of clove leaf essential oil. J. Agric. Food Chem. 54 (17): 6303–307.

Karmakar S, Choudhury M, Das AS, Maiti A, Majumdar S, Mitra C (2012). Clove (*Syzygium aromaticum* Linn) extract rich in eugenol and eugenol derivatives shows bone-preserving efficacy. Nat Prod Res. 26 (6): 500–509.

Khan MS, Zahin M, Hasan S, Husai.n FM, Ahmad I (2009). Inhibition of quorum sensing regulated bacterial functions by plant essential oils with special reference to clove oil. Lett. Appl. Microbiol. 49 (3): 354–60.

Knight KP, McKellar RC (2007). Influence of cinnamon and clove essential oils on the D- and z-values of Escherichia coli O157:H7 in apple cider. J. Food Prot. 70 (9): 2089–94.

Kuroda M, Mimaki Y, Ohtomo T, Yamada J, Nishiyama T, Mae T, Kishida H, Kawada T (2012). Sou Hypoglycaemic effects of clove (*Syzygium aromaticum* flower buds) on genetically diabetic KK-Ay mice and identification of the active ingredients. J. Nat. Med. 66 (2): 394–99.

Kurokawa M, Hozumi T, Basnet P, Nakano M, Kadota S, Namba T, Kawana T, Shiraki K (1998). Purification and characterization of eugeniin as an anti-herpesvirus compound from *Geum japonicum* and *Syzygium aromaticum*. J. Pharmacol. Exp. Ther. 284 (2): 728–35.

Lee KG, Shibamoto T (2001). Inhibition of malonaldehyde formation from blood plasma oxidation by aroma extracts and aroma components isolated from clove and eucalyptus. Food Chem. Toxicol. 39 (12): 1199–204.

Leuschner RG, Ielsch V (2003). Antimicrobial effects of garlic, clove and red hot chilli on *Listeria monocytogenes* in broth model systems and soft cheese. Int. J. Food Sci. Nutr. 54 (2): 127–33.

Liu HY, Zhu S, Komatsu K, Cai SQ, Li YH, Yu C, Jiang Y, Sa Y (2008). [Study on aqueous chemical constituents from the flower buds of *Eugenia caryophylla*]. Zhong. Yao. Cai. 31 (7): 998–1000. [Article in Chinese].

Machado M, Dinis AM, Salgueiro L, Custódio JB, Cavaleiro C, Sousa MC (2011). Anti-Giardia activity of *Syzygium aromaticum* essential oil and eugenol: effects on growth, viability, adherence and ultrastructure. Exp. Parasitol. 127 (4): 732–39.

Masteliæ J, Jerkoviæ I, Blaèeviæ I, Poljak-Blaèi M, Boroviæ S, Ivanèiæ-Baæe I, Smreèki V, Žarkoviæ N, Brèiæ-Kostiæ K, Vikiæ-Topiæ D, Mueller N (2008). Comparative Study on the Antioxidant and Biological Activities of Carvacrol, Thymol, and Eugenol Derivatives. J. Agric. Food Chem. 56: 3989–96.

Matan N, Rimkeeree H, Mawson AJ, Chompreeda P, Haruthaithanasan V, Parker M (2006). Antimicrobial activity of cinnamon and clove oils under modified atmosphere conditions. Int. J. Food Microbiol. 107 (2): 180–85.

Misharina TA, Samusenko AL (2008). [Antioxidant properties of essential oils from lemon, grapefruit, coriander, clove, and their mixtures]. Prikl. Biokhim. Mikrobiol. 44 (4): 482–86. [Article in Russian].

Mishra RK, Singh SK (2008). Safety assessment of *Syzygium aromaticum* flower bud (clove) extract with respect to testicular function in mice. Food Chem. Toxicol. 46 (10): 3333–38.

Miyazawa M, Hisama M (2001). Suppression of chemical mutagen-induced SOS response by alkylphenols from clove (*Syzygium aromaticum*) in the *Salmonella typhimurium* TA1535/pSK1002 umu test. J. Agric. Food Chem. 49 (8): 4019–25.

Miyazawa M, Hisama M (2003). Antimutagenic activity of phenylpropanoids from clove (*Syzygium aromaticum*). J. Agric. Food Chem. 51 (22): 6413–22.

Moon SE, Kim HY, Cha JD (2011). Synergistic effect between clove oil and its major compounds and antibiotics against oral bacteria. Arch. Oral Biol. 56 (9): 907–16.

Nassar MI (2006). Flavonoid triglycosides from the seeds of *Syzygium aromaticum*. Carbohydr. Res. 341 (1): 160–63.

Ngubane PS, Masola B, Musabayane CT (2011). The effects of *Syzygium aromaticum*-derived oleanolic acid on glycogenic enzymes in streptozotocin-induced diabetic rats. Ren. Fail. 33 (4): 434–39.

Nzeako BC, Al-Kharousi ZS, Al-Mahrooqui Z (2006). Antimicrobial activities of clove and thyme extracts. Sultan. Qaboos. Univ. Med. J. 6 (1): 33–39.

Panizzi L, Flamini G, Cioni PL, Morelli I (1993). Composition and antimicrobial properties of essential oils of four Mediterranean Lamiaceae. J. Ethnopharmacol. 39: 167–70.

Park MJ, Gwak KS, Yang I, Choi WS, Jo HJ, Chang JW, Jeung EB, Choi IG (2007). Antifungal activities of the essential oils in *Syzygium aromaticum* (L.) Merr. Et Perry and *Leptospermum petersonii* Bailey and their constituents against various dermatophytes. J. Microbiol. 45 (5): 460–65.

Park IS, Park SJ, Gil HW, Nam YK, Kim DS (2011). Anesthetic effects of clove oil and lidocaine-HCl on marine medaka (Oryzias dancena). Lab. Anim. (NY). 40 (2): 45–51.

Petrovic V, Marcincak S, Popelka P, Simkova J, Martonova M, Buleca J, Marcincakova D, Tuckova M, Molnar L, Kovac G (2011). The effect of supplementation of clove and agrimony or clove and lemon balm on growth performance, antioxidant status and selected indices of lipid profile of broiler chickens. J. Anim. Physiol. Anim. Nutr. (Berl). 2011 Aug 10. Epub ahead of print.

Piccaglia R, Marotti M, Giovanelli E, Deans SG, Eaglesham E (1993). Antibacterial and Antioxidant Properties of Mediterranean Aromatic Plants. Indust. Crops Prod. 2: 47–50.

Pinto E, Vale-Silva L, Cavaleiro C, Salgueiro L (2009). Antifungal activity of the clove essential oil from *Syzygium aromaticum* on *Candida, Aspergillus* and *dermatophyte* species. J. Med. Microbiol. 58 (Pt 11): 1454–62.

Prasad RC, Herzog B, Boone B, Sims L, Waltner-Law M (2005). An extract of *Syzygium aromaticum* represses genes encoding hepatic gluconeogenic enzymes. J. Ethnopharmacol. 96 (1-2): 295–301.

Prashar A, Locke IC, Evans CS (2006). Cytotoxicity of clove (*Syzygium aromaticum*) oil and its major components to human skin cells. Cell. Prolif. 39 (4): 241–48.

Raghavenra H, Diwakr BT, Lokesh BR, Naidu KA (2006). Eugenol—the active principle from cloves inhibits 5-lipoxygenase activity and leukotriene-C4 in human PMNL cells. Prostaglandins Leukot. Essent. Fatty Acids. 74 (1): 23–27.

Ranasinghe L, Jayawardena B, Abeywickrama K (2002). Fungicidal activity of essential oils of *Cinnamomum zeylanicum* (L.) and *Syzygium aromaticum* (L.) Merr et L.M. Perry against crown rot and anthracnose pathogens isolated from banana. Lett. Appl. Microbiol. 35 (3): 208–11.

Rastogi S, Pandey MM, Rawat AK (2008). High-performance thin-layer chromatography densitometric method for the simultaneous determination of three phenolic acids in *Syzygium aromaticum* (L.) Merr. and Perry. J. A.O.A.C. Int. 91 (5): 1169–73.

Rattanachaikunsopon P, Phumkhachorn P (2009). Protective effect of clove oil-supplemented fish diets on experimental *Lactococcus garvieae* infection in tilapia. Biosci. Biotechnol. Biochem. 73 (9): 2085–89.

Rodrigues TG, Fernandes A Jr, Sousa JP, Bastos JK, Sforcin JM (2009). *In vitro* and *in vivo* effects of clove on pro-inflammatory cytokines production by macrophages. Nat. Prod. Res. 23 (4): 319–26.

Saeed SA, Gilani AH (1994). Antithrombotic activity of clove oil. J. Pak. Med. Assoc. 44 (5): 112–15.

Saini A, Sharma S, Chhibber S (2009). Induction of resistance to respiratory tract infection with *Klebsiella pneumoniae* in mice fed on a diet supplemented with tulsi (*Ocimum sanctum*) and clove (*Syzgium aromaticum*) oils. J. Microbiol. Immunol. Infect. 42 (2): 107–13.

Santin JR, Lemos M, Klein-Júnior LC, Machado ID, Costa P, de Oliveira AP, Tilia C, de Souza JP, de Sousa JP, Bastos JK, de Andrade SF (2011). Gastroprotective activity of essential oil of the *Syzygium aromaticum* and its major component eugenol in different animal models. Naunyn. Schmiedebergs. Arch. Pharmacol. 383 (2): 149–58.

Santoro GF, Cardoso MG, Guimarães LG, Mendonça LZ, Soares MJ (2007). Trypanosoma cruzi: activity of essential oils from *Achillea millefolium* L., *Syzygium aromaticum* L. and *Ocimum basilicum* L. on epimastigotes and trypomastigotes. Exp. Parasitol. 116 (3): 283–90.

Sladky KK, Swanson CR, Stoskopf MK, Loomis MR, Lewbart GA (2001). Comparative efficacy of tricaine methanesulfonate and clove oil for use as anesthetics in red pacu (*Piaractus brachypomus*). Am. J. Vet. Res. 62 (3): 337–42.

Srivastava KC (1993). Antiplatelet principles from a food spice clove (*Syzygium aromaticum* L) [corrected]. Prostaglandins Leukot. Essent. Fatty Acids. 48 (5): 363–72.

Srivastava KC, Justesen U (1987). Inhibition of platelet aggregation and reduced formation of thromboxane and lipoxygenase products in platelets by oil of cloves. Prostaglandins Leukot. Med. 29 (1): 11–18.

Srivastava KC, Malhotra N (1991). Acetyl eugenol, a component of oil of cloves (*Syzygium aromaticum* L.) inhibits aggregation and alters arachidonic acid metabolism in human blood platelets. Prostaglandins Leukot. Essent. Fatty Acids. 42 (1): 73–81.

Taguchi Y, Ishibashi H, Takizawa T, Inoue S, Yamaguchi H, Abe S (2005). Protection of oral or intestinal candidiasis in mice by oral or intragastric administration of herbal food, clove (*Syzygium aromaticum*). Nihon. Ishinkin. Gakkai. Zasshi. 46 (1): 27–33.

Tajuddin, Ahmad S, Latif A, Qasmi IA (2003). Aphrodisiac activity of 50 per cent ethanolic extracts of *Myristica fragrans* Houtt. (nutmeg) and *Syzygium aromaticum* (L) Merr. and Perry. (clove) in male mice: a comparative study. BMC. Complement. Altern. Med. 3: 6.

Tajuddin, Ahmad S, Latif A, Qasmi IA (2004). Effect of 50 per cent ethanolic extract of *Syzygium aromaticum* (L.) Merr. and Perry. (clove) on sexual behavior of normal male rats. BMC. Complement. Altern. Med. 4: 17.

Uju DE, Obioma NP (2011). Anticariogenic potentials of clove, tobacco and bitter kola. Asian Pac. J. Trop. Med. 4 (10): 814–18.

Yang YC, Lee SH, Lee WJ, Choi DH, Ahn YJ (2003). Ovicidal and adulticidal effects of *Eugenia caryophyllata* bud and leaf oil compounds on *Pediculus capitis*. J. Agric. Food Chem. 51 (17): 4884–88.

Yoo CB, Han KT, Cho KS, Ha J, Park HJ, Nam JH, Kil UH, Lee KT (2005). Eugenol isolated from the essential oil of *Eugenia caryophyllata* induces a reactive oxygen species-mediated apoptosis in HL-60 human promyelocytic leukemia cells. Cancer. Lett. 225 (1): 41–52.

Yoshimura M, Amakura Y, Yoshida T (2011). Polyphenolic compounds in clove and pimento and their antioxidative activities. Biosci. Biotechnol. Biochem. 75 (11): 2207–12.

Yun SM, Lee MH, Lee KJ, Ku HO, Son SW, Joo YS (2010). Quantitative analysis of eugenol in clove extract by a validated HPLC method. J. A.O.A.C. Int. 93 (6): 1806–10.

Chapter 5

Cumin Seeds

(*Cuminum cyminum*)

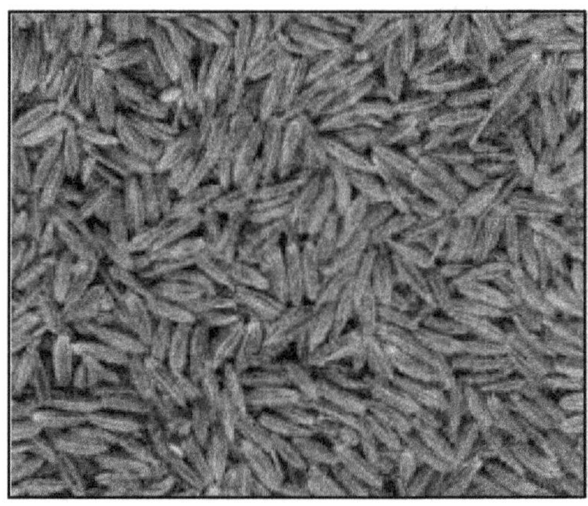

Cumin has been in use since ancient times. It is native to Egypt and has been cultivated in the Middle East, India, China and Mediterranean countries for millennia. Throughout history, cumin has played an important role as a food and medicine and has been a cultural symbol with varied attributes (Zohari and Hopf, 2000). Cumin was mentioned in the Bible not only as a seasoning for soup and bread, but also as a currency used to pay tithes to the priests.

Cumin thrives in hot and arid lands. It is the dried seed of the herb *Cuminum cyminum*, a member of the parsley family. The cumin plant grows to 30-50 cm (1-2 ft) tall and is harvested by hand. Cumin seeds resemble caraway seeds, being oblong in shape, longitudinally ridged, and yellow-brown in colour, like other members of the Umbelliferae family such as caraway, parsley and dill.

The flavour of Cumin seeds is penetrating and peppery with slight citrus overtones. This unique flavour complexity has made it an integral spice in the cuisines of Mexico, India and the Middle East. Light roasting of whole cumin seeds before using them in a recipe enhances the aroma and flavour.

Traditional Use of Cumin Seeds

Cumin seeds were highly honored as a culinary seasoning in both ancient Greek and Roman kitchens. In Iranian traditional medicine, cumin is considered stimulant, carminative and astringent and its therapeutic effects have been described on gastrointestinal, gynaecological and respiratory disorders, and also for the treatment of toothache, diarrhea and epilepsy (Zargary, 2001). In the Moroccan traditional medicine, caraway seeds are used as diuretics (Lahlou *et al.*, 2007) and given to treat diabetes and hypertension (Tahraoui *et al.*, 2007). Cumin's popularity was partly due to the fact that its peppery flavour made it a viable replacement for black pepper, which was very expensive and hard to buy. Cumin was also noted for both its medicinal and cosmetic properties. In certain Arabic traditions a paste of cumin powder, pepper and honey is thought to have aphrodisiac properties. In Siddha and Unani systems of medicine practiced in south east Asia, cumin seeds are considered carminative, eupeptic, antispasmodic, astringent and used in the treatment of mild digestive disorders, diarrhea, dyspepsia, flatulence, morning sickness, colic, dyspeptic headache and bloating, and are said to promote the assimilation of other herbs and to improve liver function. Patients suffering from lumbago and rheumatism are relieved of the symptoms from the vapors of cumin seeds. Scabies has been treated with a mixture of alcohol, castor oil and cumin seeds.

Nutritive Value of Cumin seeds

Nutrient	*Amount*	*Nutrient*	*Amount*
Energy (kcal)	375	Carbohydrates (g)	44.2
Protein (g)	17.8	Total Fat (g)	74.0
Dietary Fiber (g)	10.5	Sodium (mg)	1788
Potassium (mg)	68	Calcium (mg)	931
Copper (mg)	0.87	Iron (mg)	66.36
Magnesium (mg)	366	Manganese (mg)	3.3
Phosphorus (mg)	499	Zinc (mg)	4.8
Folates (g)	2.5	Niacin (mg)	4.6
Pyridoxine (mg)	0.44	Riboflavin (mg)	0.32
Thiamin (mg)	0.63	Vitamin A (IU)	1270
Vitamin C (mg)	7.7	Vitamin E (mg)	3.3
Vitamin K (mg)	5.4	Carotene-ß (µg)	762
Lutein-zeaxanthin (µg)	448		

USDA, (2012).

Several nutrients including starch, sugars and other carbohydrates, tannins, phytic acid and dietary fiber components have been found in cumin seeds (El-Sawi *et al.*, 2002; Al-Bataina *et al.*, 2003).Toghrol and Daneshpejouh, 1974; Uma *et al.*, 1973; Maiga *et al.*, 2005; Milan *et al.*, 2008; Cumin seeds are also very good source of iron and manganese.

Chemical Constituents

Cumin seeds are rich sources of essential oils and have been actively researched for their chemical composition and biological activities. In recent times (especially during the last 3 years) considerable progress has been made regarding validation of the acclaimed medicinal attributes of cumin by extensive experimental studies.

Major constituents in cumin seed essential oil are gamma-terpinene (15.82 per cent), 2-methyl-3-phenyl-propanal (32.27 per cent) and myrtenal (11.64 per cent) and in caraway are gamma-terpinene (24.40 per cent), 2-methyl-3-phenyl-propanal (13.20 per cent) and 2, 4(10)-thujadien (14.02 per cent) (Jalali-Heravi *et al.*, 2007). A nonspecific lipid transfer protein has been isolated from the cumin seed (Zaman and Abbasi, 2009).

Bettaieb *et al.* (2010) gives a detailed picture of the composition. Essential oil yields were 0.03 per cent in roots, 0.1 per cent in stem and leaves, and 1.7 per cent in flowers. Major components of the oils were bornyl acetate (23 per cent), α-terpinene (34 per cent), and daku-terpinene (51 per cent) in roots, stems and leaves, and flowers, respectively. In all C. cyminum organs, total phenolics content ranged from 11.8 to 19.2 mg of gallic acid equivalents per gram of dry weight (mg of GAE/g of DW). Among the polyphenols studied, 13 were identified in roots, 17 in stem and leaves, and 15 in flowers. The major phenolic compound in the roots was quercetin (26 per cent), whereas in the stems and leaves, p-coumaric, rosmarinic, trans-2-dihydrocinnamic acids and resorcinol were predominant. In the flowers, vanillic acid was the main compound (51 per cent) (Bettaieb *et al.*, 2010). Bettaieb *et al.* (2011) also observed that cumin seeds are rich in an unusual fatty acid, petroselinic acid. Besides, cumin essential oil is a rich source of many compounds, including cuminaldehyde and daku-terpinene.

Therapeutic Value

Cumin seeds have traditionally been believed to be beneficial in digestive disorders, and scientific research has shown that cumin may stimulate the secretion of pancreatic enzymes, compounds necessary for proper digestion and nutrient assimilation. It has been used in the treatment of mild digestive disorders as a carminative and eupeptic, as an astringent in bronco pulmonary disorders, and as a cough remedy, as well as an analgesic (De *et al.*, 2003). It is used to treat diabetes and hypertension (Tahraoui *et al.*, 2007). Cumin is considered a stimulant, carminative and astringent and its overall therapeutic effects have been described on gastrointestinal, gynaecological and respiratory disorders, and also for the treatment of toothache, diarrhoea and epilepsy (Zargary, 2001).

Antioxidant

Cumin oil exhibit a higher activity in each antioxidant system with a special attention for beta-carotene bleaching test (IC (50): 20 µg/ml) and reducing power (EC (50): 11 µg/ml) (Hajlaoui *et al.*, 2010). The acetone extract of cumin flowers was strongly effective as a diphenyl-2-picrylhydrazyl radical scavenger, lipid peroxidation inhibitor, and reducing agent, with IC (50) values of 4, 32, and 8 µg/ml, respectively.

The acetone extract of stems and leaves showed the highest chelating power. However, the essential oils exhibited moderate activities in the different tests (Bettaieb *et al.*, 2010).

Cumin essential oil was found best in reducing Fe^{3+} ions and can be used as potential source of natural antioxidants in foods (El-Ghorab, 2010). Cumin with a high phenolic content and good antioxidant activity can be supplemented for both nutritional purposes and preservation of foods (Allahghadri *et al.*, 2010).

Nitric oxide is a neural messenger molecule in the central nervous system that is generated from L-arginine via the nitric oxide synthase (NOS). Kermani *et al.* (2012) found some components of the *C. cyminum* L. seed attenuate the excessive effect of L-arginine on morphine-induced conditioned place preference through the NOS inhibitory mechanism. It seems that cumin fruit essential oil possibly acts as a NOS inhibitor.

Antimicrobial

There is a continuing quest for safe and effective antimicrobial agents. This need has been heightened recently by the emergence of many antimicrobial-resistant organisms such as *K. pneumonia which* is an important Gram-negative pathogen, frequently associated with nosocomially acquired infections (Maroncle, 2002). It is involved in urinary tract infections, pneumonia, bacteremia, septicemia, and infections of surgical wounds. Biofilm growth enhances resistance to antibiotic therapies, as well as host defense mechanisms (Boddicker *et al.*, 2006).

Cumin seeds showed excellent *in vitro* antibacterial activity against methicillin-resistant *S. aureus* (MRSA). The *C. cyminum* exhibited bactericidal activity at a concentration of 300 µg/ml, and *it* could be a potential anti- MRSA agent, which will also be of great benefit in combating antibiotic resistance of *S. aureus* causing serious human infections and may contribute to the development of potential antimicrobial agents for inclusion in anti- *S. aureus* regimens (Mandal *et al.*, 2011).

Fabio *et al.* (2007) reported the zone diameter of inhibition (ZDI) of 24 and 18 mm, respectively for *C. zeylanicum* and *S. aromaticum* against *S. aureus*. Agaoglu *et al.* (2007) reported *C. zeylanicum* as the most effective spice against the microorganisms tested, and the most susceptible bacterial strain to this spice was *S. aureus* (ZDI: 32 mm); the ZDIs due to the action of *S. aromaticum* and *C. cyminum* against *S. aureus* were documented as 15 mm and 10 mm, respectively. The antibacterial activity of *C. cyminum* essential oil is perhaps attributable to the high levels of cuminaldehyde (16.1 per cent), the other main component includes *a*-pinene (11.4 per cent) (Iacobellis *et al.*, 2005; Helander *et al.*, 1998).

Derakhshan *et al.* (2008) reported that the essential oil of cumin seeds has a significant antibacterial activity against *K. pneumoniae in vitro.* The essential oil decreased biofilm formation and enhanced the activity of the ciprofloxacin disk. The incubation of the R-plasmid DNA with essential oil could not induce plasmid DNA degradation. The results of this study by Derakhshan *et al.* (2010) suggested the potential use of cumin seed essential oil against *K. pneumoniae in vitro*, may contribute to the *in vivo* efficacy of the same.The mechanism by which the cumin seed essential oil acts, to enhance the activity of ciprofloxacin against *K. pneumoniae*, as indicated by an increased inhibition zone diameter, is not known; but some cell wall damage or alteration in the outer membrane proteins may be caused by the cumin seed essential oil, which sensitizes cells to ciprofloxacin as well as resists cells to trimethoprim-sulphamethoxazole (Gutmann *et al.*, 1985; Huovinen *et al.*, 1987). The enhancement of antibacterial efficacy of ciprofloxacin by the essential oil is significant.

Essential oil of *C. cyminum* L. seed in combination with nisin can inhibit growth of food-borne pathogens in food. Cumin seed showed the most bactericidal effects on *B. cereus* at 8°C.Ultrastructural studies of vegetative cells confirmed the synergistic destructive effects of the essential oil and nisin on the cell wall of *B. cereus* and *B. subtilis* (Pajohi *et al.*, 2011). *C. cyminum* oil exhibited higher antibacterial and antifungal activities against *Vibrio* spp. strains with a diameter of inhibition zones ranging from 11 to 23 mm. Thus *C. cyminum* essential oil may be considered as an interesting source of antibacterial, antifungal and antioxidant components that could be used as potent agents in food preservation and for therapeutic or nutraceutical industries (Hajlaoui *et al.*, 2010).

Keskin and Toroglu (2011) studied the antimicrobial activity of cumin seed and the inhibition zone was found to be 7-15 mm with 30 µl. All cumin oils and cuminic aldehyde exhibited a considerable inhibitory effect against all the organisms tested, (Gram-positive and Gram-negative bacteria isolated from different sources of food–pork fillet, minced meat and sausages) except *Pseudomonas* spp. (Wanner *et al.*, 2010). According to Khosravi *et al.* (2011) the essential oil of *C. cyminum*, could be used as a natural inhibitor in foods at low concentrations to protect from fungal and toxin contaminations by *A. parasiticus*.

In a study carried out by Chaudhary and Tariq (2008), cumin was found to be more effective against the gram negative bacteria as compared to the gram positive bacteria, With the largest inhibitory zone against *E. coli* (23.8mm ± 1.2SD). The aqueous decoction of cumin also exhibited significant inhibitory activity against *M. roseus* (20.8mm ± 2.3SD), *P. shigelloides* (18.5mm ± 8.3SD), *Alcaligenes* spp. (17.1mm ± 2.9SD), *Citrobacter* spp. (16.2mm ± 0.5SD), *K. pneumoniae* (15.9mm ± 0.8SD), *A. hydrophila* (15.8mm ± 1.3SD), *K. ozaenae* (15.2mm ± 1.3SD), *P. aeruginosa* (12.3mm ± 3.3SD), *E. aerogenes* (12.0mm ± 0.1SD) and *S. aureus* (8.9mm ± 5.6SD).

The antibacterial activity of 1-(2-Ethyl, 6-Heptyl) Phenol (EHP) was studied against four Gram-negative and four Gram-positive bacterial pathogens. It was effective against the gram negative bacteria but less effective in case of gram positive bacteria. The most sensitive bacterial strain was *S. aureus* where, an inhibition zone of 0.8, 1.6, 2.8, and 3.5 cm was obtained with EHP concentrations of 1, 2.5, 5.0, and 1.0 µg/ml respectively. *S. aureus* was followed by *B. subtilis, S. pneumoniae* and *B. thuringiensis*. The activity of EHP against Gram-negative bacteria was less than that against Gram-positive ones where the largest zone of inhibition in Gram-negative bacteria was observed against *E. coli*; *i.e.*, 1.5 and 1.8 cm inhibition diameters were reported at 5 and 10 µg/ml EHP concentration respectively. *E. coli* was followed by *S. typhi, S. marcescens* and least *for P. aeruginosa* (Mekawey *et al.*, 2009). Similar results were seen in another study where cumin was more effective against the gram positive bacteria as compared to the gram negative bacteria. Amongst the gram negative bacteria, the antimicrobial activity of cumin was seen in case of E.coli and not much against any other strain (Sheikh *et al.*, 2010).

Cumin oil was also found to have strong antifungal activity. Antifungal testing of the essential oil of *C. cyminum* showed that it is active in general on all fungi but in particular on the dermatophytes, and *T. rubrum* was the most inhibited fungus even at the lowest dose of 5 µL. Less sensitive to treatment were the phytopathogens (Romagnoli *et al.*, 2002). In another study conducted by Rahman *et al.* (2000) it showed highest percent inhibition for *P. boydii* (88.2 per cent) followed by *A. flavus* (66.7 per cent), *M. canis* (51.6 per cent), *T. simi* (25.0 per cent), *F. lycopersici* (19.2 per cent) and *C. albicans* (11.0 per cent). Thus spices like cumin and their volatile compounds can be used as natural preservatives in food products and may be an alternative to the use of chemical additives.

Antiviral

Studies conducted by Romeilah *et al.* (2010) and Motamedifar *et al.* (2010) showed antiviral activities of cumin oil against herpes simplex virus 1 (HSV-1) in a cell line model. However, studies *in vivo* are needed to assess the true antiviral activities of these essential oils and to determine the metabolic pathways involved in their degradation.

Immunomodulatory

Many herbs and spices are known to modulate the immune system and have been shown to restore the immunity in immunocompromised individuals. Chauhan *et al.* (2010) found cumin seeds to significantly increase T cells (CD4 and CD8) count thereby suggesting immunomodulatory activity through modulation of T lymphocytes expression. In restraint stress induced immune-suppressed animals; compound 1 countered the depleted T lymphocytes, decreased the elevated corticosterone levels and size of adrenal glands and increased the weight of thymus and spleen.

Anticarcinogenic

Medicinal plants are considered as potential sources of chemotherapeutic drugs because of their diverse phytochemicals and little or no toxic effect. Among the nine plant products tested, cumin seeds (*C. cyminum* Linn) and basil leaves (*Ocimum sanctum* Linn) significantly decreased the incidence of both B[a]P-induced neoplasia and 3'MeDAB-induced hepatomas. Thus Cumin seeds are proved to be valuable anticarcinogenic agents by Aruna and Sivaramakrishnan (1992).

Colon cancer is the second most common cancer among men and women worldwide. Nalini *et al.* (2006) confirmed that cumin or black pepper suppresses colon carcinogensis in the presence of the procarcinogen DMH as a significantly increased excretion of fecal bile acids and neutral sterols and a significantly decreased number of tumours in the colon were observed in cumin + DMH- and black pepper + DMH-administered rats.

According to Gagandeep *et al.* (2003) reduction in tumour burden and significant elevation of the specific activities of superoxide dismutase ($P < 0.01$) and catalase

($P < 0.05$) and other related observations strongly suggest the cancer chemopreventive potentials of cumin seed and could be attributed to its ability to modulate carcinogen metabolism.

Cumin seeds increased the carcinogen-detoxifying enzyme, glutathione-S-transferase activity by more than 78 per cent in the stomach, liver and oesophagus,– high enough to be considered as protective agent against carcinogenesis. Also it significantly suppressed (*in vivo*) the chromosome aberrations (CA) caused by benzo (a) pyrene in mouse bone marrow cells and considered as protective agent against carcinogenesis (Aruna and Sivaramakrishnan, 1990). Again, Aruna and Sivaramakrishnan (1992) observed that cumin seed significantly decreased the incidence of both benzo [a] pyrene P-induced neoplasia and 3'-methyl-4-dimethylaminoazobenzene -induced hepatomas and suggested that the effect could be attributed to its ability to modulate carcinogen metabolism and thus may prove to be valuable anti carcinogenic agent.

1-(2-Ethyl, 6-Heptyl) Phenol (EHP), a biologically active compound extracted by benzene from *C. cyminum* (cumin) Egyptian seeds exhibited antitumour activity against six types of tumour cell lines (HEPG2, HELA, HCT116, MCF7, HEP2, CACO2). MCF7 was the most sensitive tumour cell line where only 33 per cent of the cells survived followed by HEPG2 (41 per cent of the cells survived) and HEP2 (56 per cent of the cells survived) at an EHP concentration of 10 μg/ml.

The percentage of tumour cell survival of $CACO_2$ and HCT116 was 72 per cent and76 per cent respectively exhibiting much less activity. However, EHP activity against HELA was negligible. (Mekawey *et al.*, 2009).

Antidiabetic

Srinivasan (2005) reviewed all the available information from animal experimentation as well as clinical trials where spices, their extracts or their active principles were examined for treatment of diabetes. He found in a limited number of studies, that cumin seeds (*C. cyminum*), along with ginger (*Zingiber officinale*), mustard (*Brassica nigra*), curry leaves (*Murraya koenigii*) and coriander (*Coriandrum sativum*) have been reported to be hypoglycaemic.

Methanolic extract of seeds of *C. cyminum* (CC) when fed to diabetic rats for 28 days caused a reduction in blood glucose, glycosylated haemoglobin, creatinine, blood urea nitrogen and improved serum insulin and glycogen (liver and skeletal muscle) content when compared to diabetic control rats. Significant reduction in renal oxidative stress and AGE was also observed with CC when compared to diabetic control. and glibenclamide. CC and glibenclamide improved antioxidant status in kidney and pancreas of diabetic rats. Diabetic rats showed increase in rat tail tendon collagen, glycated collagen, collagen linked fluorescence and reduction in pepsin digestion (Jagtap and Patil, 2010).

The biologically active constituent of *C. cyminum* seed oil was characterized as cuminaldehyde. The IC (50) value of cuminaldehyde is 0.00085 mg/ml against aldose reductase and 0.5 mg/ml against alpha-glucosidase, respectively. Cuminaldehyde was about 1.8 and 1.6 times less in inhibitory activity than acarbose and quercitin, respectively. Nonetheless, cuminaldehyde may be useful as a lead compound and a new agent for antidiabetic therapeutics (Lee, 2005).

Oral administration of 0.25 g kg(-1) body weight of *C. cyminum* for 6 weeks to diabetic rats resulted in significant reduction in blood glucose and an increase in total haemoglobin and glycosylated haemoglobin. It also prevented a decrease in body weight. *C. cyminum* treatment also resulted in a significant reduction in plasma and tissue cholesterol, phospholipids, free fatty acids and triglycerides. Supplementation with *C. cyminum* to diabetic rats significantly reduced the fatty changes and inflammatory cell infiltrates. According to Dhandapani *et al.* (2002) C. cyminum supplementation was found to be more effective than glibenclamide in the treatment of diabetes mellitus.

Cardioprotective

The levels of tissue (liver and kidney) cholesterol and triglycerides decreased when cumin was given along with alcohol and thermally oxidized oil. The level of phospholipids also increased. The activity of phospholipase A and C decreased significantly in the liver of groups fed cumin seeds indicating that cumin can decrease the lipid levels in alcohol and thermally oxidized oil induced hepatotoxicity (Aruna *et al.*, 2005).

Administration to Wistar rats of the cumin essential oil could bring a 17.38 per cent decrease in WBCs count, and 25.77 per cent, 14.24 per cent, and 108.81 per cent increase in hemoglobin concentration, hematocrit, and platelet count, respectively. LDL/HDL ratio was also reduced to half, which adds to the nutritional effects of cumin (Allahghadri *et al.*, 2010).

The liver phospholipids fatty acid concentrations of 16:0, 16:1, 18:0, 18:1 and 20:4 were near normal in cumin-treated rats when *C. cyminum* was administered at a dosage of 250 mg/kg body weight for 45 days (Kode *et al.*, 2005).

Antiepileptic

Janahmadi *et al.* (2006) demonstrated that extracellular application of the essential oil of *C. cyminum* (1 per cent and 3 per cent) dramatically decreased the frequency of spontaneous activity induced by pentylenetetrazol in a time and concentration dependent manner. In addition it showed protection against pentylenetetrazol-induced epileptic activity by increasing the duration, decreasing the amplitude of after hyperpolarization potential following the action potential, the peak of action potential, and inhibition of the firing rate.

Oral Contraceptive

C. cyminum methanol extract (CcMtE) fed to male rats for 60 days did not cause any alterations in the body weight, whereas the weight of testes, epididymides, seminal vesicles and ventral prostate were significantly reduced (pd".001). Animals treated with CcMtE showed a marked reduction in sperm density in the cauda epididymis and testes and sperm motility in the cauda epididymis. Reduction in fertility was 69.0 per cent and 76.0 per cent in 100 and 200 mg/rat/day dose levels, respectively.

Thus, *C. cyminum* inhibits spermatogenesis and fertility without producing apparent toxic effects (Gupta *et al.*, 2011).

When seed extracts of *Cuminum cyminum* (50 mg/day/rat) were fed orally to male albino rats for 60 days, it clearly showed the antifertility and androgenic effect. The sperm motility of cauda epididymis and sperm count of cauda epididymis and testis declined significantly leading to negative fertility test. Androgen dependent parameters (protein, sialic acid, fructose and ascorbic acid) were lowered, revealing reduction in the circulating androgen but on the contrary there was an increase in the testicular cholesterol level. (Venkatesh *et al.*, 2002).

Analgesic

The essential Oil of *C. cyminum* at the doses ranging between 0.0125 and 0.20 ml/kg exhibited a significant and dose-dependent analgesic effect in the animal model of chronic and inflammatory pain. But the essential oil was devoid of anti-inflammatory activity. However, further studies on the effect of the essential oil in weak inflammatory models such as cotton pellet granuloma and acetic acid-induced vascular permeability are needed before any precise conclusions can be drawn (Sayyah *et al.*, 2002).

Cumin and Memory

The influence of cumin on cognition, as determined by the acquisition, retention, and recovery in rats, was observed to be dose-dependent. The extract also produced significant inhibition of lipid peroxidation in comparison with known antioxidant ascorbic acid in both rat liver and brain. Daily administration of cumin at doses of 100, 200, and 300 mg/kg body weight 1 hour prior to induction of stress inhibited the stress-induced urinary biochemical changes in a dose-dependent manner without altering the levels in normal control groups. Thus, Koppula and Choi (2011) provided scientific support for the anti stress, antioxidant, and memory-enhancing activities of cumin extract and substantiated that its traditional use as a culinary spice in foods is beneficial and scientific in combating stress and related disorders.

Other Benefits of Cumin seeds

Mahesh *et al.* (2010) showed that aqueous extract of *C. cyminum* (AEC) seeds had protective action against gentamicin induced nephrotoxicity. The AEC 200 mg/kg showed marked decrease in elevated levels of serum urea, creatinine, lipid peroxidation (markers of nephrotoxicity) and increased clearance compare to the AEC 100 mg/kg.

Cumin is also beneficial for wound healing. It was shown by Patil *et al.* (2009) that alcoholic extract and its petroleum ether fraction of cumin seed showed increased wound healing activity on excision, incision and granuloma wound models in albino rats. However, ethyl acetate fraction failed to show significant wound healing activity.

Khatibi *et al.* (2008) showed that the *C. cyminum* fruit essential oil reduces the acquisition and expression of morphine-induced conditioned place preference in mice.

Phytoestrogens and phytoestrogen-containing plants are currently under active investigation for their role in estrogen-related disorders. On administering 0.15 mg/kg estradiol and 1 g/kg of methanolic extract of *C. cyminum* fruits (MCC) in two divided doses for 10 weeks significantly reduced urinary calcium excretion and significantly increased calcium content and mechanical strength of bones in comparison to bilaterally ovariectomized control. It showed greater bone and ash densities and improved microarchitecture of bones (Shirke *et al.*, 2008).

Interestingly, cumin seed was investigated for synthesis of gold nanoparticles by Sneha *et al.*, 2011). The gold nanoparticles formed at higher pH were stable, uniform and spherical in shape. XPS analysis showed the presence of pure gold nanoparticles Laxative effect of cumin seeds was observed by (Nworgu, 2009) in rat model.

References

Agaoglu S, Dostbil N, Alemdar S (2007). Antimicrobial activity of some spices used in the meat industry. Bull. Vet. Inst. Pulawy. 51: 53–57.

Al-Bataina BA, Maslat AO, Al-Kofahil MM (2003). Element analysis and biological studies on ten oriental spices using XRF and Ames test. J Trace Elem Med Biol. 17: 85–90.

Allahghadri T, Rasooli I, Owlia P, Nadooshan MJ, Ghazanfari T, Taghizadeh M, Astaneh SD (2010). Antimicrobial property, antioxidant capacity, and cytotoxicity of essential oil from cumin produced in Iran. J. Food Sci. 75 (2): H54–61.

Aruna K, Rukkumani R, Varma PS, Menon VP (2005). Therapeutic role of *Cuminum cyminum* on ethanol and thermally oxidized sunflower oil induced toxicity. Phytother Res. 19 (5): 416–21.

Aruna K, Sivaramakrishnan VM (1990). Plant products as protective agents against cancer. Indian J. Exp. Biol. 28 (11): 1008–11.

Aruna K, Sivaramakrishnan VM (1992). Anticarcinogenic effects of some Indian plant products. Food Chem. Toxicol. 30 (11): 953–56.

Bettaieb I, Bourgou S, Sriti J, Msaada K, Limam F, Marzouk B (2011). Essential oils and fatty acids composition of Tunisian and Indian cumin (*Cuminum cyminum* L.) seeds: a comparative study. J. Sci. Food Agric. 91 (11): 2100–107.

Bettaieb I, Bourgou S, Wannes WA, Hamrouni I, Limam F, Marzouk B (2010). Essential oils, phenolics, and antioxidant activities of different parts of cumin (*Cuminum cyminum* L.). J. Agric. Food Chem. 58 (19): 10410 -18.

Boddicker JD, Anderson RA, Jagnow J, Clegg S (2006). Signature-tagged mutagenesis of *Klebsiella pneumoniae* to identify genes that influence biofilm formation on extracellular matrix material. *Infect. Immun.* 74: 4590–97.

Chauhan PS, Satti NK, Suri KA, Amina M, Bani S (2010). Stimulatory effects of *Cuminum cyminum* and flavonoid glycoside on Cyclosporine-A and restraint stress induced immune-suppression in Swiss albino mice. Chem. Biol. Interact. 185 (1): 66–72.

Chaudhry N and Tariq P (2008) *In vitro* Antibacterial Activities of Kalonji, Cumin And Poppy Seed Pak. J. Bot. 40 (1): 461–67.

De M, De AK, Mukhopadhvay R, Banerjee AB, Micro M (2003). Antimicrobial activity of *Cuminum cyminum* L. Ars.Pharmaceutica. 44: 257–69.

Derakhshan S, Sattari M, Bigdeli M (2010). Effect of cumin (*Cuminum cyminum*) seed essential oil on biofilm formation and plasmid Integrity of *Klebsiella pneumoniae.* Pharmacogn Mag. 6 (21): 57–61.

Derakhshan S, Sattari M, Bigdeli M (2008). Effect of subinhibitory concentrations of cumin (*Cuminum cyminum* L.) seed essential oil and alcoholic extract on the morphology, capsule expression and urease activity of *Klebsiella pneumoniae.* Int. J. Antimicrob. Agents. 32: 432–36.

Dhandapani S, Subramanian VR, Rajagopal S, Namasivayam N (2002). Hypolipidemic effect of *Cuminum cyminum* L. on alloxan-induced diabetic rats. Pharmacol. Res. 46 (3): 251–55.

El-Ghorab AH, Nauman M, Anjum FM, Hussain S, Nadeem M (2010). A comparative study on chemical composition and antioxidant activity of ginger (*Zingiber officinale*) and cumin (*Cuminum cyminum*). J. Agric. Food Chem. 58 (14): 8231–37.

El-Sawi SA, Mohamed MA (2002). Cumin herb as a new source of essential oils and its response to foliar spray with some micro-nutrients. Food Chem. 77: 75–80.

Fabio A, Cermelli C, Fabio G, Nicoletti P, Quaglio P (2007). Screening of the antibacterial effects of a variety of essential oils on microorganisms responsible for respiratory infections. Phytother. Res. 21 (4): 374–77.

Gagandeep, Dhanalakshmi S, Méndiz E, Rao AR, Kale RK (2003). hemopreventive effects of *Cuminum cyminum* in chemically induced forestomach and uterine cervix tumours in murine model systems. Nutr. Cancer. 47 (2): 171- 80.

Gupta RS, Saxena P, Gupta R, Kachhawa JB (2011).Evaluation of reversible contraceptive activities of *Cuminum cyminum* in male albino rats. Contraception. 84 (1): 98 -107.

Gutmann L, Williamson R, Moreau N, Kitzis MD, Collatz E, Acar JF, *et al.* (1985). Cross-resistance to nalidixic acid, trimethoprim, and chloramphenicol associated with alterations in outer membrane proteins *of Klebsiella, Enterobacter,* and *Serratia.* J. Infect. Dis. 151: 501–507.

Hajlaoui H, Mighri H, Noumi E, Snoussi M, Trabelsi N, Ksouri R, Bakhrouf A (2010). Chemical composition and biological activities of Tunisian *Cuminum cyminum* L. essential oil: a high effectiveness against Vibrio spp. strains. Food Chem. Toxicol. 48 (8-9): 2186–92.

Helander IM, Alakomi HL, Latva-Kala K, Mattila-Sandholm T, Pol I, Smid EJ, *et al.* (1998). Characterization of the action of selected essential oil components on gram-negative bacteria. J. Agric. Food Chem. 46: 3590–95.

Huovinen P (1987). Trimethoprim resistance. Antimicrob Agents Chemother. 31: 1451–56.

Iacobellis NS, Lo Cantore P, Capasso F, Senatore F (2005). Antibacterial activity of *Cuminum cyminum* L. and *Carum carvi* L. essential oils. *J. Agric. Food Chem.* 53 (1): 57–61.

Jagtap AG, Patil PB (2010). Antihyperglycemic activity and inhibition of advanced glycation end product formation by *Cuminum cyminum* in streptozotocin induced diabetic rats. Food Chem. Toxicol. 48 (8-9): 2030–36.

Jalali-Heravi M, Zekavat B, Sereshti H (2007). Use of gas chromatography-mass spectrometry combined with resolution methods to characterize the essential oil components of Iranian cumin and caraway. J. Chromatogr. A. 1143 (1-2): 215–26.

Janahmadi M, Niazi F, Danyali S, Kamalinejad M (2006). Effects of the fruit essential oil of *Cuminum cyminum* Linn. (Apiaceae) on pentylenetetrazol-induced epileptiform activity in F1 neurones of Helix aspersa. J. Ethnopharmacol. 104 (1-2): 278–82.

Johri RK (2011). *Cuminum cyminum* and *Carum carvi*: An update. Pharmacogn. Rev. 5 (9): 63–72.

Joshi SG (2000). Medicinal plants: Family Apiaceae. 1st ed. Oxford and IBH Publishing Co. Pvt. Ltd. Delhi.

Kermani M, Azizi P, Haghparast A (2012). The role of nitric oxide in the effects of cumin (*Cuminum cyminum* L.) fruit essential oil on the acquisition of morphine-induced conditioned place preference in adult male mice. Chin J Integr Med. 12. [Epub ahead of print].

Keskin D, Toroglu S (2011). Studies on antimicrobial activities of solvent extracts of different spices. J. Environ. Biol. 32 (2): 251–56.

Khatibi A, Haghparast A, Shams J, Dianati E, Komaki A, Kamalinejad M (2008). Effects of the fruit essential oil of *Cuminum cyminum* L. on the acquisition and expression of morphine-induced conditioned place preference in mice. Neurosci. Lett. 448 (1): 94–98.

Khosravi AR, Shokri H, Minooeianhaghighi M (2011). Inhibition of aflatoxin production and growth of *Aspergillus parasiticus* by *Cuminum cyminum*, *Ziziphora clinopodioides*, and *Nigella sativa* essential oils. Foodborne. Pathog. Dis. 8 (12):1275–80.

Kode A, Rajagopalan R, Penumathsa SV, Menon VP (2005). Effect of ethanol and thermally oxidized sunflower oil ingestion on phospholipid fatty acid composition of rat liver: protective role of *Cuminum cyminum* L. Ann. Nutr. Metab. 49 (5): 300–303.

Koppula S, Choi DK (2011). *Cuminum cyminum* extract attenuates scopolamine-induced memory loss and stress-induced urinary biochemical changes in rats: a noninvasive biochemical approach. Pharm. Biol. 49 (7): 702–708.

Lahlou S, Tahraoui A, Israili Z, Lyoussi B (2007). Diuretic activity of the aqueous extracts of *Carum carvi* and *Tanacetum vulgare* in normal rats. J. Ethnopharmacol. 110: 458–63.

Lee HS (2005). Cuminaldehyde: Aldose Reductase and alpha-Glucosidase Inhibitor Derived from Cuminum cyminum L. Seeds. J. Agric. Food Chem. 53 (7): 2446–50.

Mahesh C, Gowda S, Gupta A (2010). Protective action of *Cuminum cyminum* against gentamicin induced nephrotoxicity. Journal of Pharmacy Research. 3 (4): 753–57.

Maiga A, Diallo D, Bye R, Paulsen BS (2005). Determination of some toxic and essential metal ions in medicinal and edible plants from Mali. *J. Agric. Food Chem.* 53: 2316–21.

Mandal S, Mandal MD Saha K, Pal NK (2011). *In vitro* Antibacterial Activity of three Indian Spices Against Methicillin-Resistant *Staphylococcus aureus*. Oman Med. J. 26 (5): 319–23.

Mekawey A, Mokhtar M. and Farrag R (2009). Antitumour and Antibacterial Activities of [1-(2-Ethyl, 6-Heptyl) Phenol] from *Cuminum cyminum* Seeds, Journal of Applied Sciences Research, 5 (11): 1881–88.

Milan KSM, Dholakia H, Tiku PK, Vishveshwaraiah P (2008). Enhancement of digestive enzymatic activity by cumin (*Cuminum cymonum* L.) and role of spent cumin as a bionutrient. Food Chem. 110:678–83.

Maroncle N, Balestrino D, Rich C, Forestier C (2002). Identification of *Klebsiella pneumoniae* genes involved in intestinal colonization and adhesion using signature-tagged mutagenesis. Infect. Immun. 70 (8): 4729–34.

Motamedifar M, Narjes G, Shirazi T (2010). The Effect of Cumin Seed Extracts Against *Herpes Simplex Virus* Type 1 In Vero Cell Culture, Iranian Journal of Medical Sciences (I.J.M.S.). 35 (4): 304–309.

Nalini N, Manju V, Menon VP (2006). Effect of spices on lipid metabolism in 1, 2-dimethylhydrazine-induced rat colon carcinogenesis. J. Med. Food. 9 (2): 237–45.

Nworgu Z. (2002) Preliminary screening of laxative effect of cumin seeds in rats Pakistan Journal of Scientific and Industrial Research 2002, vol. 45, no 4, pp. 256–58

Pajohi MR, Tajik H, Farshid AA, Hadian M (2011). Synergistic antibacterial activity of the essential oil of *Cuminum cyminum* L. seed and nisin in a food model. J Appl Microbiol. 2011 Jan 12. doi: 10.1111j.1365-2672.2011.04946.x. [Epub ahead of print].

Patil D, Kulkarni A, Shahapurkar A, Hatappakki B (2009). Natural cumin seeds for wound healing activity in albino rats, International Journal of Biological Chemistry. 3 (4): 148–52.

Rahman A, Chaudhary I, Farooq A, Ahmed A, Iqbal Z, Demirci B, Demrici F, Baser H (2000) Antifungal activities and essential oil constituents of some spices from Pakistan. Jour. Chem. Soc. Pak. 22 (1):

Romagnoli C, Andreotti E, Maietti S, Mahendra R, Mares D (2010). Antifungal activity of essential oil from fruits of Indian *Cuminum cyminum*. Pharm. Biol. 48 (7): 834–38.

Romeilah R, Fayed S and Mahmoud G (2010). Chemical Compositions, Antiviral and Antioxidant Activities of Seven Essential Oils. Journal of Applied Sciences Research. 6 (1): 50–62

Sayyah M, Peirovi A and Kamalinejad M (2002). Anti-Nociceptive Effect of the Fruit Essential Oil of *Cuminum cyminum* L. in Rat Iranian Biomedical Journal. 6 (4): 141- 44.

Shirke SS, Jadhav SR, Jagtap AG (2008). Methanolic extract of *Cuminum cyminum* inhibits ovariectomy-induced bone loss in rats. Exp. Biol. Med. (Maywood). 233 (11): 1403–10.

Sheikh M, Islam S, Rahman A, Rahman M, Rahman M, Rahman M, Rahim A, Alam F (2010). Control of Some Human Pathogenic Bacteria by Seed Extracts of Cumin (*Cuminum cyminum* L.) Agric. conspec. sci. 75 (1):

Sneha K, Sathishkumar M, Lee SY, Bae MA, Yun YS (2011). Biosynthesis of Au nanoparticles using cumin seed powder extract. J. Nanosci. Nanotechnol. 11 (2): 1811–14.

Srinivasan K (2005). Plant foods in the management of diabetes mellitus: spices as beneficial antidiabetic food adjuncts. Int. J. Food Sci. Nutr. 56 (6): 399 -414.

Tahraoui A, El-Hilay J, Israili ZH, Lyoussi B (2007). Ethnopharmacological survey of plants used in the traditional treatment of hypertension and diabetes in south-eastern Morocco (Errachidia province) J. Ethnopharmacol. 110: 105–17.

Toghrol F, Daneshpejouh H (1974). Estimation of free amino acids, protein and amino acid compositions of cumin seed (*Cuminum cyminum*) of Iran. J. Trop. Pediatr. Environ. Child Health. 20: 109–11.

Uma PK, Geervani P, Eggum BO (1993). Common Indian spices: Nutrient composition, consumption and contribution to dietary value. Plant Foods Hum. Nutr. 44: 137–48.

USDA (2012). National Nutrient Database for Standard Reference, Release. 25.

Venkatesh V, Sharma J and Kamal R (2002). A Comparative Study of Effect of Alcoholic Extracts of *Sapindus emarginatus, Terminalia belerica, Cuminum cyminum* and *Allium cepa* on Reproductive Organs of Male Albino Rats, Asian J. Exp. Sci. 16 (1 and 2): 51- 63.

Wanner J, Bail S, Jirovetz L, Buchbauer G, Schmidt E, Gochev V, Girova T, Atanasova T, Stoyanova A (2010). Chemical composition and antimicrobial activity of cumin oil (*Cuminum cyminum*, Apiaceae). Nat. Prod. Commun. 5 (9): 1355–58.

Zaman U, Abbasi A (2009). Isolation, purification and characterization of a nonspecific lipid transfer protein from *Cuminum cyminum*. Phytochemistry. 70: 979–87.

Zargary A (2001). Medicinal Plants. 5th ed. Tehran: Tehran University Publications.

Zohary D, Hopf M (2000). Domestication of plants in the Old World, third edition. Oxford: University Press. p. 206.

Chapter 6

Curry Leaves

(*Murraya koenigii*, Rutaceae)

Coriander Leaves and Seeds

(*Coriandrum sativum* L.)

A. CURRY LEAVES (*Murraya koenigii*, Rutaceae)

Curry leaf is one of the spices used in Indian and other Asian cuisines for its distinct flavour and aroma. Curry leaf has many herbal medicinal properties and it is a most prominently used herb in south India. The species name commemorates the botanist Johann König. The colloquial name for curry leaves is curry patta in Hindi and Kariveppilai in Tamil.

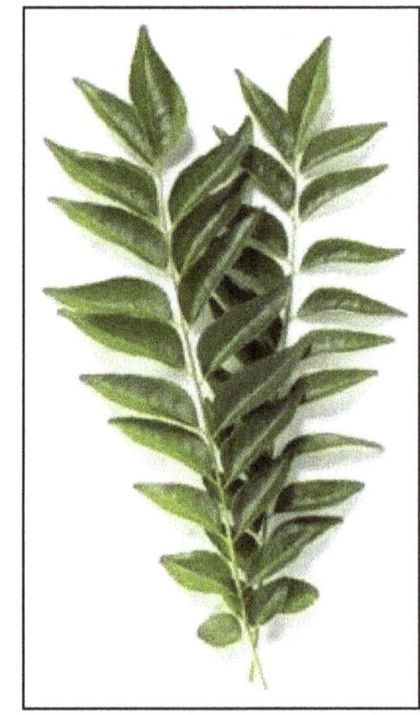

Curry leaf tree grows in the warm climates of India, about 4–6 m tall, with a trunk up to 40 cm. diameter. The leaves are pinnate, with 11 – 21 leaflets, each leaflet 2–4 cm long and 1–2 cm. broad. The leaves are slightly bitter and aromatic. The curry leaves tree is a native of India and Sri Lanka. The flowers are small white and fragrant. The berries which are small, black and shiny are edible.

Nutritional and Phytochemical Composition

The fresh curry leaves obtained from the New England states contained 9744 ng of lutein, 212 ng of alpha-tocopherol and 183 ng of beta-carotene per gram fresh weight (Palaniswamy *et al.*).

Curry leaves contain 2.5 per cent of oil. The major compounds of the essential oil extracted from curry leaves are: alpha-copaene (44.3 per cent), beta-gurjunene (25.5 per cent), isocaryophyllene (12.1 per cent), beta-caryophyllene (8.7 per cent) and germacrene D (2.9 per cent). alpha-selinene, beta-bisabolene, beta-cadinene, beta-caryophyllene, beta-elemene, beta-gurjenene, beta-phellandrene, beta-thujene and beta-transocimene. These ingredients give curry leaves it typical aroma (Erkan *et al.*, 2012).

The plant is reported to contain carbazole alkaloids (Narasimhan *et al.*, 1968), having antioxidant (Rao *et al.*, 2007; Arulselvan and Subramanian, 2007; Gupta and Sharma, 2010; Gupta *et al.*, 2011), anti-inflammatory, and antitumour activities (Muthumani *et al.*, 2009).

Nutritional Values of Curry leaves

Nutrient	*Amount*	*Nutrient*	*Amount*
Energy (kcals)	108	Calcium (mg)	830
Carbohydrate (gm)	18.7	Iron (mg)	0.93
Protein (gm)	6.1	Magnesium (mg)	44
Fat (gm)	1.0	Phosphorus (mg)	57
Thiamine (mg)	0.08	Sodium (mg)	81
Riboflavin (mg)	0.21	Zinc (mg)	0.20
Niacin (mg)	2.3		
Carotene (µg)	7560		
Vitamin C (mg)	4		

Gopalan *et al.*, 2000.

A carbazole alkaloid, mahanimbine [3, 5-dimethyl-3-(4- methylpent-3-enyl)-11H-pyrano [5, 6-a] carbazole], inhibitor of acetylcholinesterase was isolated from the petroleum ether extract of the leaves of *M. koenigii* (Kumar *et al.*, 2010). Three bioactive carbazole alkaloids, mahanimbine (1), murrayanol (2), and mahanine (3) were identified in the acetone extract of the fresh leaves of *M. koenigii* by Ramsewak *et al.* (1999).

A new carbazole alkaloid, designated as murrayakoeninol, was isolated by Chakraborty *et al.* (2009) from the leaves of *M. koenigii* (Linn) Spreng, along with four known carbazole alkaloids, *viz.* mahanimbine, koenimbine, O-methylmurrayamine-A and murrayazolinine and one from the bark *viz.* girinimbine.

M. koenigii (L.) Spreng leaves (Rutaceae) exhibited antilipase activity greater than 80 per cent. Further, bioactivity guided fractionation of the EtOAc extract led to the isolation of four alkaloids, namely mahanimbin, koenimbin, koenigicine and clausazoline-K, with IC50 values of 17.9 μM, 168.6 μM, 428.6 μM and <500 μM, respectively (Birari *et al.*, 2009).

Traditional Therapeutic Beliefs of Curry Leaves

Curry leaf has been used in folk medicine in China and other Asian countries as an analgesic, astringent, antidysenteric, antioxidant, febrifuge, hypolipidemic, hypoglycaemic, vision improver, nightblindness correction as well as fertility regulation. Traditionally, the plant is used as tonic, stomachic, and carminative (Muthumani *et al.*, 2009). Leaves, fruits, roots and bark of this plant are a rich source of carbazole alkaloids. These alkaloids have been reported for their various pharmacological activities such as antitumour, antiviral, anti-inflammatory, antidiarrhoeal, diuretic and antioxidant activities (Gupta *et al.*, 2011).

Curry leaves are believed to be beneficial in constipation, stomach problems, vomiting, nausea, snake bite, spots and rashes and in improving stomach and small intestine functioning. It is believed that their smell, taste and visual impression stimulates the salivary secretion and initiates the peristaltic wave. They are mildly laxative and in case of a digestive upset, buttermilk enriched with the paste of curry leaves, common salt and cumin seed powder is recommended. This combination is also useful in problems such as loss of appetite, tastelessness of mouth as in case of fever etc. Curry leaves are also said to have some role in the treatment of diarrhoea, dysentery and idiopathic loose motions. Traditional healers in villages use these leaves with a few other medicinal leaves applied externally in poultice form for the treatment of insect bites.

Ayurvedic research confirms that curry leaves have some role in controlling non-insulin dependent diabetes mellitus. Many people have also reported weight loss desired in diabetics. Few studies are available on curry leaves for treatment of minor burns, bruises, abrasions, etc. and claim benefits of the treatment. More clinical trials are necessary to prove effectiveness. The bark or root of this plant also has medicinal properties. One ayurvedic school recommends powdered root/bark for relief from kidney/biliary pain. Traditional healers have observed some effects on premature graying of hair. Regular intake of these leaves with buttermilk is advised. Few have tried curry leaves for treatment of minor burns, bruises, abrasions, etc. and claim benefits of the treatment.

Some of the therapeutic benefits of curry leaves are highlighted below.

Anticarcinogenic

Anticarcinogenic potential of curry leaf was evaluated by Dasgupta *et al.* (2003) adopting the protocol of Benzo(a)pyrene induced fore-stomach and 7,12 imethylbenz(a) anthracene (DMBA) induced skin papillomagenesis. Chemo-preventive response was measured by tumour burden (papillomas/mouse), and by the percentage of tumour bearing animals. Both the investigated dose levels of curry leaf showed a significant reduction in tumour burden ($P < 0.001$) as well as tumour incidence at both the tumour model system studied. Our studies strongly suggest that the curry leaf can be useful for the prevention of human stomach and skin cancers.

Khanum *et al.* (2000) reported that curry leaves have high potential as reducer of the toxicity of dimethylhydrazine hydrochloride (DMH). The antioxidant potential of curry leaves in rats treated with a known chemical carcinogen, DMH was investigated. Food intake reduced in the rats fed curry leaf-supplemented diet but the body and the organ weights were not affected. Vitamin A content in the liver significantly increased whereas glutathione (GSH) content did not alter. A 50 per cent reduction in the micronuclei induced by DMH and a 30 per cent reduction in the activity of gamma-glutamyl transpeptidase were also observed. These results indicate that curry leaves have high potential of reducing the toxicity of dimethylhydrazine hydrochloride.

Antioxidant

When ghee is stored under ambient temperature, it undergoes oxidative deterioration. The oxidation of unsaturated fatty acids produces hydroperoxides and their subsequent breakdown products *viz.* aldehydes, ketones, low molecular weight acids and oxy acids. These components are responsible for the development of off flavours in ghee. In ancient days, betel leaves and curry leaves were usually added to the butter during the clarification process. But it is now recognized that these substances indeed possess antioxidant properties, which will not only improve the shelf life and taste of the product but also they are safe to the consumers. It is observed that the plant leaves (curry and betel leaves) contain phenolic compounds such as hydroxychavicol, eugenol, and certain amino acids such as aspargine, glycine, serine, aspartic acid, glutamic acid, threonine, alanine, proline, and tryptophan which might possess antioxidant properties and help to improve the shelf life of ghee. Dasgupta *et al.* (2003) also reported that the betel and curry leaves can serve as a potent antioxidant at 1 per cent concentration without any adverse effect on the organoleptic properties of the ghee and help replace the BHA and BHT to extend the shelf life of ghee.

Nor *et al.* (2009) found that the leaf extract *M. koenigii* had a polyphenol content of 109.5±0.3 mg gallic acid equivalents/g extract and contain a heat-stable antioxidant. They suggested that *M. koenigii* could be a natural alternative to synthetic antioxidants for the industry. DPPH radical scavenging activities of essential oils were relatively low (10 per cent -24 per cent) (Erkan *et al.*, 2012).

The antioxidative properties of the leaves extracts of *M. koenigii* using different solvents were evaluated by Tachibana *et al.* (2001) based on the oil stability index (OSI) together with their radical scavenging ability against 1-1-diphenyl-2-picrylhydrazyl (DPPH). The OSI value of carbazoles at 110° C decreased in the order 1 and 3 > alpha-tocopherol > BHT > 2 > 4, 5 and control. It is assumed that compounds 1 and 3 contributed to the high OSI value of the CH (2) Cl (2) extract of *M. koenigii*. The DPPH radical scavenging activity for these carbazoles was in the order ascorbic acid > 2 > 1, 3 and alpha-tocopherol > BHT > 4 and 5. Again the anti-oxidative properties of 12 carbazole alkaloids isolated from leaves of curry leaves was reported by Tachibana *et al.* (2003) who found that an aryl hydroxyl substituent on the carbazole rings plays a role in stabilizing the thermal oxidation and rate of reaction against DPPH radical.

Ramsewak *et al.* (1999) observed that the compound 1 (mahanimbine) isolated by the bioassay guided fractionation of the acetone extract of the fresh leaves of *M. koenigii* displayed antioxidant activity at 33.1 mcg/ml.

Anti-Inflammatory Effect

Paul *et al.* (2011) found anti-inflammatory response by the oral doses of around 200mg of curry leaves extract as it was evident by interleukin (IL)-2, 4, 10, and tumour necrosis factor alpha (TNF-α) expression. In addition, the reduction of apoptosis in pancreatic cells was found in extract-treated diabetic mice. The compound murrayanol isolated from the acetone extract of the fresh leaves showed an IC-50 of 109 mcg/ml against hPGHS-1 and an IC-50 of 218 mcg/ml against hPGHS-2 in anti-inflammatory assays (Ramsewak *et al.*, 1999).

Antidiabetic Effect

Significant decrease in the blood glucose level was observed at the 30th and 60th day of administration (300 and 500 mg/kg) of curry leaves to diabetic rats. Tembhurne and Sakarkar (2011) and Arulselvan *et al.* (2006) reported that curry leaves had protective effect against gastrointestinal disturbances in diabetes by controlling glucose level as well as defending against peripheral damage of cholinergic neurons by providing antioxidant shelter.

Dusane and Joshi (2012) demonstrated the significance of chloroform and aqueous extract in glucosidase inhibition and islet protection in the murine diabetic model suggesting the potential use of curry leaves extract in adjuvant therapy for the treatment of diabetes and the possible development of potential neutraceuticals. Paul *et al.* (2011) observed that the aqueous and 50 per cent methanol extract of curry leaves not only have hypoglycaemic property but also have certain effects to regulate mice immunology related to oxidative stress metabolism. Moreover, aqueous extract was found to be better than methonolic extract thus revealing the immunomodulatory property of the curry leaf extracts of on diabetes and diabetes-related pathology in mice.

Lawal *et al.* (2008) observed that aqueous extract of curry leaves when administered at the dose levels of 100 mg/kg, 150 mg/kg and 200 mg/kg bodyweight to normal and alloxan-induced diabetic rats, the glucose lowering effect was more pronounced in the alloxan-induced diabetic rats than in control rats. When compared with chlorpropamide, the glucose lowering effect of the curry leaves extract was significantly lower at the dose levels administered in both normal and alloxan-induced diabetic rats.

Yankuzo *et al.* (2011) observed that the aqueous extract of curry leaves administered orally for 30 days at different dose levels in diabetic rats produced significant dose dependant decrease in serum urea and creatinine and marked increase in the plasma antioxidant capacity compared to the non-diabetic ones. These observations scientifically support the traditional belief that curry leaves, as an adjuvant help in the treatment of pain disorders related to renal impairments among diabetics. Fresh juice of the *M. koenigii* root is taken to relieve pain associated with kidney (Nayak *et al.*, 2010).

Analgesic

Methanolic extract of curry leaf possess antinociceptive and anti-inflammatory effect in dose dependent manner when compared with the control and standard drug diclofenac sodium (10mg/kg, p.o) (Gupta *et al.*, 2010).

Intra-peritoneal administration of the extract at doses of 100 and 200 mg/kg produced significant dose-dependent activity in all of the nociceptive models evaluated ($p < 0.05$). The study suggested the presence of potent antinociceptive and anti-inflammatory principles in the extract, supporting its folkloric use for the treatment of these conditions (Shaik *et al.*, 2009).

The abdominal constriction response produced by acetic acid is a sensitive procedure for peripheral analgesic agents. Acetic acid causes an increase in peritoneal fluid levels of prostaglandins (PGE2 and PGF2α), involving in part peritoneal receptors (Deraedt *et al.*, 1980) and inflammatory pain by inducing capillary permeability (Amico-Roxas *et al.*, 1984). In acute stage, petroleum ether extract of curry leaves and the alkaloids separated from the ether extract significantly and dose-dependently reduced the number of acetic acid-induced writhing, significantly increased the latency of paw licking in hot plate method, and significantly increased the basal reaction time in tail immersion method. In chronic stage, highest activity was observed on day 9 in acetic acid-induced writhing model. The degree of antinociception produced by Petroleum ether extraction of curry leaves and the alkaloids separated from the same at the end of 15 days suggested that curry leaf is a potential analgesic (Patil *et al.*, 2012).

Antibacterial Property

The studies on the anti- bacterial property of curry leaves seem to be scanty. Erkan *et al.* (2012) reported that the essential oil from curry leaves (Solvent-free microwave extraction) at 300 mcg/mL provided 92 per cent inhibition of L. innocua, a non pathogenic food contaminant.

Hepatoprotective

Based on the effects on protein content, liver metabolizing enzymes *viz.*, glutathione, superoxide dismutase, catalase and the morphology of the cells, antioxidant activity with anti-lipid peroxidation potential, the tannins and the carbazole alkaloids from the aqueous extract of curry leaves exhibited excellent hepato-protective activity (Sathaye *et al.*, 2011). Desai *et al.* (2012) demonstrated that hydro-ethanolic leaf extract possesses hepatoprotective potentials as pretreatment with curry leaves extract showed significant decrease in activity levels of alanine aminotransferase, aspartate aminotransferase, alkaline phosphatase, total protein, and bilirubin in CCl_4 treated hepatotoxic rats and a dose dependent increase in hepatic super oxide dismutase, catalase, reduced glutathione and ascorbic acid, and a decrease in lipid peroxidation and related toxic manifestations.

At a dose of 300 mg/kg/day to the high fat diet induced obese rats for 2 weeks the dichloromethane and ethyl acetate extracts of curry leaves significantly reduced the body weight gain, plasma total cholesterol and triglyceride levels. The observed antiobesity and antihyperlipidemic activities of these extracts are correlated with the carbazole alkaloids, mahanimbine present in them (Birari *et al.*, 2010).

Other Benefits

Patil *et al.* (2011) concluded from their study that curry leaves could be screened as a potential drug for the prevention or treatment of neuroleptic-induced orofacial dyskinesia (a late complication of prolonged neuroleptic treatment characterized by involuntary movements of the oral region). They co-administered alcohol extract of curry leaves (EEMK) (100 and 300mg/kg, p.o.) and its alkaloid fraction AMK (30 and 100mg/kg, p.o.) along with haloperidol that significantly reversed the effect on locomotion. The mechanism involved significant reversal of the haloperidol-induced decrease in forebrain superoxide dismutase and catalase levels in rats and significant reduction in the lipid peroxidation potential and restoration of GSH levels.

Interestingly all the three bioactive carbazole alkaloids, (1) mahanimbine, (2) murrayanol and (3) mahanine, isolatesd by fractionation of the acetone extract of fresh curry leaves were mosquitocidal, antimicrobial and exhibited topoisomerase I and II inhibition activities (Ramsewak *et al.*, 1999).

Conclusion

Presently curry leaves are used mainly as a flavouring agent in cooking and there is a need to educate the common man on the use of the leaves in the form of ground paste or powder before adding to the food in order to get the full value of curry leaves.

References

Amico-Roxas M, Caruso A, Trombadore S, Scifo R, Scapagnini U (1984). Gangliosides antinociceptive effects in rodents. Arch. Int. Pharmacodyn. Ther. 272: 103–17.

Arulselvan P, Senthilkumar GP, Sathish Kumar D, Subramanian S (2006). Antidiabetic effect of *Murraya koenigii* leaves on streptozotocin induced diabetic rats. Pharmazie. 61 (10): 874–77.

Arulselvan P, Subramanian SP (2007). Beneficial effects of *Murraya koenigii* leaves on antioxidant defense system and ultra structural changes of pancreatic beta-cells in experimental diabetes in rats. Chem. Biol. Interact. 165 (2): 155–64.

Birari R, Javia V, Bhutani KK (2010). Antiobesity and lipid lowering effects of *Murraya koenigii* (L.) Spreng leaves extracts and mahanimbine on high fat diet induced obese rats. Fitoterapia. 81 (8): 1129–33.

Birari R, Roy SK, Singh A, Bhutani KK (2009). Pancreatic lipase inhibitory alkaloids of *Murraya koenigii* leaves. Nat Prod Commun. 4 (8): 1089–92.

Chakraborty M, Saha S, Mukhapadhyay S (2009). Murrayakoeninol—a new carbazole alkaloid from *Murraya koenigii* (Linn) Spreng. Nat. Prod. Commun. 4 (3): 355–58.

Dasgupta T, Rao, A.R, Yadava P.K (2003). Chemomodulatory action of curry leaf (*Murraya koenigii*) extract on hepatic and extrahepatic xenobiotic metabolising enzymes, antioxidant levels, lipid peroxidation, skin and forestomach papillomagenesis. Nutrition Research 23 (10): 1427–46.

Deraedt R, Jougney S, Delevalcee F, Falhout M (1980). Release of prostaglandin E and F in an algogenic reaction and its inhibition. Eur J Pharmacol. 51: 17–24.

Desai SN, Patel DK, Devkar RV, Patel PV, Ramachandran AV (2012). Hepatoprotective potential of polyphenol rich extract of *Murraya koenigii* L.: an *in vivo* study. Food Chem. Toxicol. 50 (2): 310–14.

Dusane MB, Joshi BN (2012). Islet protective and insulin secretion property of *Murraya koenigii* and *Ocimum tenuflorum* in streptozotocin-induced diabetic mice. Can J Physiol. Pharmacol. 90 (3): 371–78.

Erkan N, Tao Z, Rupasinghe HP, Uysal B, Oksal BS (2012). Antibacterial activities of essential oils extracted from leaves of *Murraya koenigii* by solvent-free microwave extraction and hydro-distillation. Nat. Prod. Commun. 7 (1): 121–24.

Gopalan C, Rama Sastri BV, Balasubramanian SC. (Revised and Updated by) Narasinga Rao BS, Deosthale, YG, Pant KC (2000). NIN, ICMR, Hyderabad, India.

Gupta P, Nahata A, Dixit VK (2011). An update on *Murraya koenigii* spreng: a multifunctional Ayurvedic herb. Zhong Xi Yi Jie He Xue Bao. 9 (8): 824–33.

Gupta S, George M, Singhal M, Sharma G, Garg V (2010). Leaves extract of Murraya koinigii Linn for Anti-inflammatory Analgesic and activity in animal models. J. Adv. Pharm. Tech. Res. 1: 68–77.

Gupta V, Sharma M (2010). Protective effect of *Murraya koenigii* on lipid peroxide formation in isolated rat liver homogenate. Int. J. Pharma. Biosci. 1: 1–6.

Khanum F, Anilakumar KR, Sudarshana Krishna KR, Viswanathan KR, Santhanam K (2000). Anticarcinogenic effects of curry leaves in dimethylhydrazine-treated rats. Plant Foods Hum. Nutr. 55 (4): 347–55.

Kumar NS, Mukherjee PK, Bhadra S, Saha BP, Pal BC (2010). Acetylcholinesterase inhibitory potential of a carbazole alkaloid, mahanimbine, from *Murraya koenigii*. Phytother. Res. 24 (4): 629–31.

Lawal HA, Atiku MK, Khelpai DG, Wannang NN (2008). Hypo-glycaemic and hypolipidaemic effect of aqueous leaf extract of *Murraya koenigii* in normal and alloxan-diabetic rats. Niger J Physiol Sci. 23 (1-2): 37–40.

Muthumani P, Venkatraman S, Ramseshu KV, Meera R, Devi P, Kameswari B (2009). Pharmacological studies of anticancer, anti inflammatory activities of *Murraya koenigii* (Linn) Spreng in experimental animals. J. Pharm. Sci. Res. 1: 137–41.

Narasimhan NS, Paradhar MV, Chitguppi VP (1968). Structure of Mahanimbin and Koenimbin. Tetrahedron. Lett. 53: 5501–504.

Nayak A, Banerji J, Banergy A, Mandal S (2010). Review on chemistry and pharmacology of *Murraya koenigii* Spreng (Rutaceae) J. Chem. Pharm. Res. 2: 286–99.

Nor FM, M, Suhaila, Nor IA, Razali I (2009). Antioxidative properties of *Murraya koenigii* leaf extracts in accelerated oxidation and deep-frying studies. International Journal of Food Sciences and Nutrition. 60: (S2): 1–11.

Palaniswany UR, CaporuscioC, Stuart JD (2009). A chemical analysis of antioxidant vitamins in fresh curry leaf (Murreya koenigii) by reversed phase HPLC with UV detection. ISHS Acta Horticulturae 620. XXVI International Horticultural Congress: Asian Plants with Unique Horticultural Potential: Genetic Resources, Cultural Practices, and Utilization.

Patil R, Hiray Y, Shinde S, Langade P (2011). Reversal of haloperidol-induced orofacial dyskinesia by *Murraya koenigii* leaves in experimental animals. Pharm. Biol. Dec 2. [Epub ahead of print].

Patil RA, Langade PM, Dighade PB, Hiray YA (2012). Antinociceptive activity of acute and chronic administration of *Murraya koenigii* L. leaves in experimental animal models. Indian J. Pharmacol. 44 (1): 15–19.

Paul S, Bandyopadhyay TK, Bhattacharya A (2011). Immunomodulatory effect of leaf extract of *Murraya koenigii* in diabetic mice. Immunopharmacol. Immunotoxicol. 33 (4): 691–99.

Ramsewak RS, Nair MG, Strasburg GM, DeWitt DL, Nitiss JL (1999). Biologically active carbazole alkaloids from *Murraya koenigii*. J. Agric. Food Chem. 47 (2): 444–47.

Rao LJ, Ramalakshmi K, Borse B, Raghavan B (2007). Antioxidant and radical-scavenging carbazole alkaloids from the oleoresin of curry leaf (*Murraya koenigii* Spreng) Food Chem. 100: 742–47.

Sathaye S, Bagul Y, Gupta S, Kaur H, Redkar R (2011). Hepatoprotective effects of aqueous leaf extract and crude isolates of *Murraya koenigii* against *in vitro* ethanol-induced hepatotoxicity model. Exp. Toxicol. Pathol. 63 (6): 587–91.

Shaik MWM, Sulaiman MR, Tengku MTA, Chiong HS, Zakaria ZA, Jabit ML, Baharuldin MT, Israf DA (2009). Anti-inflammatory and anti-nociceptive effects of *Mitragyna speciosa* Korth methanolic extract. Med Princ Pract. 18 (5): 378–84.

Tachibana Y, Kikuzaki H, Lajis NH, Nakatani N (2001). Antioxidative activity of carbazoles from *Murraya koenigii* leaves. J. Agric. Food Chem. 49 (11): 5589–94.

Tachibana Y, Kikuzaki H, Lajis NH, Nakatani N (2003). Comparison of anti-oxidative properties of carbazole alkaloids from *Murraya koenigii* leaves. J. Agric. Food Chem. 51 (22): 6461–67.

Tembhurne SV, Sakarkar DM (2011). Effects of *Murraya koenigii* leaf extract on impaired gastrointestinal motility in streptozotocin-induced diabetic rats. Zhong. Xi. Yi. Jie. He. Xue. Bao. 9 (8): 913–19.

Yankuzo H, Ahmed QU, Santosa RI, Akter SF, Talib NA (2011). Beneficial effect of the leaves of *Murraya koenigii* (Linn.) Spreng (Rutaceae) on diabetes-induced renal damage *in vivo*. J Ethnopharmacol. 135 (1): 88–94.

B. CORIANDER LEAVES (*Coriandrum sativum* L.)

Coriander leaves or dhania, is an annual herb in the family of Apiaceae. It is a soft, hairless plant growing to 50 centimetres (20 in) tall. The leaves are variable in shape, broadly lobed at the base of the plant, and slender and feathery at the end. All parts of the plant are edible, but the fresh leaves and the dried seeds are the parts most commonly used in cooking. Coriander is common in South Asian, Middle Eastern, Central Asian, Mediterranean, Indian, Latin American, Portuguese, Chinese, African, and Scandinavian cuisine.

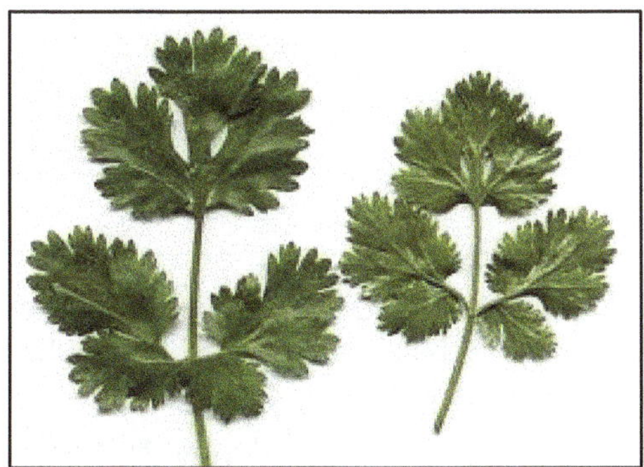

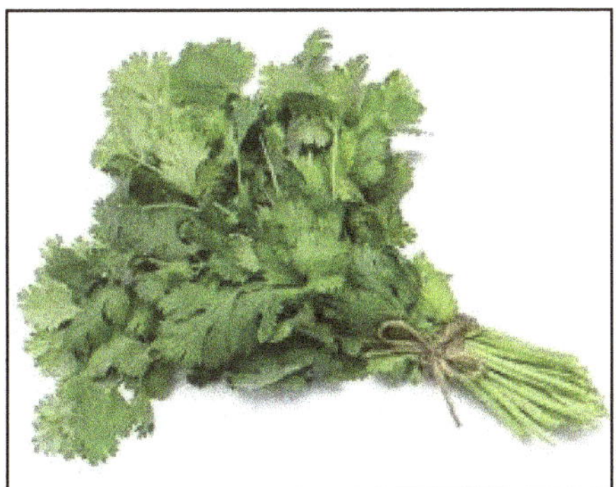

Coriander has been in use for thousands of years, even as far back as 5000 BC. It is native to southern Europe, North Africa and the Middle East; and was used in cooking by the ancient Egyptians, Romans and Greeks. Romans used coriander to flavour their bread and to preserve their meat whilst traveling. The fresh leaves are an ingredient in many South Asian foods (such as chutneys and salads), Chinese and Mexican recipes, particularly in salsa and guacamole; and as a garnish, in salads in Russia and other countries. While in the English-speaking world (except in U.S.) the leaves and seeds are known as coriander, dhania pattha, kothmir, kothamalli or kothmira etc., and in American culinary usage the leaves are generally referred to by the Spanish word cilantro.

Coriander has also been used for thousands of years in medicine, to mask the naturally unpleasant taste of some medicines, as well as for medicinal purposes.

Nutritive Value of Coriander Leaves

Fresh coriander is particularly rich in Vitamins A and K, but also contains plenty of Vitamins B, C and E. It is also a good source of minerals such as potassium, calcium, magnesium and phosphorous. The leaves of the cilantro (coriander) plant contains many phyto-chemical compounds; phenolics, flavonoids, antioxidants like quercitin.

Therapeutic Uses of Dhania

Coriander has traditionally been used to treat all kinds of stomach and digestive problems. It is said to help regain a loss of appetite and therefore is beneficial for sufferers of anorexia. It reduces flatulence and helps relieving spasms within the gut

Nutritive Value of Coriander Leaves

Nutrient	*Amount*	*Nutrient*	*Amount*
Energy (kcals)	23	Calcium (mg)	67
Carbohydrate (g)	3.67	Iron (mg)	1.77
Protein(g)	2.13	Magnesium (mg)	26
Fat (g)	0.52	Phosphorus (mg)	48
Thiamine (mg)	0.067	Potassium (mg)	521
Riboflavin (mg)	0.162	Sodium (mg)	46
Niacin (mg)	1.114	Zinc (mg)	0.50
Vitamin A (IU)	6748	Vitamin C (mg)	27.0
Vitamin B6 (mg)	0.149	Folate (µg)	62

USDA (2012).

and counters the effects of nervous tension. In Chinese medicine, the seeds are used to treat stomach disorders, whilst the leaves can be chewed in order to combat bad breath. It is applied externally as a lotion for rheumatic pain.

Coriander has been used as a folk medicine for the relief of anxiety and insomnia in Iran. Experiments in mice support its use as an anxiolytic (Emamghoreishi *et al.*, 2005).

The essential oil of coriander leaves has been found useful in many traditional medicines as analgesic, antiseptic, aphrodisiac, stimulant, antispasmodic, carminative, depurative, deodorant, digestive, fungicidal, lipolytic and stomachic agent.

Antioxidant

Coriander, like many spices, contains antioxidants, which can delay or prevent the spoilage of food seasoned with this spice. Wangensteen *et al.* (2004) found that both the leaves and seeds to contain antioxidants, with the effect being stronger in the leaves.

Antimicrobial Agent

Chemicals derived from coriander leaves were found to have antibacterial activity against Salmonella choleraesuis possibly caused in part by acting as nonionic surfactants (Kubo *et al.*, 2004). Coriander essential oil showed a delay in *E. coli* growth, suggesting possible agricultural antibacterial applications.

Antidiabetic

Coriander has been documented as a traditional treatment for diabetes. A study on mice found coriander extract had both insulin-releasing and insulin-like activity (Grey and Flatt, 2007).

Hypolipidemic Agent

Coriander seeds were found to have a significant hypo-lipidaemic effect in rats, resulting in lowering of total cholesterol and triglyceride levels, and increasing high-density lipoprotein levels. This effect appeared to be caused by increasing synthesis of bile by the liver and increasing the breakdown of cholesterol into other compounds (Chitra and Leelamma, 1997).

References

Chithra V, Leelamma, S (1997). Hypolipidemic effect of coriander seeds (Coriandrum sativum): Mechanism of action. Plant Foods for Human Nutrition 51 (2): 167–72.

Emamghoreishi M, Khasaki M, Aazam MF (2005). Coriandrum sativum: evaluation of its anxiolytic effect in the elevated plus-maze. Journal of Ethnopharmacology. 96 (3): 365–70.

Gray AM, Flatt PR (2007). Insulin-releasing and insulin-like activity of the traditional antidiabetic plant Coriandrum sativum (coriander). British Journal of Nutrition. 81 (3): 203.

Kubo I, Fujita KI, Kubo A, Nihei KI, Ogura T (2004). Antibacterial Activity of Coriander Volatile Compounds againstSalmonella choleraesuis. Journal of Agricultural and Food Chemistry. 52 (11): 3329–32.

USDA (2012). National Nutrient Data base for standard reference, release 25.

Wangensteen H, Samuelsen AB, Malterud KE (2004). Antioxidant activity in extracts from coriander. Food Chemistry. 88 (2): 293.

Chapter 7
Fenugreek
(*Trigonella foenum-graecum*)

Trigonella foenum-graecum, commonly known as fenugreek/methi is a traditional Indian as well as Iranian medicinal plant. It is a native of Indian subcontinent and Eastern Mediterranean region belonging to the family of leguminacae and is an annual herb. The name of the species foenum graecum means 'Greek hay' while the genus name Trigonella means little triangle referring to the shape of the leaf. The leaves and seeds of methi are widely used in India, Egypt, Southern Europe and other regions (Nadkarni, 1954; Grieve 1959).

India is the largest producer as well as exporter of Methi in the world where Rajasthan, Gujarat, Uttarakhand, Uttar Pradesh, Maharashtra, Haryana and Punjab are the major methi producing states. Rajasthan produces the lion's share of India's production, accounting for over 80 per cent of the nation's total methi output.

The dried seeds of Methi are used as a spice while the leaves are used as a vegetable in the Indian culinary arts. Methi seeds are a rich source of protein (Aykroyd *et al.*, 1956), iron (Ranganathan, 1938), fibre and ω-3 fatty acids while the leaves are sources of beta-carotene, iron, calcium, magnesium, potassium and vitamin C. (Krishnaswamy, 2008). The seeds are rich in Lysine (Kolousek and Coulson, 1955) and the germinated ones in Methionine (Picci, 1960).

Traditional Uses

In India, it is commonly believed that methi promotes good digestion. The main reason for this is the high fiber content which acts as a scrub brush on the digestive tract. Indigestion, flatulence, diarrhoea, dysentery, peptic ulcers and colic are all complaints that may be relieved with the use of methi. In addition, people who suffer from biliousness or a sluggish liver may derive benefit. Methi has been used effectively in the treatment of ulcers, boils, arthritis and sinusitis (an inflammation of the mucous membranes of the nasal passages and sore throat). A strong methi brew is consumed to relieve a sore throat. The seeds or the leaves are eaten to soothe internal inflammation or swelling. Fenugreek seed powder mixed with warm water provides soothing relief for a raw throat. This is also said to enhance and speed up the healing process of a sore throat (Passsano, 1995). Methi leaves are used externally on burns or boils to prevent infection and aid in quick healing. Moreover, Methi in the form of gruel has been found to increase the flow of milk in nursing mothers.

Srinivasan (2006) also reported that methi is used as a good hypoglycaemic, hypocholestrolemic, galactogouge, laxative, stimulant, carminative, stomachic, anti-acidic, anti-ulcerative, antibacterial, antihypertensive, antithrombotic, anti-carcinogenic, antioxidant and diuretic in Indian homes.

Nutrient Composition of Methi

Nutritional value per 100 g

Nutrient	*Amount*	*Nutrient*	*Amount*
Thiamine (Vit. B1) (mg)	0.332	Riboflavin (Vit.B2) mg)	0.366
Niacin (Vit. B3) (mg)	1.640	Vitamin B6 (mg)	0.600
Folate (Vit. B9) (μg)	57	Vitamin C (mg)	3.0
Vitamin A (IU)	60	Energy (kcal)	323
Carbohydrates (g)	58.35	Dietary fiber (g)	24.6
Fat (g)	6.41	Protein (g)	23
Calcium (mg)	176	Iron (mg)	33.53
Magnesium (mg)	191	Phosphorus (mg)	296
Potassium (mg)	770	Sodium (mg)	67
Zinc (mg)	2.50		

USDA (2012).

Active Components in Methi

Methi seeds are rich source of the polysaccharide Galactomannan. 4-hydroxy isoleucine has found to be a major free amino acid in the seeds. They are also a source of saponins such as gitogenin, tigogenin and neotigogens. Other bioactive constituents of methi include mucilage, volatile oils and alkaloids such as choline and trigonelline, sotolone and pyrazines. Bitterness of methi seeds is mainly due to the oil, steroidal saponins and alkaloids which are all non-toxic on consumption (Rao *et al.*, 1996). Fenugreek seeds contain diosgenin which is found in certain types of steroids. This is not harmful, but it acts as an anti-inflammatory agent and even relieves pains much like an Advil or Excedrin.

Therapeutic Benefits of Methi

In Ayurveda, the seed and leaves are known for their cholesterol-reducing, anti-inflammatory, anticancer, carminative, demulcent, emollient, expectorant, febrifuge, galactogogue (milk producing), hypoglycaemic, laxative, parasiticidal, restorative and uterine tonic effects.

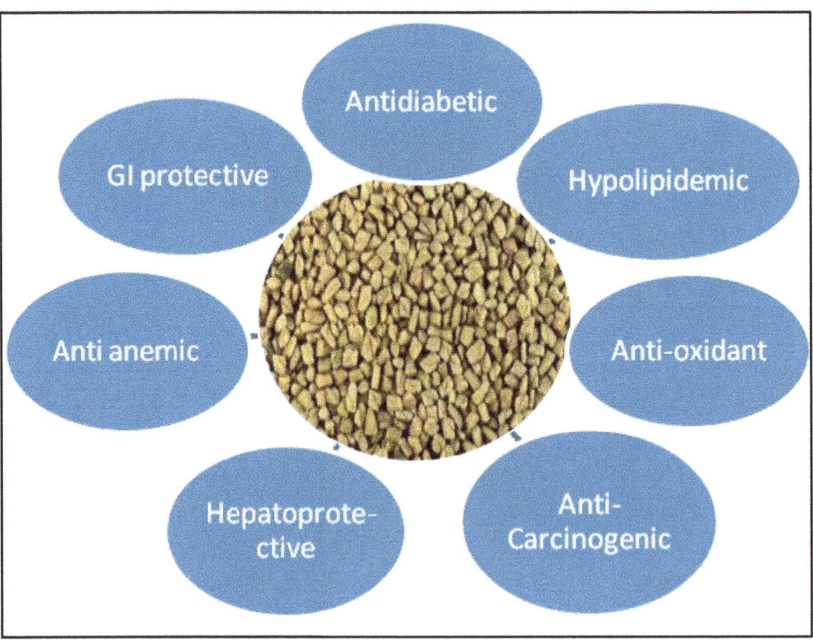

Methi as an Antioxidant

Methi seeds when germinated show significant antioxidant activity. It increases the activity of key antioxidant enzymes like Superoxide dismutase (SOD), Catalase (CAT), Glutathione-s-transferase (GST) and glutathione (GSH). This may be attributed to the presence of flavonoids and polyphenols in the seeds (Dixit *et al.*, 2005; Tripathi and Chandra, 2009).

Analgesic and Anti-inflammatory Activities of Methi

The phytochemical composition of *Trigonella foenum-graecum* leaves extract revealed that alkaloids, cardiac glycosides, and phenols are the major components in the extract responsible for its anti-inflammatory, analgesic and antipyretic effects. Ahmadiani *et al.* (2001) felt that a NSAID-like mechanism must be involved in the existence of these properties. But the presence of alkaloids, the absence of other effective compounds such as flavonoids, saponins, steroids, etc., and also its analgesic effect on tail-flick test that usually is not produced by NSAIDs, suggest possibility of another mechanism that must be working, thus increasing the possibility of alkaloids as effective agent in this extract,

Parvizpur *et al.* (2004 and 2006) attributed the analgesic effect of *Trigonella foenum-graecum* extract to the blocking of spinal purinoceptors. The mechanisms involved are (1) the response of rabbit platelets to ADP induced aggregation, (2) the contraction of mouse vas deferens induced by alpha,beta-Me-ATP (a P(2) receptor agonist; this receptor mediates the rapid phase of ADP- and ATP-evoked influx of Ca^{2+} through a non-specific cation channel in platelets), (3) alpha, beta-Me-ATP induced hyperalgesia in tail flick test in male rats and (4) the specific inhibition of COX-1 and COX-2,

Javan *et al.* (1997) observed that the extract of fenugreek leaves produces anti-nociceptive effects through central and peripheral mechanisms and 2000 mg/kg of the extract is more potent than 300 mg/kg of sodium salicylate.

Trigonella foenum-graecum seed extract (40 mg/kg) when compared with the standard analgesics pentazocine (PTZ, 5 mg/kg p.o.) and diclofenac sodium (DIS, 5 mg/kg p.o.) showed highly significant, analgesic activity against thermally as well as chemically induced pain ($p < 0.001$). Also the extract showed anti-inflammatory activity in carrageenan-induced rat paw edema model at the doses 10 and 20 mg/kg i.p. and compared well with diclofenac sodium (5 mg/kg i.p.). Further investigations are, however, necessary to explore mechanism(s) of action involved in these pharmacological activities (Vyas *et al.*, 2008).

Antidiabetic Effect

India is soon going to be a diabetes capital and the incidence of other non-communicable diseases is also increasing rampantly. Methi seeds have been known since a long time for their antidiabetic action. It was first Fourier who observed in 1948 that coarsely ground methi seeds improved severe diabetes in human subjects. Since then a number of studies have been conducted and effects have been well documented. Initially the antidiabetic properties were linked to the high fibre content of the methi seeds but now several other active ingredients in methi are also thought to have hypoglycaemic effect.

Ali *et al.* (1995) confirmed the involvement of soluble dietary fiber (SDF) in the hypoglycaemic effect of T. foenum graecum seeds. However, compound(s) other than SDF are also involved in the hypoglycaemic activity. The findings of Hannan *et al.* (2003) found the SDF of fenugreek seeds to have a beneficial effect on dyslipidemia and has a tendency to inhibit platelet aggregation in Type 2 model diabetic rats. Hannan *et al.* (2007) also indicated that the antidiabetic effect is mediated through inhibition of carbohydrate digestion and absorption, and enhancement of peripheral insulin action. According to Gad *et al.* (2006) the hypoglycaemic effect of Fenugreek is mediated through insulinomimetic effect as well as inhibition of intestinal alpha-amylase activity.

Sharma *et al.* (1990) confirmed that fenugreek diet significantly reduced fasting blood sugar and improved the glucose tolerance test. There was a 54 per cent reduction in 24-h urinary glucose excretion. Serum total cholesterol, LDL and VLDL cholesterol; and triglycerides were also significantly reduced. The HDL cholesterol fraction, however, remained unchanged.

Gupta *et al.* (2001) reported the adjunct use of fenugreek seeds improves glycaemic control and decreases insulin resistance in mild type-2 diabetic patients along with a favourable effect on hypertriglyceridemia.

Oxidative stress plays a key role in the complications of diabetes. Fenugreek seeds known for their antioxidant property. Fenugreek administration to diabetic animals showed a reversal of the disturbed antioxidant levels and peroxidative damage. Lu *et al.* (2008) found the combined therapy of *Trigonella foenum-graecum* L. total saponins with sulfonylureas (hypoglycaemic drug) could lower the blood glucose level and ameliorate clinical symptoms in the treatment of type 2 Diabetes Mellitus and the therapy was relatively safe.

In depth studies on the phytochemicals further established therapeutic efficacy of methi in diabetes. The active ingredients in Methi *i.e.,* 4-hydroxyisoleucine and galactomannan, increase pancreatic insulin secretion and inhibits sucrose α-D-glucosidase and α-amylase (Sauvaire, 1998; Ajabnoor, 1988; Amin 1987). Therefore it helps to reduce fasting and postprandial blood glucose levels in diabetic patients by increasing the erythrocyte insulin receptors and peripheral glucose utilization that contribute to an improvement in glucose tolerance. Thus, Methi may exert its hypoglycaemic effect by acting at the insulin receptor as well as at the gastrointestinal level. Trigonelline, another component is suggested to exert hypoglycaemic effect in healthy patients without diabetes (Raghuram *et al.,* 1994; Sharma *et al.,* 1996). Thus the best documented medical use of methi is to control blood sugar in both insulin-dependent (type 1) and noninsulin–dependent (type 2) diabetics. These effects are proved in animal studies as well (Zia *et al.,* 2001; Raju *et al.,* 2001).

Fenugreek seed powder administered for 30 days at a dosage of 2 g/kg body weight to alloxan-diabetic rats decreased lipid peroxidation and susceptibility to oxidative stress associated with depletion of antioxidants in liver, kidney and pancreas. Ravikumar and Anuradha (1999) showed that disrupted free radical metabolism in diabetic animals may be normalized by fenugreek seed supplementation in the diet. In normal rats, supplementation resulted in increased antioxidant status with reduction in peroxidation. Ca^{2+} ATPase activity in liver was protected by the aqueous extract to nearly 80 per cent of the initial activity (Anuradha and Ravikumar, 2001).

According to Annida *et al.* (2005) even the fenugreek leaf powder supplementation significantly lowered lipid peroxidation and significantly increased the antioxidant system in diabetic rats. The effect at a dose of 1 g/kg of body weight of fenugreek leaf powder was similar to that of glibenclamide. Thus, fenugreek leaf powder reduces oxidative stress in experimental diabetes.

Xue *et al.* (2007) concluded from their experiments that *Trigonella foenum-graecum* extract can lower kidney/body weight ratio, blood glucose, blood lipid levels and improve haemorheological properties in experimental diabetic rats following repeated treatment for 6 weeks. Further, the seed extract could also protect the kidneys against functional and morphologic injuries by increasing antioxidant activities and inhibiting accumulation of oxidized DNA in the kidney, suggesting methi as a potential drug for the prevention and therapy of diabetic nephropathy (Xue *et al.,* 2011).

Vanadate treatment to diabetic rats has been reported to correct the altered carbohydrate metabolism and antioxidant status. However, Mohammed *et al.* (2004)

proved that doses of vanadate could be lowered when used in combination with fenugreek seed powder to effectively counter diabetic alterations without any toxic side effects. Thus, fenugreek seeds showed an encouraging antioxidant property and can be valuable candidates in the treatment of the reversal of the complications of diabetes (Genet *et al.*, 2002).

Losso *et al.* (2009) developed a fenugreek bread formula that was produced in a commercial bakery by incorporating fenugreek flour into a standard wheat bread formula. They found the bread to maintain fenugreek's functional property of reducing insulin resistance. Similar baked products can be prepared with added fenugreek to improve the taste, which will reduce insulin resistance and treat type 2 diabetes.

Hypolipidemic Effect

Studies on Methi have shown significant reduction in total cholesterol, LDL cholesterol and Triglycerides concentrations without any change in HDL-cholesterol concentrations. The steroidal saponins (diosgenin, yamogenin, tigogenin and neotigogenin) are thought to inhibit cholesterol absorption and synthesis and hence its potential role in arteriosclerosis. The saponins also help to increase the cholesterol and bile acid excretion. (Sharma and Raghuram, 1990; 1991; Sharma *et al.*, 1991). Thus it helps in maintaining overall cardiovascular health.

Maintenance of Gut Integrity

Methi seeds are helpful in maintaining a healthy digestive system, thus the continuous and daily use of this spice may improve the digestibility and absorbability of food consumed for the best metabolic use in the body cells (Doshi *et al.*, 2012).

Gastroprotective Effect

Pandian *et al.* (2002) observed the seeds to show significant ulcer protective effects probably not only due to the anti-secretory action but also to the effects on mucosal glycoproteins. The seeds also prevented the rise in lipid peroxidation induced by ethanol presumably by enhancing antioxidant potential of the gastric mucosa thereby lowering mucosal injury.

Antianemic Agent

Methi has good potential to raise blood hemoglobin due to the presence of essential amino acids (lysine and threonine), iron, folate and ascorbate. (Doshi *et al.*, 2012). Rats fed with biscuits prepared from wheat flour supplemented by germinated fenugreek seed flour at 10 per cent level exhibited extremely higher ($P<0.05$) values of blood hemoglobin, hematocrit, serum iron, liver weights and liver minerals content (Fe, Ca and Zn) as compared to rats fed on wheat biscuit diet. Thus Ibrahim and Hegazy (2009) demonstrated that, 10 per cent germinated Fenugreek seed flour considerably improves bioavailability iron.

Anticarcinogenic

The ethanolic extract of methi leaves show anticancer activity against mice inoculated with Ehrlich ascites carcinoma cells (Prabhu and Krishanmoorthy, 2010).

Methi seeds were shown to protect against experimental cancers of breast (Amin *et al.*, 2005) and colon (Raju *et al.*, 2004). Surprisingly, Shabbeer's (2009) studies showed that death of cancer cells occurs despite growth stimulatory pathways being simultaneously upregulated (phosphorylated) by fenugreek extract. Thus, these studies add another biologically active agent to the armamentarium of naturally occurring agents with therapeutic potential.

In recent years, Akt signaling (Protein Kinase B (PKB) is a serine/threonine-specific protein kinase) has gained recognition for its functional role in more aggressive, therapy-resistant malignancies. As it is frequently constitutively active in cancer cells, several drugs are being investigated for their ability to inhibit Akt signaling. *In vivo* tumour studies indicated that diosgenin significantly inhibits tumour growth in both MCF-7 and MDA-231 xenografts in nude mice thus suggesting that diosgenin might prove to be a potential chemotherapeutic agent for the treatment of breast cancer (Srinivasan *et al.*, 2009).

Hepatoptoective Effects

The hepatoprotective properties of methi seeds have been reported in experimental models (Kaviarasan, 2006; Meera *et al.*, 2009). Administration of fenugreek seed polyphenol extract had a positive influence on both lipid profile and on the quantitative and qualitative properties of collagen in alcoholic liver disease. The protective effect is presumably due to the bioactive phytochemicals in fenugreek seeds (Kaviarasan *et al.*, 2007). However further studies are needed to explore the hepatoprotective and reproductive role of Methi in humans.

As a Galactogogue

Methi has been used for centuries as an excellent galactagogue. The oil of the seeds has been found to promote lactation in rats (El Ridi *et al.*, 1944; El Ridi and Shahat 1954). In a study with ten women, fenugreek significantly increased volume of breastmilk (Swafford 2000). It can be used either short-term to boost milk production or long-term both augment production and/or pumping yields. Use of methi may be warranted after considering risks versus benefits (Gabay, 2002). There are no studies indicating problems with long-term usage. Most mothers have found that the herb can be discontinued once milk production is stimulated to an appropriate level. Adequate production is usually maintained as long as sufficient breast stimulation and emptying continues.

Methi on Weight Management

Chevassus *et al.* (2009) observed that the repeated administration of a fenugreek seed extract specifically decreases dietary fat consumption in normal healthy individuals. In overweight subjects, dietary fat consumption decreased slightly but significantly in a short-term study. But no significant effect was observed on weight, appetite/satiety scores or oxidative parameters (Chevassus *et al.*, 2010).

Use of Methi in Cataract

Lens, an insulin-independent tissue, is affected in severe diabetes showing visual signs of cataract. *T. foenum-graecum* protects against experimental cataract by virtue of its antioxidant properties. The activities of antioxidant enzymes such as superoxide dismutase ($P < 0.01$), catalase, ($P < 0.01$), glutathione peroxidase ($P < 0.01$), and glutathione-S-transferase ($P < 0.01$) could be restored in the *T. foenum-graecum* supplemented group as compared to control. *In vivo*, none of the eyes was found with nuclear cataract in treated group as opposed to 72.5 per cent in the control group (Gupta *et al.*, 2010). But they warrant further studies to explore its role in human cataract.

Preet *et al.* (2005) found that lowered doses of vanadate administered in combination with methi was the most effective in controlling the altered glucose metabolism and antioxidant status in diabetic lenses, which are significant factors involved in the development of diabetic complications, that reflects in the reduced lens opacity.

Other Roles

Protection against Ethanol

The seed extract could prevent iron-induced lipid peroxidation in experimental ethanol toxicity in rats. The seeds exhibited appreciable antioxidant property *in vitro* which was comparable with that of reduced glutathione and alpha-tocopherol. Further, histopathological examination of liver and brain revealed that, aqueous extract of fenugreek seeds could offer a significant protection against ethanol toxicity (Thirunavukkarasu *et al.*, 2003). Kaviarasan *et al.* (2006) from their study suggested that the polyphenolic compounds of fenugreek seeds can be considered cytoprotective during ethanol-induced liver damage.

Protection against Pesticide Toxicity

Cypermethrin (CM) is an important type II pyrethroid pesticide used extensively in pest control and is reported to cause hepatic and renal toxicity. Oxidative stress and lipid peroxidation (LPO) has been implicated in the toxicology of pyrethroids. Fenugreek is known for its antitoxic and antioxidant potential. Phytochemicals present in fenugreek could play an important role in ameliorating the pesticide-induced toxicity (Sushma and Devasena, 2010).

Complementary Protein Value

Methi improves the quality of protein in foods due to its lysine content. Rice-blackgram dal diet supplemented with raw or germinated fenugreek seeds at 10 per cent level showed better weight gain in rats as compared to the unsupplemented rice-blackgram dal diet and also the gain in weight in the supplemented group compared well with the food mixture supplemented with skim milk powder (Rajalakshmi and Subbulakshmi, 1963).The nitrogen balance improved and increased the biological value of the food mixture.

Estrogenic Effect

Methi has also shown positive effects in male and female reproductive system in animal models. (Sharma and Bhinda, 2005; Aswar *et al.*, 2010). Earlier reports show that fenugreek seeds provide a mastogenic effect resulting in enhanced breast size.

However, very little is known about its estrogenic effect. Sreeja *et al.* (2010) provided the evidence for estrogenic activities of fenugreek seeds. Further *in vitro* and *in vivo* studies could demonstrate its suitability as an alternative to Hormone Replacement Therapy.

Conclusions

The evidence to date suggests that methi could be a potential natural health product for the prevention and treatment of several problems like diabetes, dyslipidemia, etc. Thus it is important to popularize and create awareness about the beneficial effects of Methi. Since methi has a very bitter taste, food products masking the bitter flavour should be developed leading to enhanced consumer acceptance. The biological effects should be firmly established through well controlled clinical trials.

References

Ahmadiani A, Javan M, Semnanian S, Barat E, Kamalinejad M (2001). Anti-inflammatory and antipyretic effects of *Trigonella foenum-graecum* leaves extract in the rat. J. Ethnopharmacol. 75 (2-3): 283–86.

Ajabnoor M, Tilmisany A (1988). Effect of *Trigonella foenum-graceum* on blood glucose levels in normal and alloxan-diabetic mice. J. Ethnopharmacol 22 (1): 45–49.

Ali L, Azad Khan AK, Hassan Z, Mosihuzzaman M, Nahar N, Nasreen T, Nur-e-Alam M, Rokeya B (1995). Characterization of the hypoglycaemic effects of *Trigonella foenum-graceum* seed. Planta. Med. 61 (4): 358–60.

Amin A, Alkaabi A, Falasi SA, Sayel A (2005). Chemopreventive activities of *Trigonella foenum-graceum* (Methi) against breast cancer. Cell. Biol. Int. 29: 687–94.

Amin R, Abdul-Ghani A, Suleiman M (1987). Effect of *Trigonella foenum-graceum* on intestinal absorption. Proc. of the 47th Annual Meeting of the American Diabetes Assocation (Indianapolis U.S.A.). Diabetes. 36 (Suppl. 1): 211a.

Annida B, Stanely Mainzen Prince P (2005). Supplementation of fenugreek leaves reduces oxidative stress in streptozotocin-induced diabetic rats. J. Med. Food. 8 (3): 382–85.

Anuradha CV, Ravikumar P (2001). Restoration on tissue antioxidants by fenugreek seeds (*Trigonella foenum-graceum*) in alloxan-diabetic rats. Indian J. Physiol. Pharmacol. 45 (4): 408–20.

Aswar U, Bodhankar S, Mohan V, Thakurdesai P (2010). Effect of Furostanol Glycosides from *Trigonella foenum-graceum* on the Reproductive System of Male Albino Rats. Phytotherapy. Research, 24: 1482–88.

Aykroyd W R, Patwardhan V N, Ranganathan S (1956). Health Bulletin No. 23. Indian Council of Medical Research. New Delhi.

Chevassus H, Molinier N, Costa F, Galtier F, Renard E, Petit P (2009). A fenugreek seed extract selectively reduces spontaneous fat consumption in healthy volunteers. Eur. J. Clin. Pharmacol. 65 (12): 1175–78.

Chevassus H, Gaillard JB, Farret A, Costa F, Gabillaud I, Mas E, Dupuy AM, Michel F, Cantié C, Renard E, Galtier F, Petit P (2010). A fenugreek seed extract selectively reduces spontaneous fat intake in overweight subjects. Eur. J. Clin. Pharmacol. 66 (5): 449–55.

Dixit P, Ghaskadbi S, Mohan H, Devasagayam T (2005). Antioxidant properties of germinated methi seeds. Phytotherapy. Research, 19 (11): 977–83.

Doshi M, Mirza A, Umarji B, Karambelkar R (2012). Effect of *Trigonella foenum-graceum* (Methi) on Hemoglobin Levels in Females of Child Bearing Age. Biomedical Research. 23 (1): 47–50.

El Ridi. MS.Azouz WM, El Ayyadi M (1954). Chem. Abstr. 48: 2325.

El Ridi MS, Shahat M (1944). Chem. Abstr. 39: 301, 304.

Gabay MP (2002). Galactogogues: medications that induce lactation. J. Hum. Lact. 18 (3): 274–79.

Gad MZ, El-Sawalhi MM, Ismail MF, El-Tanbouly ND (2006). Biochemical study of the antidiabetic action of the Egyptian plants fenugreek and balanites. Mol. Cell. Biochem. 281 (1-2): 173–83.

Genet S, Kale RK, Baquer NZ (2002). Alterations in antioxidant enzymes and oxidative damage in experimental diabetic rat tissues: effect of vanadate and fenugreek (*Trigonella foenum-graceum*). Mol. Cell. Biochem. 236 (1-2): 7–12.

Gupta A, Gupta R, Lal B (2001). Effect of *Trigonella foenum-graceum* (fenugreek) seeds on glycaemic control and insulin resistance in type 2 diabetes mellitus: a double blind placebo controlled study. J. Assoc. Physicians India 49: 1057–61.

Gupta SK, Kalaiselvan V, Srivastava S, Saxena R, Agrawal SS (2010). *Trigonella foenum-graceum* (Fenugreek) protects against selenite-induced oxidative stress in experimental cataractogenesis. Biol. Trace Elem. Res. 136 (3): 258–68.

Grieve M (1959). A Modern Herbal. Hafner Publishing Co. New York.

Hannan JM, Ali L, Rokeya B, Khaleque J, Akhter M, Flatt PR, Abdel-Wahab YH (2007). Soluble dietary fibre fraction of *Trigonella foenum-graceum* (fenugreek) seed improves glucose homeostasis in animal models of type 1 and type 2 diabetes by delaying carbohydrate digestion and absorption, and enhancing insulin action. Br. J. Nutr. 97 (3): 514–21.

Hannan JM, Rokeya B, Faruque O, Nahar N, Mosihuzzaman M, Azad Khan AK, Ali L (2003). Effect of soluble dietary fibre fraction of *Trigonella foenum-graceum* on glycemic, insulinemic, lipidemic and platelet aggregation status of Type 2 diabetic model rats. J. Ethnopharmacol. 88 (1): 73–77.

Ibrahim MI and Hegazy AI (2009). Iron Bioavailability of Wheat Biscuit Supplemented by Fenugreek Seed Flour. World Journal of Agricultural Sciences. 5 (6): 769–76.

Javan M, Ahmadiani A, Semnanian S, Kamalinejad M (1997). Antinociceptive effects of *Trigonella foenum-graceum* leaves extract. J. Ethnopharmacol. 58 (2): 125–29.

Kaviarasan S, Ramamurty N, Gunasekran P, Varalakshmi E, Anuradha CV (2006). Fenugreek (*Trigonella foenum-graceum*) seed extract prevents ethanol-induced toxicity and apoptosis in Chang liver cells. Alcohol Alcohol. 41 (3): 267–73.

Kaviarasan S, Viswanathan P, Anuradha CV (2007). Fenugreek seed (*Trigonella foenum-graceum*) polyphenols inhibit ethanol-induced collagen and lipid accumulation in rat liver. Cell. Biol. Toxicol. 23 (6): 373.-.83.

Kolousek J, Coulson CH (1955). Chem. Abstr. 48: 1138.

Krishnaswamy K (2008). Traditional Indian spices and their health significance. Asia Pac. J. Clin. Nutr, 17 (S1): 265–68.

Losso JN, Holliday DL, Finley JW, Martin RJ, Rood JC, Yu Y, Greenway FL (2009). Fenugreek bread: a treatment for diabetes mellitus. J. Med. Food. 12 (5): 1046–49.

Lu FR, Shen L, Qin Y, Gao L, Li H, Dai Y (2008). Clinical observation on *Trigonella foenum-graceum* L. total saponins in combination with sulfonylureas in the treatment of type 2 diabetes mellitus. Chin. J. Integr. Med. 14 (1): 56–60.

Meera R, Devi P, Kameswari B, Madhumita B, Merlin N (2009). Antioxidant and hepato-protective activities of *Ocimum basilicum* Linn.and *Trigonella foenum-graceum* Linn. Against H_2O_2 and CCl_4 induced hepatotoxicity in goat liver, Indian journal of experimental biology. 47: 584–90.

Mohammad S, Taha A, Bamezai RN, Basir SF, Baquer NZ (2004). Lower doses of vanadate in combination with trigonella restore altered carbohydrate metabolism and antioxidant status in alloxan-diabetic rats. Clin. Chim. Acta. 342 (1-2): 105–114.

Nadkarni KM (1954). Indian Materia Medica. Vol.I. Popular Book Depot, Mumbai.

Pandian RS, Anuradha CV, Viswanathan (2002). Gastroprotective effect of fenugreek seeds (*Trigonella foenum-graceum*) on experimental gastric ulcer in rats. J. Ethnopharmacol. 81 (3): 393–97.

Parvizpur A, Ahmadiani A, Kamalinejad M (2004). Spinal serotonergic system is partially involved in antinociception induced by (TFG) leaf extract. J. Ethnopharmacol. 95 (1): 13–17.

Parvizpur A, Ahmadiani A, Kamalinejad M (2006). Probable role of spinal purinoceptors in the analgesic effect of *Trigonella foenum* (TFG) leaves extract. J. Ethnopharmacol. 104 (1-2): 108–112.

Passano P (1995). The many uses of Methi, Nutrition, No- 91: 31-35.

Picci G (1960). Chem. Abstr. 54: 17564.

Prabhu A and Krishnamoorthy M (2010). Anticancer activity of *Trigonella foenum-graceum* on ehrlich ascites carcinoma in mus musculus system. J. Pharm. Res, 3: 1183–86.

Preet A, Gupta BL, Yadava PK, Baquer NZ (2005). Efficacy of lower doses of vanadium in restoring altered glucose metabolism and antioxidant status in diabetic rat lenses. J. Biosci. 30 (2): 221–30.

Raghuram T, Sharma R, Sivakumar B, Sahay B (1994). Effect of methi seeds on intravenous glucose disposition in non-insulin dependent diabetic patients. Phytotherapy Research, 8 (2): 83–86.

Rajalakshmi R, Subbulakshmi G (1964). Effect of Fenugreek (*Trigonella foenum-graceum* Linn.) Supplementation on the Biological Value of Rice and Black Gram (Phaseolus mungo) Diet. Ind. Jour. Biochem. 1 (2): 104–106.

Raju J, Patlolla J, Swamy M, Rao C (2004). Diosgenin, a steroid saponin of *Trigonella foenum-graceum* (Methi), inhibits azoxymethane-induced aberrant crypt foci formation in F344 rats and induces apoptosis in HT-29 human colon cancer cells. Cancer Epidemiol. Biomarkers Prev, 13: 1392–98.

Raju J, Gupta D, Rao A, Yadava P and Baquer N (2001). *Trigonella foenum-graceum* (methi) seed powder improves glucose homeostasis in alloxan diabetic rat tissues by reversing the altered glycolytic, gluconeogenic and lipogenic enzymes, Molecular And Cellular Biochemistry 224 (1-2): 45–51.

Ranganathan S (1938). Indian Journal of Medical Research, 25: 677.

Rao U, Sesikiran B, Rao S, Naidu N, Rao V, Ramchandran E (1996). Short term nutritional and safety evaluation of methi, Nutrition Research, 16: 1495–1505.

Ravikumar P, Anuradha CV (1999). Effect of fenugreek seeds on blood lipid peroxidation and antioxidants in diabetic rats. Phytother. Res. 13 (3): 197–201.

Sauvaire Y, Petit P, Broca C, Manteghetti M, Baissac Y, Fernandez-Alvarez J, Gross R, Roye M, Leconte A, Gomis R, Ribes G (1998). 4-Hydroxyisoleucine: a novel amino acid potentiator of insulin secretion. Diabetes. 47 (2): 206–210.

Shabbeer S, Sobolewski M, Anchoori RK, Kachhap S, Hidalgo M, Jimeno A, Davidson N, Carducci MA, Khan SR (2009). Fenugreek: a naturally occurring edible spice as an anticancer agent. Cancer Biol. Ther. 8 (3): 272–78.

Sharma J and Bhinda A (2005). Antifertility Activity of Steroidal Extract of *Trigonella foenum-graceum* (seeds) in Female Rats. Asian J. Exp. Sci. 19 (1): 115–20.

Sharma RD Raghuram T (1990). Hypoglycaemic effect of methi seeds in non-insulin dependant diabetic subjects. Nutr. Res, 10: 731–39.

Sharma RD, Raghuram TC, Rao NS (1990). Effect of fenugreek seeds on blood glucose and serum lipids in type I diabetes. Eur. J. Clin. Nutr. 44 (4): 301–306.

Sharma RD, Raghuram T, Rao V (1991). Hypolipidaemic effect of methi seeds. A clinical study. Phytotherapy Research. 5 (3): 145–47.

Sharma RD Sarkar A, Hazara D, Mishra B, Singh J, Sharma S, Maheshwari B, Maheshwari P (1996). Use of Fenuqreek seed powder in the management of non-insulin dependent diabetes mellitus. Nutr. Res. 16 (8): 1331–39.

Sreeja S, Anju VS, Sreeja S (2010). *In vitro* estrogenic activities of fenugreek *Trigonella foenum-graceum* seeds. Indian J. Med. Res. 131: 814–19.

Srinivasan K (2006). Methi (*Trigonella foenum-graceum*) A review of health beneficial physiological effects. Food reviews international. 22: 203–24.

Srinivasan S, Koduru S, Kumar R, Venguswamy G, Kyprianou N, Damodaran C (2009). Diosgenin targets Akt-mediated prosurvival signaling in human breast cancer cells. Int. J. Cancer. 125 (4): 961–67.

Sushma N, Devasena T (2010). Aqueous extract of *Trigonella foenum-graceum* (fenugreek) prevents cypermethrin-induced hepatotoxicity and nephrotoxicity. Hum. Exp. Toxicol..29 (4): 311–19.

Swafford S, Berens B (2000). Effect of fenugreek on breast milk production. ABM News and Views. 6 (3): Annual meeting abstracts Sept. 11–13, 2000.

Thirunavukkarasu V, Anuradha CV, Viswanathan P (2003). Protective effect of fenugreek (*Trigonella foenum-graceum*) seeds in experimental ethanol toxicity. Phytother. Res. 17 (7): 737–43.

Tripathi U and Chandra D (2009). The plant extracts of *Momordica charantia* and *Trigonella foenum-graceum* have antioxidant and anti-hyperglycemic properties for cardiac tissue during diabetes mellitus. Oxidative Medicine and Cellular Longevity. 2 (5): 290–96.

USDA (2012). National Nutrient Database for Standard Reference, Release 25.

Vyas S, Agrawal RP, Solanki P, Trivedi P (2008). Analgesic and anti-inflammatory activities of *Trigonella foenum-graceum* (seed) extract. Acta. Pol. Pharm. 65 (4): 473–76.

Xue WL, Li XS, Zhang J, Liu YH, Wang ZL, Zhang RJ (2007). Effect of *Trigonella foenum-graceum* (fenugreek) extract on blood glucose, blood lipid and hemorheological properties in streptozotocin-induced diabetic rats. Asia Pac. J. Clin. Nutr. 16 Suppl 1: 422–26.

Xue W, Lei J, Li X, Zhang R (2011). *Trigonella foenum-graceum* seed extract protects kidney function and morphology in diabetic rats via its antioxidant activity. 31 (7): 555–62.

Zia T, Hasnain N, Hasan S (2001). Evaluation of the oral hypoglycaemic effect of *Trigonella foenum-graceum* L. (methi) in normal mice. Journal of Ethnopharmacology, 75 (2-3): 191–95.

Chapter 8

Garlic

(*Allium sativum*)

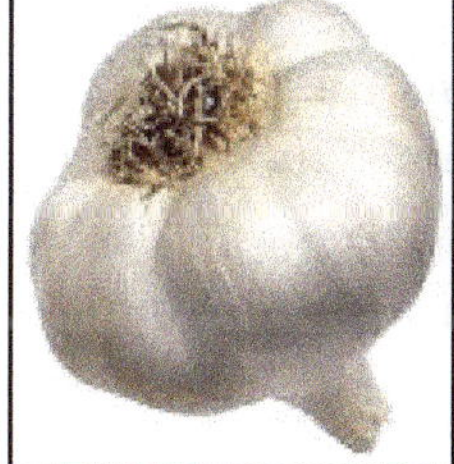
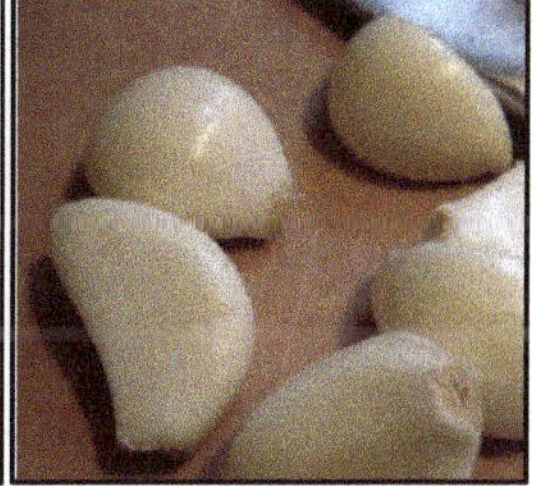

Garlic has been used as both food and medicine in many cultures for thousands of years. It formed part of the diet of the Israelites in Egypt and of the labourers employed by Khufu in constructing his pyramid. Garlic is still grown in Egypt, but the Syrian variety is the kind most esteemed now. It was consumed by ancient Greek and Roman soldiers, sailors.

Garlic is a spice used for centuries as a seasoning and is considered one of the most relevant traditional remedies for small ailments. The medicinal use of garlic dates back to thousands of years, but there was little scientific support of its therapeutic and pharmacologic properties. Recently, a wide range of biological activities of garlic have been verified *in vitro* and *in vivo*; and its therapeutic properties/benefits in CVD, diabetes, infections and cancer have been proved.

Production

Garlic has its beginnings in Central Asia and has been cultivated for 6,000 years. Although wild garlic grows in North America, the cultivated varieties come via Europe. Though different varieties of garlic are available round the year in India, In the US, the California variety is regularly available where as the Washington garlic is available only from September through March. Though garlic is grown globally, China is by far the largest producer of garlic, with approximately 10.5 billion kilograms (23 billion pounds) annually, accounting for over 77 per cent of world output followed by India (4.1 per cent), South Korea (2 per cent), Russia (1.6 per cent) and the least in United States (grown primarily as a cash crop in every state except for Alaska) (1.4 per cent) (1.4 per cent) (USDA, 2006).

Colours of garlic include brilliant white, tan, cream, purple and dark wine, but the most popular varieties are white. Good quality garlic will be large, very firm, evenly-shaped (no missing cloves) and the sheath will be tight and unbroken. Garlic that is soft, spongy, cloves missing or that has green sprouts growing from the tip is generally avoided.

Food Uses

"Garlic is one of the most versatile flavours to ever grace a kitchen."

Garlic is an essential component in most recipes all over the world including eastern Asia, south Asia, Southeast Asia, the Middle East, northern Africa, southern Europe, and parts of South and Central America. The commonly used part of the plant is the bulb which is divided into many sections called cloves. The cloves are consumed raw as well as cooked. The leaves along with the tender fresh garlic are used in cooking but the roots attached to the bulb and the thin skin of the cloves is not considered to be edible.

Garlic is widely used around the world for its pungent flavour as a seasoning or condiment. The flavour varies in intensity and aroma with the different cooking methods. It is often combined with onion, tomato, or ginger. In Japan and Korea, garlic cloves are fermented at high temperature; the resulting product, called black garlic, which is sweet and syrupy, is sold as an additive.

At the household level, garlic is stored in warm (above 18°C [64°F]) and dry conditions to keep it dormant (to avoid sprouting). It is traditionally hung; soft neck varieties are often braided in strands, called 'plaits' or 'grappes'. Commercially, garlic is stored dry at –3°C.

Chemical Composition of Garlic

Garlic contains many sulfur containing active principles mainly in the form of cysteine derivatives, *viz.* S-alkyl cysteine sulfoxides (which decompose into a variety of thiosulfinates and polysulfides by the action of an enzyme allinase on extraction), ajoene, diallylsulfide, dithiin, S-allylcysteine; and non-sulfur containing compounds such as enzymes, saponins, flavonoids, and maillard reaction products. Furthermore a phytoalexin called allixin (3-hydroxy-5-methoxy-6-methyl-2-penthyl-4*H*-pyran-4-one) was also found in garlic along with a non-sulfur compound possesing a γ-pyrone skeleton structure. Allicin is a highly unstable molecule and, during processing, is rapidly transformed into a variety of organosulfur components (Lanzotti, 2006).

The major sulfur-containing compounds in intact garlic are γ-glutamyl-*S*-allyl-L-cysteines and *S*-allyl-L-cysteine sulfoxides (alliin). Both are abundant as sulfur compounds, and alliin is the primary odorless, sulfur-containing amino acid, a precursor of allicin (Stoll and Seebeck, 1948), methiin, (+)-*S*-(*trans*-1-propenyl)-L-cysteine sulfoxide, and cycloalliin (Fujiwara *et al.*, 1958). These sulfoxides, except cyloalliin, are converted into thiosulfinates (such as allicin) through enzyme reactions when raw garlic is cut or crushed. Thus, no thiosulfinates are found in intact garlic (Amagase, 2006). Diallyl disulphide was identified as the major component in garlic oil (36.51 per cent) (Kiralan *et al.*, 2012).

The enzyme alliinase, which is responsible for the conversion of alliin to allicin, is irreversibly destroyed at the acidic environment of stomach. This is the reason why most garlic supplements contain garlic powder or granules, but do not contain allicin itself. Garlic alliinase could be encapsulated and coated with materials which would protect it in the harsh conditions of the stomach (Touloupakis and Ghanotakis 2011). There are many garlic supplements commercially available, *e.g.*, dehydrated garlic powder, garlic oil, garlic oil macerate and aged garlic extract (AGE).

A large number of sulfur compounds contribute to the smell and taste of garlic. Diallyl disulfide is believed to be an important odor component. Allicin has been found to be the compound most responsible for the "hot" sensation of raw garlic. The process of cooking garlic removes allicin, thus mellowing its spiciness (Amagase *et al.*, 2001). Garlic's strong-smelling sulfur compounds are metabolized, forming allyl methyl sulfide which is not digested but is passed into the blood to be carried to the lungs and the skin to be excreted.

The white garlic cultivars and Chinese garlic cultivars contain higher contents of total phenolics and ferulic acid than the purple garlic cultivars. However, the differences in the total phenolic content between the purple and white garlic cultivars were not significant (Beato *et al.*, 2011).

Nutritional Value of Garlic

Garlic is a good source of protein, vitamin C and minerals (calcium, zinc etc.). Selenium and amino acids (cysteine, glutamine, isoleucine and methionine) along with bioflavonoids such as quercetin, cyanidin, allistatin I and allistatin II, and vitamins C, E and A in garlic help to protect cells from the risks of oxidative stress (Ayaz and Alpsoy 2007).

Nutritional Values of garlic (per 100 g)

Nutrient	*Amount*	*Nutrient*	*Amount*
Calcium (mg)	31.2	Phosphorus (mg)	153
Potassium (mg)	401	Iron (mg)	1.2
Magnesium (mg)	25	Zinc (mg)	1.16
Energy (kcal)	149	Protein (g)	6.3
Fat (g)	0.5	Carbohydrates (g)	33.06
Fibre (g)	2.1	Thiamine (mg)	0.2
Riboflavin (mg)	0.110	Niacin (mg)	0.700
Vitamin C (mg)	31.2	Vitamin B6 (mg)	1.235

USDA (2012).

The therapeutic benefits of garlic are due to its very low saturated fat, no cholesterol, very low sodium, low sugar, high calcium, manganese, phosphorus, selenium, vitamin B6 and vitamin C content, besides its phytochemicals.

Traditional Therapeutic Uses

Considerable anecdotal evidence supports the invaluable role that garlic has in the therapy of many diseases (Bolton *et al.*, 1982). Over the centuries, garlic has acquired a special position in the folklore of many cultures as a prophylactic and therapeutic medicinal agent. It is cited in the *Egyptian Codex Ebers*, a 35-century-old document, as useful in the treatment of heart disorders, tumours, worm infestations, bites and other ailments. Charak (ca. 3000 BC), the father of Ayurvedic medicine, claimed that garlic maintains the fluidity of blood and strengthens the heart (Fenwick and Hanley 1985). Early in the 20th century, garlic is said to have been used in the treatment of pulmonary tuberculosis. Over the last 20 years, this important and exciting role of garlic has been confirmed by basic and clinical research reports from around the world (Rahman, 2001).

Garlic is used as a home remedy to help speedy recovery from sore throat or other minor ailments because of its antibiotic properties. The sulphur compound allicin, and other phytochemicals in garlic have been confirmed to be responsible for its antibiotic, antioxidant, anti-tumour, antitoxic (inhibition of aflatoxin) and neurotrophic effects.

Garlic and garlic supplements are consumed in many cultures for their hypolipidemic, antiplatelet and procirculatory effects. In addition to these proclaimed beneficial effects, some garlic preparations also appear to possess hepatoprotective, immune-enhancing, anticancer and chemopreventive activities ((Amagase *et al.*, 2006). Some preparations appear to be antioxidative, whereas others may stimulate oxidation. These additional biological effects attributed to AGE may be due to compounds, such as S-allylcysteine, S-allylmercaptocysteine, N(alpha)-fructosyl arginine and others, formed during the extraction process (Amagase *et al.*, 2001).

Antioxidant and Anti-inflammatory Effect

One of major proteins of garlic which has been isolated and purified is the 14 kDa protein. This protein has been shown to have immunomodulatory effects (Ahmadabad *et al.*, 2011). Administration of Garlic and onion to Fructose-fed rats reduced oxidative stress, increased endothelial nitric oxide synthase activity, and also attenuated vascular cell adhesion molecule-(VCAM-1) expression. Thus, Vazquez-Prieto *et al.* (2011) provided new evidence showing the anti-inflammatory and antioxidant effect of garlic.

Antibacterial Property of Garlic

Garlic is known to have antimicrobial activity against several spoilage and pathogenic bacteria. Allicin from garlic is a powerful antibacterial and antifungal compound. In 1858, Louis Pasteur observed garlic's antibacterial activity, and it was used as an antiseptic to prevent gangrene during World War I and World War II (Ellen, 2005). Groppo *et al.* (2002) compared the antimicrobial activity of tea tree oil, garlic, and chlorhexidine solutions against oral microorganisms on thirty subjects. Chlorhexidine and garlic groups showed antimicrobial activity against mutans streptococci, but not against other oral microorganisms. Maintenance of reduced levels of microorganisms was observed only with garlic and tea tree oil during the two consecutive weeks (fourth and fifth). More recently, it has been found from a clinical trial that a mouthwash containing 2.5 per cent fresh garlic shows good antimicrobial activity, although the majority of the participants reported an unpleasant taste and bad breath (Groppo *et al.*, 2007).

Park *et al.* (2008) found garlic and onion in enhanced meats to show an antioxidant activity as effective as that of sodium ascorbate and also an antimicrobial effect to inhibit the growth of total bacteria and Enterobacteriaceae. But Lu *et al.* (2011) found *L. monocytogenes* to be more resistant to garlic extract and diallyl compounds treatment than *E. coli* O157:H7. Fourier transform infrared (FT-IR) spectroscopy indicated that diallyl constituents contributed more to the antimicrobial effect than phenolic compounds.

With or without garlic added (20 per cent, wt/wt), *Salmonella*, *E. coli* O157:H7, and *L. monocytogenes* did not grow in unsalted butter, when inoculated products were stored at 4.4, 21, and 37°C for up to 48 h. The inactivation of Salmonella and *L. monocytogenes* was more rapid in jumbo garlic butter than in elephant or small-cloved garlic butter (Alder *et al.*, 2002).

Aqueous garlic extract (1 ml/kg, i.p., corresponding to 250 mg/kg) was administered for 28 days to male Wistar albino rats with liver fibrosis induced in by bile duct ligation and scission alleviated the oxidative injury of the liver and improved the hepatic structure and function indicating its potential therapeutic value in protecting the liver fibrosis and oxidative injury due to biliary obstruction (Gedik *et al.*, 2005).

In 2007, the BBC reported that *Allium sativum* may have beneficial properties, such as preventing and fighting the common cold. This assertion has the backing of long tradition in herbal medicine, which has used garlic for hoarseness and coughs. The Cherokee also used it as an expectorant for coughs and croup (or laryngotracheobronchitis) (Hamel and Chitoskey, 1975).

In modern naturopathy, garlic is used as a treatment for intestinal worms and other intestinal parasites, both orally and as an anal suppository. Garlic cloves are used as a remedy for chest infections, digestive disorders, and fungal infections such as thrush.

Emergence of multi-drug resistant (MDR) and extensively drug resistant (XDR) TB throughout the developing world is very disturbing in the present scenario of TB management. Hannan *et al.* (2011) investigated the minimum inhibitory concentration of garlic extract to range from 1 to 3 mg/ml against both non-MDR and MDR M. tuberculosis isolates. The use of garlic against MDR-TB may be of great importance regarding public health in order to decrease the burden of drug resistance and cost in the management of diseases. But Fani *et al.* (2007) found that all isolates, MDR and non-MDR of S. mutans were sensitive to garlic extract. Thus on the basis of the *in vitro* data, they suggested that mouthwashes or toothpaste containing optimum concentration of garlic extract could be used for prevention of dental caries.

Bakri and Douglas (2005) studied the effects of garlic against oral bacterial species particularly putative periodontal pathogens or their enzymes. Time-kill curves for *Streptococcus mutans* and *P. ginigvalis*, showed that killing of the latter started almost immediately, whereas there was a delay before *S. mutans* was killed. The garlic extract also inhibited the trypsin-like and total protease activity of *P. gingivalis* by 92.7 per cent and 94.88 per cent, respectively. These data indicate that garlic extract inhibits the growth of oral pathogens and certain proteases and so may have therapeutic value, particularly for periodontitis.

CVD

Garlic is claimed to help prevent heart disease (including atherosclerosis, high cholesterol, and high blood pressure) and cancer. Evidence from numerous studies points to the fact that garlic can bring about the normalization of plasma lipids, enhancement of fibrinolytic activity, inhibition of platelet aggregation and reduction of blood pressure and glucose.

Garlic supplements have been associated with a blood pressure (BP)-lowering effect of clinical significance in hypertensive patients (Ried *et al.*, 2008; 2010; Reinhart *et al.*, 2008). The antihypertensive properties of garlic have been linked to stimulation of intracellular nitric oxide and hydrogen sulphide production, and blockage of angiotensin II production, which in turn promote vasodilation and thus reduction in BP (Suetsuna, 1998; Castro *et al.*, 2010). Ried *et al.* (2013) demonstrated that a daily dosage of two capsules of the high potency formula of aged garlic extract is effective.

Animal studies, and some early investigational studies in humans, have suggested possible cardiovascular benefits of garlic. The cardiovascular effects of garlic have been documented in several older publications too (May 1926, Schlesinger 1926, Taubmann 1934). However, only in late 70s Sainani *et al.* (1976) found that people who regularly eat larger amounts of garlic and onions have lower lipid and cholesterol levels than people who refrain from eating these. Later, Agarwal (1996) demonstrated that garlic ingestion could bring down the blood cholesterol and triglyceride levels significantly.

A Czech study by Sovova and Sova (2004) found that garlic supplementation reduced accumulation of cholesterol on the vascular walls of animals. Another study had similar results, with garlic supplementation significantly reducing aortic plaque deposits of cholesterol-fed rabbits (Durak *et al.*, 2002). Another study by Durak *et al.* (2004) showed that supplementation with garlic extract inhibited vascular calcification in human patients with high blood cholesterol. The known vasodilative effect of garlic is possibly caused by catabolism of garlic-derived polysulfide to hydrogen sulfide in red blood cells, a reaction that is dependent on reduced thiols in or on the RBC membrane. Hydrogen sulphide is an endogenous cardio protective vascular cell-signaling molecule.

According to Yeh and Yeh (1994) and Yeh and Liu (2001), the hypocholesterolemic effect of garlic stems, in part, from decreased hepatic cholesterogenesis, whereas the triacylglycerol-lowering effect appears to be due to inhibition of fatty acid synthesis. They also proved the primary hepatocyte cultures to be useful as tools for screening the anticholesterogenic properties of garlic principles. Gebhardt, (1991) also demonstrated that water-soluble garlic extracts diminish hepatic cholesterol biosynthesis, thus contributing to the reduction of blood cholesterol. The main target site seems to be HMGCoA-reductase.

The complete depression of cholesterol synthesis by diallyl disulfide (DADS), diallyl trisulfide (DATS), and dipropyl disulfide (DPDS) was found to be associated with cytotoxicity by Liu and Yeh (2000; 2001) as indicated by marked increase in cellular LDH release. Judging from maximal inhibition and IC50 (concentration required for 50 per cent of maximal inhibition), SAC, SEC, and SPC are equally potent in inhibiting cholesterol synthesis.

Chang *et al.* (2011) reported that treatment with Garlic oil significantly inhibits the up-regulation in MAPK (*e.g.*, p38, JNK and ERK1/2) and IL-6/MEK5/ERK5 signaling pathways in the diabetic rat hearts, reducing the levels of cardiac pathologic hypertrophy markers such as ANP and BNP, and improving the cardiac contractile function. His study demonstrates that garlic oil is a potential cardioprotective agent from diabetic cardio-myopathy.

Rahman (2007), Chan *et al.* (2007), Borrelli *et al.* (2007), Steiner and Lin (1998) have found garlic to reduce platelet aggregation (and hyperlipidemia (Kojuri *et al.*, 2007, Mader 1990). However, a randomized clinical trial funded by the National Institutes of Health (NIH) in the United States and published in the Archives of Internal Medicine in 2007 found that the consumption of garlic in any form did not reduce blood cholesterol levels in patients with moderately high baseline cholesterol levels.

Silagy and Neil (1994) reviewed16 trials with data from 952 subjects and compared the pooled mean difference in the absolute change (from baseline to final measurement in mmol/l) of total serum cholesterol, triglycerides, and high-density lipoprotein (HDL)-cholesterol between subjects treated with garlic therapy against those treated with placebo or other agents. The mean difference in reduction of total cholesterol between garlic-treated subjects and those receiving placebo (or avoiding garlic in their diet) was -0.77 mmol/l (95 per cent CI: -0.65, -0.89 mmol/l). These changes represent a 12 per cent reduction with garlic therapy beyond the final levels achieved with placebo alone. Dried garlic powder preparations also significantly lowered serum triglyceride by 0.31 mmol/l compared to placebo.

Alder *et al.* (2003) on reviewing ten studies found 6 of them to be effective. The average drop in total cholesterol was 24.8 mg/dL (9.9 per cent), LDL 15.3 mg/dL (11.4 per cent), and triglycerides 38 mg/dL (9.9 per cent). The overall average MQI score was 39.6 per cent (18–70 per cent). Major shortcomings of many of the RCTs included short duration, lack of power analysis and intention to treat analysis, as well as lack of control of diet as a confounding variable.

Gebhardt and Beck (1996) demonstrated that different garlic-derived organosulfur compounds interfere differently with cholesterol biosynthesis and, thus, may provoke multiple inhibition of this metabolic pathway in response to garlic consumption.

Diallyl disulfide, diallyl trisulfide and dipropyl disulfide depressed cholesterol synthesis by 10 to 25 per cent at low concentrations (< or =0.5 mmol/l), and abolished the synthesis at high concentrations (> or =1.0 mmol/L (Liu and Yeh, 2000).

Monascus Garlic Fermented Extract attenuates hyper-lipidemia, suggesting that MGFE is a potent agent for preventing arteriosclerotic diseases (Sumioka *et al.*, 2006). Matsuura (2001) found that the saponin fractions from garlic lowered plasma total and LDL cholesterol concentrations without changing HDL cholesterol levels in a hyper-cholesterolemic animal model. Several steroid saponins occur in both garlic and AGE. These results suggest that special consideration should be given to steroid saponins, as well as organosulfur compounds, in biological and pharmacologic studies of garlic and its preparations. The intake of garlic fermented with Monascus pilosus decreased triglyceride and cholesterol in serum with no appreciable adverse effects in normal to mildly hyper-lipidemic individuals, suggesting that it may be effective to improve and prevent the metabolic syndrome (Higashikawa *et al.*, 2011).

Recently, it has been observed that aged garlic extract, but not the fresh garlic extract, exhibited radical scavenging activity. Just how much garlic should be consumed to achieve any health benefits is unknown. It takes at least 10 cloves to inhibit blood clotting to the same degree as a daily aspirin. Also, practitioners disagree as to whether cooked or dried garlic confers the same benefits imparted by eating it raw.

Garlic in Diabetes

Allicin, the sulfur-containing compound in garlic has been shown to have significant hypoglycaemic activity (Sheela and Augusti, 1992). This effect is thought to be due to increased hepatic metabolism, increased insulin release from pancreatic beta cells and/or insulin sparing effect (Bever *et al.*, 1979). Aqueous homogenate of garlic (10 ml/kg/day) administered orally to sucrose fed rabbits (10 g/kg/day in water for two months) significantly increased hepatic glycogen and free amino acid content, decreased fasting blood glucose, and triglyceride levels in serum in comparison to sucrose controls (Zacharias *et al.*, 1980). S-allyl cystein sulfoxide (SACS), the precursor of allicin and garlic oil, which controlled lipid peroxidation better than glibenclamide and insulin. It also improved diabetic conditions. SACS also stimulated *in vitro* insulin secretion from beta cells isolated from normal rats (Augusti and Sheela, 1996).

Regular and prolonged use of therapeutic amounts of aged garlic extracts lower blood homocysteine levels and has shown to prevent some complications of diabetes mellitus. Padiya *et al.* (2011) observed significant ($p < 0.05$) reduction in body weight gain and serum glycated haemoglobin levels along with improvement in both hepatic TBARS and GSH levels in fructose fed rats after administration of raw garlic homogenate and thus concluded that garlic is effective in improving insulin sensitivity while attenuating metabolic syndrome and oxidative stress.

Garlic was able to reduce blood glucose significantly compared with the control group of alloxan induced diabetic rats but the histomorphometric study of the pancreas of the treated group didn't show a significant change of the pancreatic tissue and hence the effect might be due to the action of allyle propyl disulphide or diallyle disulphide and thereby an increase in the insulin response (Jelodar *et al.*, 2005). Garlic is proved to be a good supplement in the management of patients with diabetes and hyperlipidemia. Garlic (300 mg), in combination with typical anti diabetic remedy *i.e.* Metformin (500 mg) has shown to improve glycemic control. In addition there was a considerable decrease in mean total cholesterol and triglycerides and a significant increase in HDL cholesterol as compared to placebo group (Metformin 500 mg alone) (Ashraf *et al.*, 2005; 2011).

El-Demerdash *et al.* (2005) also found garlic and onion juices to exert antioxidant and antihyperglycemic effects and they also expected the same foods to alleviate liver and renal damage caused by alloxan-induced diabetes. However, Jung *et al.* (2011) suggested that the bioactivities of black Yeast (Saccharomyces cerevisiae)-fermented aged black garlic (FBG) showed favourable hepatoprotective, nephroprotective, hypolipidemic, and antiobesity effects compared with the control, but no hypoglycaemic effects.

Garlic in Cancer

In the past decade, the cancer-protective effects of garlic have been well established by epidemiologic studies and animal experiments. Epidemiological studies have shown that higher intake of allylsulfides and flavonoids particularly quercetin is associated with reduced risk of several types of cancers. Allixin showed an anti-tumour promoting effect *in vivo*, inhibiting skin tumour formation by12-O-tetradecanoylphorbol-13-acetate in 7,12-dimethylbenz [a] anthracene initiated mice. It is believed to promote cardiovascular activity and a beneficial, soothing action on the respiratory system. Several mechanisms have been proposed to explain the cancer-preventive effects of Allium vegetables and related organosulfur compounds (Thomson and Ali 2003). These include inhibition of mutagenesis, modulation of enzyme activities, inhibition of DNA adduct formation, free-radical scavenging, and effects on cell proliferation and tumour growth.

In tumour-bearing mice, significant anti tumour effects of aged black garlic extracts (ABGE) were observed, such as growth inhibition of inoculated tumours. Further investigation of serum superoxide dismutases, glutathione peroxidase, interleukin-2 and the increased indices of spleen and thymus indicated that the anticancer action of ABGE may be partly due to its antioxidant and immunomodulative effects (Wang *et al.*, 2012).

Allixin and/or its analogs may be expected to be useful in cancer prevention and/or chemotherapy. Several mechanisms have been reviewed by Butt *et al.* (2009) including activation of detoxification phase-I and II enzymes, reactive oxygen species (ROS) generation, and reducing DNA damage. Garlic could be useful in preventing the suppression of immune response associated with increased risk of malignancy as it stimulates the proliferation of lymphocytes, macrophage phagocytosis, release of interleukin-2, tumour necrosis factor-alpha and interferon-gamma, and enhances natural killer cells.

The two major compounds in aged garlic, S-allylcysteine and S-allylmercapto-L-cysteine, had the highest radical scavenging activity. In addition, some organosulfur compounds derived from garlic, including S-allylcysteine, have been found to retard the growth of chemically induced and transplantable tumours in several animal models. Therefore, the consumption of garlic may provide some kind of protection from cancer development (Thomson and Ali, 2003). Diallyl disulfide could be a promising anticancer agent for both hormone-dependent and independent breast cancers, and may harmonize with polyunsaturated fatty acids known as modulators of breast cancer cell growth (Nakagawa *et al.*, 2001).

Garlic components have been found to block covalent binding of carcinogens to DNA, enhance degradation of carcinogens, have anti-oxidative and free radical scavenging properties and to regulate cell proliferation, apoptosis and immune responses. There are a number of mechanisms at work which jointly are responsible for eliciting the anticarcinogenic effects noted in laboratory studies in a wide range of experimental systems (Das, 2002).

Seki *et al.* (2008) also confirmed on the basis of their study that diallyl trisulfide is responsible, at least in part, for the epidemiologically proven anticancer effect for garlic eaters. Tsubura *et al.* (2011) found Diallyl disulfide to be more effective than water-soluble compounds in suppressing breast cancer. Mechanisms of action include the activation of metabolizing enzymes that detoxify carcinogens, the suppression of DNA adduct formation, the inhibition of the production of reactive oxygen species, the regulation of cell-cycle arrest and the induction of apoptosis. Selenium-enriched garlic or organoselenium compounds provide more potent protection against mammary carcinogenesis in rats and greater inhibition of breast cancer cells in culture than natural garlic or the respective organosulfur analogues.

Miroddi *et al.* (2011) found the oil-soluble sulfur compounds to be responsible for anticancer effects exerted through multiple mechanisms such as: inhibition of metabolic carcinogenic activation, arrest of cell cycle, antioxidant and pro-apoptotic action. Zhang *et al.* (2010) observed allicin to reduce cell viability in a dose- and time-dependent manner, partly through induction of apoptosis in gastric cancer cells. At the molecular level, allicin induced cytochrome c release from the mitochondria and increased caspase-3, -8, and -9 activation, with concomitant upregulation of expression of the genes bax and fas expression in the tumour cells. Allicin treatment inhibited proliferation and induced apoptosis in SGC-7901 cancer cells. Both intrinsic mitochondrial and extrinsic Fas/FasL-mediated pathways of apoptosis occur simultaneously in SGC-7901 cells following allicin treatment.

Both water- and lipid-soluble allyl sulfur compounds are effective in blocking a myriad of chemically induced tumours. Milner (2001) reviewing the available epidemiological and laboratory studies suggested the probable mechanisms of action for anticarcinogenic potential of garlic as 1. blocking nitrosamine formation and metabolism, 2. altering several phase I and II enzymes. Changes in DNA repair and in immunocompetence may also account for some of this protection. Some, but not all, allyl sulfur compounds can also effectively retard tumour proliferation and induce apoptosis. Changes in cellular thiol and phosphorylation stains may account for some of these antitumourigenic properties. The anticarcinogenic potential of garlic can be influenced by several dietary components including specific fatty acids, selenium, and vitamin A.

Currently, immunotherapy with Bacillus Calmette-Guerin (BCG) is the most effective treatment for superficial bladder carcinoma, but treatment-related toxicity may limit its use in some patients. Riggs and his colleagues (1997) have reported that mice that received 50 mg oral Allium sativum (AS) had significant reductions in tumour volume ($P < 0.05$) when compared with animals that received the saline control, and mice that received 500 mg oral AS had significant reductions in both tumour volume and mortality.

According to Lamm and Riggs (2001) garlic may be useful in preventing the suppression of immune response that is associated with increased risk of malignancy. Their data suggest that maintenance of immune stimulation can significantly reduce the risk of cancer. Clinical trials should be initiated to test the hypothesis that the immune stimulation and other beneficial effects of garlic are able to reduce the incidence of cancer.

Milner (1996) suggests that in spite of the evidence supporting the benefits of oil-soluble compounds of garlic diallyl disulfide are effective in reducing the proliferation of neoplasms, additional evidence is needed to determine the quantity needed by humans to minimize cancer risk. Also, Sengupta *et al.* (2004) pined that though there is a large body of evidence supporting anticarcinogenic mechanisms of garlic, they are still speculative, and further research is needed to support causality between such properties and cancer-preventive activity in experimental animals.

Other Uses

Combinations of promoters of iron and zinc bioavailability such as allium spices (1.5 g/10 g), amchur (0.75 g/10 g) and β-carotene-rich vegetables (2.5 g/10 g) were found to show a positive influence on the bioaccessibility of iron by Gautam *et al.* (2011). The specific combinations were amchur-carrot, amchur-garlic, onion-carrot, and onion-amaranth in a few specific grains.

Chronic renal failure (CRF) induced oxidative tissue injury occurs via the activation of pro-inflammatory mediators and by neutrophil infiltration into tissues. Deniz *et al.* (2011) attributed from his study, the protective effects of garlic on CRF-induced injury to its ability to inhibit neutrophil infiltration and pro-inflammatory mediators.

El-Shenawy and Hassan (2008) concluded from their experiment that oral administration of either selenium or garlic produces a significant protection against liver and kidney damage induced by the $HgCl_2$ injection, but garlic appears to be more protective. Nwokocha *et al.* (2011) demonstrated that raw garlic (7 per cent w/w) offers more hepatoprotective effect to cadmium (200 ppm) followed by mercury (10 ppm) and least protection to lead (100 ppm) through the processes of uptake, assimilation and elimination of these metals.

Garlic has been used reasonably successfully in AIDS patients to treat cryptosporidium in an uncontrolled study in China (Fareed *et al.*, 2007). It has also been used by at least one AIDS patient to treat toxoplasmosis, another protozoal disease (James, 2007). Garlic supplementation in rats, along with a high protein diet, has been shown to boost testosterone levels (Oi *et al.*, 2001).

Yang *et al.* (2011a, b) observed that some of the sulfur compounds unique to garlic or onion interacted with common sulfur compounds detected in irradiated meat and masked or changed the odor characteristics of irradiated raw ground beef. So they concluded that >0.5 per cent onion or <0.01 per cent garlic would be needed to mask or prevent irradiation aroma in irradiated raw ground beef.

To avoid environmental pollution and health problems caused by the use of traditional synthetic pesticides, there is a trend to search for naturally occurring toxicants from plants. Among the compounds discussed for antifungal and insecticidal activity, the natural extracts from garlic and horseradish have attracted considerable attention. Garlic extracts at the same concentration provided a good fungicidal activity against *Botrytis cinerea* Pers. and *S. rolfsii*. *A. rusticana* and *A. sativum* preparations also showed an interesting and significant insecticidal activity against larvae of *A. albopictus* (Tedeschi *et al.*, 2011).

Cytokines involved in inflammatory bowel disease (IBD) direct a predominantly cell-mediated T- helper-1 (Th1) immune response. The nonspecific anti-inflammatory treatment being used in the management of patients with IBD has not changed much since the 1970s and new therapeutic agents are keenly sought. Hodge *et al.* (2002) in his review article said that several compounds isolated from garlic modulate leukocyte cell proliferation and cytokine production. Twenty to fifty per cent of the immunomodulatory activity of garlic extract on cytokine production was acid labile. The inhibitory activity of methylprednisolone, a commonly used anti-inflammatory in inflammatory bowel disease with garlic on leukocyte cytokine production was additive. Thus by inhibiting Th1 and inflammatory cytokines while upregulating IL-10 production, treatment with garlic extract may help to resolve inflammation associated with IBD.

Conclusions

Garlic is proved to be effective in infections (bacterial, viral, mycotic and parasitic infections) having the properties of empowering immune system along with antitumour and antioxidant effects (Goncagul and Ayaz, 2010). Garlic plants may also play an important role in the ecological control of pathogenic microorganisms in nature (Adetumbi and Lau (1983). Thus, Garlic is one of the most versatile ready remedy for prevention and cure for various avoidable illnesses.

References

Adetumbi MA, Lau BH (1983). *Allium sativum* (garlic)–a natural antibiotic. Med. Hypotheses. 12 (3): 227–37.

Agarwal K C (1996). Therapeutic actions of garlic constituents. Med. Res. Rev. 16: 111–24.

Ahmadabad HN, Hassan ZM, Safari E, Bozorgmehr M, Ghazanfari T, Moazzeni SM (2011). Evaluation of the immunomodulatory effect of the 14 kDa protein isolated from aged garlic extract on dendritic cells. Cell Immunol. 269 (2): 90–95.

Adler BB, Beuchat LR (2002). Death of *Salmonella, Escherichia coli* O157:H7, and *Listeria monocytogenes* in garlic butter as affected by storage temperature. J Food Prot. 65 (12): 1976–80.

Alder R, Lookinland S, Berry JA, Williams M (2003). A systematic review of the effectiveness of garlic as an anti-hyperlipidemic agent. J. Am. Acad. Nurse. Pract. 15 (3): 120–29.

Amagase H (2006). Clarifying the real bioactive constituents of garlic. J. Nutr. 136 (3 Suppl): 716S–725S.

Amagase H, Petesch BL, Matsuura H, Kasuga S, Itakura Y. (2001) Intake of garlic and its bioactive components. J. Nutr. 131 (3s): 955S–62S.

Ashraf R, Aamir K, Shaikh AR, Ahmed T (2005). Effects of garlic on dyslipidemia in patients with type 2 diabetes mellitus. J Ayub Med Coll Abbottabad. 17 (3): 60–64.

Ashraf R, Khan RA, Ashraf I (2011). Garlic (*Allium sativum*) supplementation with standard antidiabetic agent provides better diabetic control in type 2 diabetes patients. Pak. J. Pharm. Sci. 24 (4): 565–70.

Augusti KT (1996) Therapeutic values of onion (*Allium cepa* L.) and garlic (*Allium sativum* L.). Indian J Exp Biol. 34 (7): 634-40.

Augusti KT, Sheela CG (1996). Antiperoxide effect of S-allyl cysteine sulfoxide, an insulin secretagogue in diabetic rats. Experientia. 52: 115–20.

Ayaz E, Alpsoy HC (2007). Garlic (*Allium sativum*) and Traditional Medicine. Turkiye Parzytoloji Dergisi 31 (2): 145–49.

Bakri IM, Douglas CW (2005). Inhibitory effect of garlic extract on oral bacteria. Arch. Oral Biol. 50 (7): 645–51.

Beato VM, Orgaz F, Mansilla F (2011). Montaño AChanges in phenolic compounds in garlic (*Allium sativum* L.) owing to the cultivar and location of growth. Plant Foods Hum. Nutr. 66 (3): 218–23.

Bever BO, Zahnd GR (1979). Plants with oral hypoglycaemic action. Quart. J. Crude Drug Res. 17: 139–46.

Bolton S, Null G, Troetal W M (1982). The medical uses of garlic-fact and fiction. Am. Pharm. 22: 40–43.

Borrelli F, Capasso R, Izzo AA (2007). Garlic (*Allium sativum* L.): adverse effects and drug interactions in humans. Mol. Nutr. Food Res. 51(11): 386–97.

Butt MS, Sultan MT, Butt MS, Iqbal J. (2009). Garlic: nature's protection against physiological threats. Crit. Rev. Food Sci. Nutr. 49 (6): 538–51.

Castro C, Lorenzo AG, Gonzalez A, Cruzado M (2010). Garlic components inhibit angiotensin II-induced cell-cycle progression and migration: involvement of cell-cycle inhibitor p27 (Kip1) and mitogen-activated protein kinase. Mol. Nutr. Food Res. 54: 781–87.

Chan KC, Yin MC, Chao WJ (2007). Effect of diallyl trisulfide-rich garlic oil on blood coagulation and plasma activity of anticoagulation factors in rats. Food Chem Toxicol 45 (3): 502–507.

Chang SH, Liu CJ, Kuo CH, Chen H, Lin WY, Teng KY, Chang SW, Tsai CH, Tsai FJ, Huang CY, Tzang BS, Kuo WW (2011). Garlic Oil Alleviates MAPKs- and IL-6-mediated Diabetes-related Cardiac Hypertrophy in STZ-induced DM Rats. Evid. Based Complement. Alternat. Med. 2011: 950150.

Das S (2002). Garlic–A Natural Source of Cancer Preventive Compounds. Asian Pac. J. Cancer Prev. 3 (4): 305–311.

Deniz M, ªener G, Ercan F, Yeðen BÇ (2011). Garlic extract ameliorates renal and cardiopulmonary injury in the rats with chronic renal failure. Ren Fail. 33 (7): 718–25.

Durak A, Ozturk HS, Olcay E, Guven C (2002). Effects of garlic extract supplementation on blood lipid and antioxidant parameters and atherosclerotic plaque formation process of cholesterol-fed rabbits. J. Herb. Pharmcother. 2 (2): 19–32.

Durak I, Kavutcu M, Aytac B, *et al.* (2004). Effects of garlic extract consumption on blood lipid and oxidant/antioxidant parameters in humans with high blood cholesterol. J. Nutr. Biochem. 15 (6): 373–77.

El-Demerdash FM, Yousef MI, El-Naga NI (2005). Biochemical study on the hypoglycaemic effects of onion and garlic in alloxan-induced diabetic rats. Food Chem. Toxicol. 43 (1): 57–63.

El-Shenawy SM, Hassan NS (2008) Comparative evaluation of the protective effect of selenium and garlic against liver and kidney damage induced by mercury chloride in the rats. Pharmacol Rep. 60 (2): 199-208.

Ellen Tattelman (American Family Physician) July 1, (2005). Health effects of Garlic.

Fani MM, Kohanteb J, Dayaghi M (2007) Inhibitory activity of garlic (*Allium sativum*) extract on multidrug-resistant Streptococcus mutans. J Indian Soc Pedod Prev Dent. 25 (4): 164–68.

Fareed G, Scolaro M, Jordan W, Sanders N, Chesson C, Slattery M, Long D, Castro C. (2007). The use of a high-dose garlic preparation for the treatment of *Cryptosporidium parvum diarrhea*. NLM Gateway. Retrieved on December 7.

Fenwick GR, Hanley AB (1985). The genus *Allium*. Crit. Rev. Food Sci. Nutr. 22: 199 - 271.

Fujiwara M, Yishimura M, Tsuno S, Murakami F (1958). "Allithiamine," a newly found derivative of vitamin B1. IV. on the alliin homologues in the vegetables. J. Biochem. (Tokyo). 45: 141–49.

Gautam S, Platel K, Srinivasan K (2011). Promoting influence of combinations of amchur, β-carotene-rich vegetables and *Allium* spices on the bioaccessibility of zinc and iron from food grains. Int J Food Sci Nutr. 62 (5): 518–24.

Gebhardt R (1991). Inhibition of cholesterol biosynthesis by a water-soluble garlic extract in primary cultures of rat hepatocytes. Arzneimittelforschung. 41 (8): 800–804.

Gebhardt R, Beck H (1996). Differential inhibitory effects of garlic-derived organosulfur compounds on cholesterol biosynthesis in primary rat hepatocyte cultures. Lipids. 31 (12): 1269–76.

Gedik N, Kabasakal L, Sehirli O, Ercan F, Sirvanci S, Keyer-Uysal M, Sener G (2005). Long-term administration of aqueous garlic extract (AGE) alleviates liver fibrosis and oxidative damage induced by biliary obstruction in rats. Life Sci. 76 (22): 2593-606.

Goncagul G, Ayaz E (2010). Antimicrobial effect of garlic (*Allium sativum*). Recent Pat. Anti-infect. Drug Discov. 5 (1): 91–93.

Groppo FC, Ramacciato JC, Simões RP, Flório FM, Sartoratto A (2002). Antimicrobial activity of garlic, tea tree oil, and chlorhexidine against oral microorganisms. Int. Dent. J. 52 (6): 433–37.

Groppo, F. Ramacciato, J. Motta, R. Ferraresi, P. Sartoratto, A (2007). Antimicrobial activity of garlic against oral streptococci. Int. J. Dent. Hyg. 5 (2): 109–115.

Hannan A, Ikram Ullah M, Usman M, Hussain S, Absar M, Javed K (2011). Anti-mycobacterial activity of garlic (*Allium sativum*) against multi-drug resistant and non-multi-drug resistant *Mycobacterium tuberculosis*. Pak. J. Pharm. Sci. 24(1): 81–85.

Hamel, PB, Chiltoskey MU (1975). Cherokee Plants and Their Uses — A 400 Year History. Sylva, N.C. Herald Publishing Co. (p. 35).

Higashikawa F, Noda M, Awaya T, Ushijima M, Sugiyama M (2011). Reduction of serum lipids by the intake of the extract of garlic fermented with Monascus pilosus: A randomized, double-blind, placebo-controlled clinical trial. Clin. Nutr. 2011 Oct 29. [Epub ahead of print].

Hodge G, Hodge S, Han P (2002). *Allium sativum* (garlic) suppresses leukocyte inflammatory cytokine production *in vitro*: potential therapeutic use in the treatment of inflammatory bowel disease. Cytometry. 48 (4): 209–15.

James JS (1988). Treatment Leads on Cryptosporisiosis: Preliminary Report on Opportunistic Infection, Aids Treatment News No. 049–January 29, Retrieved December 7, 2007.

Jelodar GA, Maleki M, Motadayen MH, Sirus S (2005). Effect of fenugreek, onion and garlic on blood glucose and histopathology of pancreas of alloxan-induced diabetic rats. Indian J.Med. Sci. 59 (2): 64–9.

Jung YM, Lee SH, Lee DS, You MJ, Chung IK, Cheon WH, Kwon YS, Lee YJ, Ku SK (2011). Fermented garlic protects diabetic, obese mice when fed a high-fat diet by antioxidant effects. Nutr. Res. 31 (5): 387–96.

Kiralan M, Bayrak A, Abdulaziz OF, Ozbucak T (2012). Essential oil composition and antiradical activity of the oil of Iraq plants. Nat. Prod. Res. 26 (2): 132 – 29.

Kojuri J, Vosoughi AR, Akrami M (2007). Effects of anethum graveolens and garlic on lipid profile in hyperlipidemic patients. Lipids Health Dis 1 (6): 5.

Lamm DL, Riggs DR (2001) Enhanced immunocompetence by garlic: role in bladder cancer and other malignancies. J Nutr. 131 (3s): 1067S-70S.

Lanzotti V (2006). The analysis of onion and garlic. J Chromatogr A. 1112 (1-2): 3-22.

Liu L, Yeh YY (2000). Inhibition of cholesterol biosynthesis by organosulfur compounds derived from garlic. Lipids. 35 (2): 197–203.

Liu L, Yeh YY (2001). Water-soluble organosulfur compounds of garlic inhibit fatty acid and triglyceride syntheses in cultured rat hepatocytes. Lipids. 36 (4): 395–400.

Lu X, Rasco BA, Kang DH, Jabal JM, Aston DE, Konkel ME (2011) Infrared and Raman spectroscopic studies of the antimicrobial effects of garlic concentrates and diallyl constituents on foodborne pathogens. Anal. Chem. 83 (11): 4137–46.

Mader FH (1990). Treatment of hyperlipidaemia with garlic-powder tablets. Evidence from the German Association of General Practitioners' multicentric placebo-controlled double-blind study. Arzneimittelforschung 40 (10): 1111–16.

Matsuura (2001). Saponins in Garlic as Modifiers of the Risk of Cardiovascular Disease. *J. Nutri.* 131: 1000S–1005S.

May S (1926). Zur Behandlung arteriosklerotischer Beschwerden. Fortschr. Ther. 2: 762-764.

Milner JA (1996). Garlic: its anticarcinogenic and antitumourigenic properties. Nutr. Rev. 54 (11 Pt 2): S82–86.

Milner JA (2001). A historical perspective on garlic and cancer. J. Nutr. 131 (3s): 1027S–31S.

Miroddi M, Calapai F, Calapai G (2011). Potential beneficial effects of garlic in oncohematology. Mini Rev. Med. Chem. 11 (6): 461–72.

Nakagawa H, Tsuta K, Kiuchi K, Senzaki H, Tanaka K, Hioki K, Tsubura A.(2001). Growth inhibitory effects of diallyl disulfide on human breast cancer cell lines. Carcinogenesis. 22 (6): 891–97.

Nwokocha CR, Owu DU, Nwokocha MI, Ufearo CS, Iwuala MO (2012). Comparative study on the efficacy of *Allium sativum* (garlic) in reducing some heavy metal accumulation in liver of wistar rats. Food Chem. Toxicol. 50 (2): 222–26.

Oi Y, Imafuku M, Shishido C, Kominato Y, Nishimura S, Iwai K. (2001). Garlic supplementation increases testicular testosterone and decreases plasma corticosterone in rats fed a high protein diet. Journal of Nutrition 131 (8): 2150–56.

Padiya R, Khatua TN, Bagul PK, Kuncha M, Banerjee SK (2011). Garlic improves insulin sensitivity and associated metabolic syndromes in fructose fed rats. Nutr. Metab. (Lond). 27; 8: 53.

Park SY, Yoo SS, Shim JH, Chin KB (2008). Physico-chemical properties, and antioxidant and antimicrobial effects of garlic and onion powder in fresh pork belly and loin during refrigerated storage. J. Food Sci. 73 (8): C577–84.

Rahman K (2001). Historical Perspective on Garlic and Cardiovascular Disease *Journal of Nutrition.* 131: 977S–979S.

Rahman K (2007). Effects of garlic on platelet biochemistry and physiology. Mol. Nutr. Food Res. 51 (11): 1335–44.

Reinhart KM, Coleman CI, Teevan C, Vachhani P, White CM (2008). Effects of garlic on blood pressure in patients with and without systolic hypertension: a meta-analysis. Ann. Pharmacother. 42: 1766–71.

Ried K, Frank OR, Stocks NP, Fakler P, Sullivan T (2008). Effect of garlic on blood pressure: a systematic review and meta-analysis. BMC Cardiovasc. Disord. 8:.13.

Ried K, Frank OR, Stocks NP (2010). Aged garlic extract lowers blood pressure in patients with treated but uncontrolled hypertension: a randomised controlled trial. Maturitas. 67: 144–50.

Ried K, Frank OR, Stocks NP (2013).Aged garlic extract reduces blood pressure in hypertensives: a dose–response trial. Eur. J. Clin. Nutr. 67 (1): 64–70.

Riggs DR, DeHaven JI, Lamm DL (1997) *Allium sativum* (garlic) treatment for murine transitional cell carcinoma. Cancer. 79 (10): 1987–94.

Sainani GS, Desai DB, More KN (1976). Onion, garlic and atherosclerosis. Lancet. 2: 575–76.

Seki T, Hosono T, Hosono-Fukao T, Inada K, Tanaka R, Ogihara J, Ariga T (2008). Anticancer effects of diallyl trisulfide derived from garlic. Asia Pac. J. Clin. Nutr. 17 Suppl. 1: 249–52.

Sengupta A, Ghosh S, Bhattacharjee S (2004). *Allium* vegetables in cancer prevention: an overview. Asian Pac. J. Cancer Prev. 5 (3): 237–45.

Schlesinger K (1926). Knoblauch (*Allium sativum*) als Heilmittel bei Arteriosklerose. Wien. Med. Wochenschr. 76: 1076–77.

Sheela CG, Augusti KT (1992). Antidiabetic effects of S-allyl cysteine sulphoxide isolated from garlic *Allium sativum* Linn. Indian J. Exp. Biol. 30: 523–26.

Silagy C, Neil A (1994). Garlic as a lipid lowering agent—a meta-analysis. J. R. Coll. Physicians Lond. 28 (1): 39–45.

Sovova M, Sova P (2004). Pharmaceutical importance of *Allium sativum* L. 5. Hypolipemic effects *in vitro* and *in vivo*. Ceska. Slov.Farm. 53 (3): 117–23.

Steiner M, Lin RS (1998). Changes in platelet function and susceptibility of lipoproteins to oxidation associated with administration of aged garlic extract. J. Cardiovasc. Pharmacol. 31 (6): 904–908.

Stoll A, Seebeck E (1948). Allium compounds. I. Alliin the true mother compound of garlic oil. Helv. Chim. Acta. 31: 189–210.

Suetsuna K (1998). Isolation and characterization of angiotensin I-converting enzyme inhibitor dipeptides derived from *Allium sativum* L. (garlic) J. Nutr. Biochem. 9: 415–19.

Sumioka I, Hayama M, Shimokawa Y, Shiraishi S, Tokunaga A. (2006). Lipid-lowering effect of monascus garlic fermented extract (MGFE) in hyperlipidemic subjects. Hiroshima J. Med. Sci. 55 (2): 59–64.

Taubmann G (1934). Therapie mit Drogen. Med. Klin. 32: 1067–69.

Tedeschi P, Leis M, Pezzi M, Civolani S, Maietti A, Brandolini V (2011). Insecticidal activity and fungitoxicity of plant extracts and components of horseradish (*Armoracia rusticana*) and garlic (*Allium sativum*). J. Environ. Sci. Health. B. 46 (6): 486–90.

Thomson M, Ali M (2003). Garlic (*Allium sativum*): A review of its potential use as an anti-cancer agent. Curr. Cancer Drug Targets. 3 (1): 67–81.

Touloupakis E, Ghanotakis DF (2011). Nutraceutical use of garlic sulfur-containing compounds. Adv.Exp. Med. Biol. 698: 110–21.

Tsubura A, Lai YC, Kuwata M, Uehara N, Yoshizawa K (2011). Anticancer effects of garlic and garlic-derived compounds for breast cancer control. Anticancer Agents Med. Chem. 11 (3): 249–53.

USDA (2012). National Nutrient Database for Standard Reference, Release 25.

Vazquez-Prieto MA, Rodriguez Lanzi C, Lembo C, Galmarini CR, Miatello RM (2011). Garlic and onion attenuates vascular inflammation and oxidative stress in fructose-fed rats. J. Nutr. Metab. 475216.

Wang X, Jiao F, Wang QW, Wang J, Yang K, Hu RR, Liu HC, Wang HY, Wang YS (2012). Aged black garlic extract induces inhibition of gastric cancer cell growth *in vitro* and *in vivo*. Mol. Med. Report. 5 (1): 66–72.

Yang HS, Lee EJ, Moon SH, Paik HD, Nam K, Ahn DU (2011a). Effect of garlic, onion, and their combination on the quality and sensory characteristics of irradiated raw ground beef. Meat Sci. 89 (2): 202–208.

Yang HS, Lee EJ, Moon SH, Paik HD, Ahn DU (2011b). Addition of garlic or onion before irradiation on lipid oxidation, volatiles and sensory characteristics of cooked ground beef. Meat Sci. 88 (2): 286–91.

Yeh YY, Liu L (2001). Cholesterol-lowering effect of garlic extracts and organosulfur compounds: human and animal studies. J. Nutr. 131 (3s): 989S–93S.

Yeh YY, Yeh SM (1994). Garlic reduces plasma lipids by inhibiting hepatic cholesterol and triacylglycerol synthesis. Lipids. 29 (3): 189–93.

Zacharias NT, Sebastian KL, Philip B, Augusti KT (1980). Hypoglycaemic and hypolipidaemic effects of garlic in sucrose fed rabbits. Ind. J. Physiol. Pharmacol. 24: 151–54.

Zhang W, Ha M, Gong Y, Xu Y, Dong N, Yuan Y (2010). Allicin induces apoptosis in gastric cancer cells through activation of both extrinsic and intrinsic pathways. Oncol Rep. 24 (6): 1585–92.

Chapter 9
Ginger
(*Zingiber officinale*)

The word ginger is derived from the Sanskrit word 'stringa-vera', which means horn-like body. This is because it resembles the antlers of a deer. An ancient Sanskrit saying about ginger "Adrakam sarva kandanaam" means every good quality is found in the ginger. It is the underground stem of the ginger plant. This spice is mentioned in the writings of Confucius, the famous Chinese philosopher. It also finds a place in the Koran, which is the sacred book of the followers of Islam. It was one of the earliest known spices in Western Europe, with its use dating back to the ninth century A.D. Ginger has been used for centuries for cooking and medicinal purposes. It has been written about in early Sanskrit and Chinese texts and also in ancient Greek and

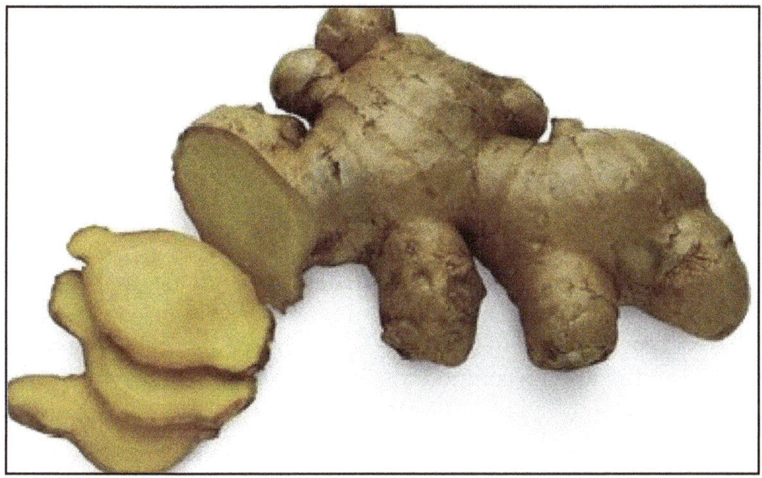

Roman literature. The ancient Greeks ate ginger wrapped in bread to prevent nausea after a lavish feast. Chinese sailors chewed ginger to prevent seasickness.

Ginger seems to originate from Southern China. Today, it is cultivated all over tropic and subtropical Asia (50 per cent of the world's harvest is produced in India), in Brazil, Jamaica whence the best quality is exported and Nigeria, whose ginger is rather pungent, but lacks the fine aroma of other provenances. Initial G in most of the European names of ginger is due to a Late Latin form gingiber.

Ginger is a major crop cultivated in India. It is a small grassy plant grown in all seasons throughout the year. Indian Ginger is famous for its flavour, texture and taste. More than a spice, ginger is considered as a taste maker, a drug, an appetizer and a flavourant. Superior quality of ginger is produced in Kerala though it is grown throughout the country. The congenial climate and the fertile soil are responsible for production of quality ginger. India has a predominant position in ginger production and export. The principal buyers are the Middle East, USA, UK and Netherlands. In the world market Indian ginger is popularly known as 'cochin ginger' and 'calicut ginger'.

Ginger has been used to treat heartburn, vomiting, stomach cramps, loss of appetite and as a digestive aid. It is also used to treat cold, cough and respiratory problems; to relieve toothache and as an antioxidant as well. Qidwai *et al.* (2003) conducted a study on 270 patients, visiting the Family Practice Center, the Aga Khan University, Karachi on the use of folk remedies which included ginger along with many others for medicinal uses conditions such as common cold, cough and flu to more serious conditions such as asthma, jaundice and heat stroke.

Varieties of Ginger

"Tongling White Ginger" enjoys a reputation for being one of the top gingers in China for its thin white peel, tender flesh, rich juice, and flavour (Feng *et al.*, 2011). Some other varieties are African ginger; Black ginger; Jamaican ginger.

Chemical Constituents of Ginger

Ginger is known to contain a number of potentially bioactive substances, mainly gingerols and their related dehydration products, the shogaols, as well as volatile oils including sesquiterpenes, such as b-bisabolene and (-)-zingiberene, and monoterpenes, mainly geranial and neral (Chevallier, 1996; Ursell, 2000). In particular, gingerols have been shown to inhibit both prostaglandin and leukotriene biosynthesis (Kiuchi *et al.*, 1992) and angiogenesis (Kim *et al.*, 2005a). In addition, several ginger components exhibit serotonin receptor-blocking activity (Huang *et al.*, 1991; Abdel-Aziz *et al.*, 2005).

Feng *et al.* (2011) isolated and identified two novel gingerdione dimers, bisgingerdiones A (1) and B (2); two new gingerol derivatives, (5R)-5-acetoxy-1,7-bis(4-hydroxy-3-methoxyphenyl)heptan-3-one (3) and methyl (Z)-neral acetal-[6]-gingerdiol (4); and 38 known compounds (5-42) from Tongling White Ginger.

Gingerol, shogaol, zingerone, and paradol are the pungent principles in ginger (Connell and McLachlan, 1978). The pungent gingeroles degrade to the milder shoagoles during storage; high gingerole content and good pungency thus indicate freshness and quality.

The main aroma-defining component is zingiberol (Varma *et al.*, 1962). The crude extract of ginger showed the presence of saponins, flavonoids, and alkaloids while other classes of compounds did not test positive (Ghayur and Gilani, 2005a).

The essential oil (1 to 3 per cent of the fresh rhizome) contains mostly sesquiterpenes, *e.g.*, (-)-zingiberene (up to 70 per cent), (+)-ar-curcumene β-sesquiphellandrene, bisabolene and farnesene. Monoterpenoids occur in traces (β-phelladrene, cineol, citral).

Nutritive Value of Ginger

Nutritional value per 100 g

Nutrient	*Amount*	*Nutrient*	*Amount*
Energy (kcal)	20	Carbohydrates (g)	17.8
Sugars (g)	1.7	Dietary fiber (g)	2.0
Fat (g)	0.75	Protein (g)	1.8
Calcium (mg)	16	Iron (mg)	0.6
Magnesium (mg)	43	Phosphorus (mg)	34
Potassium (mg)	415	Zinc (mg)	0.34
Thiamine (Vit. B1) (mg)	0.025	Riboflavin (Vit.B2) mg)	0.034
Niacin (Vit. B3) (mg)	0.75	Vitamin B6 (mg)	0.16
Folate (Vit. B9) (μg)	11	Vitamin C (mg)	5

USDA (2012).

Traditional Therapeutic Uses of Ginger

An ethno botanical exploration undertaken in Jawadhu Hills of Thiruvannamalai district, Tamilnadu, India, brought under notice various plants and their extracts used by the people for treating various disorders. Personal interviews conducted with village dwellers, herbal medicine practitioners and other traditional healers reported the use of ginger by the people to relieve cold and cough. Tea brewed with ginger is a folk remedy for cold. Also, 3-4 tulsi leaves taken along with a piece of ginger on an empty stomach are considered an effective cure for congestion, cold and cough by the locals (Ranganatha *et al.*, 2012). The local people, experienced aged rural folk, traditional herbal medicine practitioners and local herb drug sellers of the forest areas of Villupuram district, Tamilnadu, India, also made use of ginger for treating cold and cough. Dried ginger is boiled with palm sugar candy and is internally useful in the case of chronic cough and cold (Sankaranarayanan *et al.*, 2010). A semi-structured questionnaire survey conducted among 45 Vaidyas to document their knowledge on preparing various herbal formulations in Ukhimath block, Uttarkhand, found the use of mixture of rhizome extract of ginger and honey to relieve cough, cold and throat pain (Semwal *et al.*, 2010).

Fresh ginger has been used for cold-induced diseases, nausea, asthma, cough, colic, heart palpitation, swelling, dyspepsia, loss of appetite and rheumatism. In nineteenth century, ginger served as a popular remedy for cough and asthma when the juice of fresh ginger was mixed with a little juice of fresh garlic and honey. Ginger has also been known to possess various other interesting pharmacological and physiological properties. For instance, it acts as an anti-inflammatory, analgesic, antipyretic, antihepatotoxic and cardiotonic substance (Surh *et al.*, 1998).

The medicinal properties attributed to ginger include antiarthritic (Srivastava and Mustafa, 1989; 1992; Bliddal *et al.*, 2000), antimigraine (Mustafa and Srivastava, 1990; Cady *et al.*, 2005), antithrombotic (Bordia *et al.*, 1997; Thomson *et al.*, 2002), anti-inflammatory (Thomson *et al.*, 2002, Penna *et al.*, 2003), hypolipidaemic (Bordia *et al.*, 1997; Thomson *et al.*, 2002; Bhandari *et al.*, 2005), hypocholesterolaemic (Furhman *et al.*, 2000) and antinausea properties (Ernst and Pittler, 2000; Portnoi *et al.*, 2003).

The main pharmacological actions of ginger include immunomodulatory, antitumourigenic, anti-inflammatory, antiapoptotic, antihyperglycemic, antilipidemic and antiemetic actions. Ginger is a strong antioxidant substance and may either mitigate or prevent generation of free radicals. It is considered a safe herbal medicine with only few and insignificant adverse/side effects (Ali *et al.*, 2008). A randomized double-masked, placebo-controlled trail conducted on pregnant women for 4 days using 1gram ginger daily found ginger to be very effective in reducing the severity of nausea and vomiting, thus providing relief to pregnant women (Vutyavanich *et al.*, 2001). On treatment with ginger capsules, the nausea and vomiting of experimental group subsided compared to the control group thus confirming that ginger is an effective remedy for decreasing nausea and vomiting during pregnancy (Ozgoli *et al.*, 2009b).

The disease specific benefits of ginger are presented below.

Ginger as Antioxidant and Anti-inflammatory Agent

Ghasemzadeh *et al.* (2010) validated the medicinal potential of the leaves and young rhizome of *Zingiber officinale* (Halia Bara) and the positive relationship between total phenolics content and antioxidant. Halia Bara had higher antioxidant activities as well as total contents of phenolic and flavonoid in comparison with Halia Bentong (another variety of ginger). Ginger oil has dominantly protective effect on DNA damage induced by H_2O_2. Ginger oil might act as a scavenger of oxygen radical and might be used as an antioxidant (Lu *et al.*, 2003).

Oral administration of aqueous extract of Zinziber officinale (3 mg/animal/day) along with paraben for thirty days caused significant amelioration of lipid peroxidation in liver and kidney homogenates (Verma and Asnani, 2007; and (Asnani and Verma, 2007); and increased significantly the activities of enzymatic (superoxide dismutase, glutathione peroxidase, catalase) and non-enzymatic (glutathione and ascorbic acid) antioxidants in the liver of mice (Asnani and Verma, 2009).

Ginger is reported to possess anti-inflammatory, effect along with several other benefits (Langner, 1998). The volatile oil of ginger influences both cell-mediated immune response and nonspecific proliferation of *T. lymphocytes* and may exert beneficial effects in a number of clinical conditions, such as chronic inflammation and autoimmune diseases (Zhou *et al.*, 2006).

Dugasani *et al.*, (2010) found 6-Shogaol to exhibit the most potent antioxidant and anti-inflammatory properties which they attributed to the presence of alpha,beta-unsaturated ketone moiety. The carbon chain length also must have played a significant role in making 10-gingerol as the most potent among all the gingerols. This study justifies the use of dry ginger in traditional systems of medicine.

Ginger as Antibacterial

Two highly alkylated gingerols, [10]-gingerol and [12]-gingerol effectively inhibited the growth of oral pathogens. The ethanol and n-hexane extracts of ginger exhibited antibacterial activities against three anaerobic Gram-negative bacteria, *P. gingivalis* ATCC 53978, *P. endodontalis* ATCC 35406 and *P. intermedia* ATCC 25611, causing periodontal diseases, at a minimum inhibitory concentration (MIC) range of 6-30 µg/mL. These ginger compounds also killed the oral pathogens at a minimum bactericidal concentration (MBC) range of 4-20 µg/mL, but not the other ginger compounds 5-acetoxy-[6]-gingerol, 3,5-diacetoxy-[6]-gingerdiol and galanolactone (Park *et al.*, 2008).

Throat swabs were collected from 333 individuals with running nostrils, cough and/or catarrh and *S. aureus, S. pyogenes, S. pneumoniae* and *H. influenzae* were isolated from the specimens using standard microbiological procedures. Ginger extracts exhibited antibacterial activity against the pathogens. The Minimum Inhibitory Concentration ranged from 0.0003 µg/ml to 0.7 mcg/ml while Minimum Bactericidal Concentration ranged from 0.1.35 mcg/ml to 2.04 µg/ml (Akoachere *et al.*, 2002).

Lin *et al.* (2010) found 10-Gingerol to be much more effective as a larvicide and found greater loss of spontaneous movement than 10-shogaol and albendazole. In addition, these constituents of *Zingiber officinale* showed effects against 2, 2-diphenyl-1-picrylhydrazyl (DPPH) and peroxyl radicals. Thus these constituents of Zingiber officinale have been proved to be responsible for its larvicidal activity against A. simplex.

Ginger extract has been found to be effective against various antibiotic resistant pathogens causing respiratory tract infections. A study aimed at evaluating the antibacterial activity of ginger and bitter kola against 288 clinical isolates of respiratory tract pathogens commonly affecting individuals of all ages found that plant extracts of ginger and bitter kola to show antibacterial activity against the isolates with zones of inhibition ranging from 1 mm to 9 mm. *Staphylococcus aureus* among the isolates was most susceptible to ginger.

Some of the chemical compounds from *Zingiber officinale* collected from Tongling, China showed weak cytotoxic and anti-HIV-1 activities. And also inhibitory activities against human and mouse 11β-HSD1 (11β-hydroxysteroid dehydrogenases) with IC (50) values between 1.09 and 1.30 µM (Feng *et al.*, 2011).

Ginger on Respiratory Tract Infections

Fresh ginger has been used for cold-induced diseases, nausea, asthma, cough, colic, heart palpitation, swelling, dyspepsia, loss of appetite and rheumatism. In nineteenth century, ginger served as a popular remedy for cough and asthma when the juice of fresh ginger was mixed with a little juice of fresh garlic and honey.

Ginger extract has been found to be effective against various antibiotic resistant pathogens causing respiratory tract infections. A study aimed at evaluating the antibacterial activity of ginger and bitter kola against 288 clinical isolates of respiratory tract pathogens commonly affecting individuals of all ages found that plant extracts of ginger and bitter kola showed antibacterial activity against the isolates with zones of inhibition ranging from 1 mm to 9 mm. *S. aureus* among the isolates was most susceptible to ginger extract with an inhibition zone diameter of 6 mm, concluding that ginger extract could be a better option to some of the antibiotics commonly used for treating respiratory tract infections (Akoachere *et al.*, 2002).

Ginger in Indigestion

The use of ginger the ancient medicine for gastrointestinal problems (stimulation of digestion) has been given scientific approval. Today, medicinal ginger is used mainly for prevention of the symptoms of travel sickness (Langer *et al.*, 1998).

Dietary ginger aids in the digestion of lipids and carbohydrates by enhancing the activity of intestinal lipase and disaccharidases, sucrase and maltase (Platel and Srinivasan, 1996). Platel *et al.* (2002) found the combination of spices brought about a pronounced stimulation of bile flow and of bile acid secretion. The activities of pancreatic lipase, amylase and chymotrypsin were elevated. The higher secretion of bile especially with an elevated level of bile acids and a beneficial stimulation of pancreatic digestive enzymes, particularly of lipase could probably be the two mechanisms by which these combinations of spices aid in digestion.

Emesis

The efficacy of ginger rhizome for the prevention of nausea, dizziness, and vomiting as symptoms of motion sickness (kinetosis), as well as for postoperative vomiting and vomiting of pregnancy, has been well documented and proved beyond doubt in numerous high-quality clinical studies (Langner *et al.*, 1998; Apariman *et al.*, 2006).

In a prospective, randomised, double-blind trial Phillips *et al.* (1993) compared the effect of powdered ginger root on the incidence of postoperative nausea and vomiting with metoclopramide and placebo. The incidence of nausea and vomiting was similar in patients given metoclopramide and ginger (27 per cent and 21 per cent) and less than in those who received placebo (41 per cent). The requirement for postoperative antiemetics was lower in those patients receiving ginger. Thus, the authors confirmed that ginger is an effective and promising prophylactic antiemetic and can be especially useful for day case surgery. The effectiveness of ginger as an antiemetic agent was proved by statistically significant fewer incidences of nausea recorded in 60 women who had major gynaecological surgery when compared with placebo and metoclopramide (Bone *et al.*, 1990; Fischer-Rasmussen *et al.*, 1991). Chaiyakunapruk *et al.* (2006) conducted a systematic review and meta-analysis of selected studies and concluded that a dose at least 1 g of ginger is more effective than placebo for the prevention of postoperative nausea and vomiting and post-operative vomiting.

The ginger users demonstrated a higher rate of reduction in nausea and vomiting than the placebo users did (85 per cent versus 56 per cent ; $p < 0.01$) and also during pregnancy. Willetts *et al.* (2003) observed the nausea experience score to be significantly less for the ginger extract group relative to the placebo group after the first day of treatment and this difference was present for each treatment day. Retching was also reduced by the ginger extract although to a lesser extent. But they did not find any significant effect on vomiting.

However, conventional antiemetics are burdened with the potential of teratogenic effects during the critical embryogenic period of pregnancy. Sripramote and Lekhyananda (2003) had reported that there was no significant difference between ginger and Vitamin B6 and on the other hand, Ensiyeh and Sakineh (2009) proved that ginger is more effective than Vitamin B6 as an antiemetic.

Borrelli *et al.* (2005) on reviewing the literature found ginger to be as effective as the reference drug (vitamin B6) in relieving the severity of nausea and vomiting episodes. The observational study including follow-up periods showed the absence of significant side effects or adverse effects on pregnancy outcomes. There were no spontaneous or case reports of adverse events during ginger treatment in pregnancy. However, they feel more observational studies, with a larger sample size, are needed to confirm the encouraging preliminary data on ginger safety.

Abdel-Aziz *et al.* (2006) concluded that gingerol and shogaol exert their antiemetic effect at least partly by acting on the 5-HT(3) receptor ion-channel complex, probably by binding to a modulatory site distinct from the serotonin binding site. Pertz *et al.* (2011) observed that this antiemetic effect may be based on a weak inhibitory effect of gingerols and shogaols at M (3) and 5-HT (3) receptors. But 5-HT (4) receptors, which play a role in gastroduodenal motility, appear not to be involved in the action of these compounds.

Ginger has been found effective in multiple studies for treating nausea caused by seasickness, morning sickness and chemotherapy (Ernst and Pittler, 2000), though it was not found superior over a placebo for post-operative nausea. Bryer (2005) reviewed 4 recent well-controlled, double-blind, randomized clinical studies and observed that these studies provided convincing evidence for the effectiveness of ginger in treating nausea and vomiting of pregnancy along with a dosage update for the various forms of ginger.

Diarrhea

Ginger compounds are active against a form of diarrhea which is the leading cause of infant death in developing countries. Zingerone is likely to be the active constituent against enterotoxigenic *E. coli* heat-labile enterotoxin-induced diarrhea (Chen *et al.*, 2007). Ghayur and Gilani (2005a) indicated that ginger contains a cholinergic, spasmogenic component evident in stomach fundus preparations which provides a sound mechanistic insight for the prokinetic action of ginger. In addition, the presence of a spasmolytic constituent(s) of the calcium antagonist type may explain its use in hyperactive states of gut like colic and diarrhea.

Ginger on Diabetes

A few isolated studies about the hypoglycaemic properties of ginger in animals have reported variable results. Akhani *et al.* (2004) observed that ginger juice exhibits hypoglycaemic activity in both normal and streptozotocin (STZ)-induced diabetic rats. Al-Amin *et al.* (2006) suggested that ginger may be of great value in managing the effects of diabetic complications in human subjects as they found raw ginger to possess hypoglycaemic, hypocholesterolaemic and hypolipidaemic potential. Additionally, raw ginger was found to be effective in reversing the diabetic proteinuria observed in the diabetic rats. Gonlachanvit *et al.* (2003) reported that ginger prevented the gastric slow wave dysrhythmias evoked by acute hyperglycemia. As there was no effect on dysrhythmias elicited by a prostaglandin E (1) analog, it is possible that ginger probably blunts the production of prostaglandins rather than inhibiting their action.

Mascolo *et al.* (1989) reported a significant hypoglycaemic activity in normal rabbits at different times after a variety of administration schedules and doses. Weidner and Sigwart (2000) reported that an ethanolic extract of ginger had no effect on blood glucose levels in normal rats. The variability of the results in these studies may be due to the use of different ginger preparations. According to Zainab *et al.* (2006) ginger may be of great value in managing the effects of diabetic complications in human subjects as they observed raw ginger to possess hypoglycaemic, hypocholesterolaemic and hypolipidaemic potential. Additionally, they found raw ginger to be effective in reversing the diabetic proteinuria observed in the diabetic rats.

Hypertension and CVD

Ginger is now exciting considerable interest for its potential to treat many aspects of cardiovascular disease. Koo *et al.* (2001) and Nurtjahja-Tjendraputra *et al.* (2003) showed that gingerol compounds and their derivatives are more potent anti-platelet agents than aspirin. [8]-Paradol, a natural constituent of ginger, was found to be the most potent COX-1 inhibitor and anti platelet aggregation agent. The mechanism underlying arachidonic acid-induced platelet aggregation inhibition may be related to attenuation of COX-1/Tx synthase enzymatic activity. Dosages of 5 g or more demonstrated significant anti-platelet activity. More human trials are needed using an appropriate dosage of a standardised extract. If found positive, ginger has the potential to offer not only a cheaper natural alternative to conventional agents but one with significantly lower side effects (Nicoll and Henein, 2009).

Rats fed with ethanolic extract of ginger (200 mg/kg, p.o along with cholesterol showed a significantly lower degree of atherosclerosis as compared to gemfibrozil, a standard orally effective hypolipidaemic drug. indicating that ginger is definitely an antihyperlipidaemic agent (Bhandari *et al.*, 1998).

Herbalists prescribe ginger after dinner to hypertensive patients. Interestingly, a few studies have been carried out to explore the BP-lowering potential of ginger extract. Previously, Weidner and Sigwart (2000) have observed that the standardized ethanol extract of dried ginger was not active on the systolic BP or heart rate in conscious rats when given orally. On the contrary, the ginger pungent principles, gingerol and shogaol, have been studied for their cardiovascular effects in laboratory animals (Suekawa *et al.*, 1984; 1986a) and the precise mode of action remains to be elucidated. Ghayur and Gilani (2005b) observed that the blood pressure lowering effect is mediated through blockade of voltage-dependent calcium channels. Fresh ginger crude extract, when injected intravenously in rats under anesthesia, evoked a dose-dependent fall in arterial BP (Ghayur and Gilani, 2005b) which is in line with its traditional use in hypertension (Duke, 2002).

Ginger might delay blood clotting. Taking ginger along with medications that slower clotting might increase the chances of bruising and bleeding (Backon, 1986). However, there is conflicting evidence related to the effect of ginger constituents on human platelets suggesting that recommended doses (less than 5 g) of ginger do not affect platelet aggregation (Bordia, 1997; Verma *et al.*, 1993; Weidner and Sigwart 2000). Similarly, no significant effect was found by Jiang *et al.* (2005), on platelet aggregation and coagulation in healthy human subjects who received a daily dose of 3.6 g of ginger for 5 days. The authors also suggested that the co-administration of ginger at recommended doses is unlikely to cause problems in healthy persons because, ginger administered in herbal medicine products at recommended doses were found to affect the pharmacokinetics or pharmacodynamics of either S-warfarin or R-warfarin in humans, nor did they affect coagulation status.

In the United States, ginger is used to prevent motion and morning sickness. It is recognized as safe by the Food and Drug Administration and is sold as an unregulated dietary supplement.

Ginger on Cancer

Studies conducted in cultured cells as well as in experimental animals revealed that the anticancer properties of ginger are attributed to the presence of certain pungent phenolic compounds (Kundu *et al.*, 2009; Park *et al.*, 1998) such as vallinoids, *viz.* [6]-gingerol and [6]-paradol, as well as some other constituents like shogaols, zingerone etc. Surh *et al.* (1999) observed that the pungent vanilloids found in ginger possess potential chemopreventive activities. Wang *et al.* (2003) observed that 6-gingerol from fresh ginger induced cell death in promyelocytic leukemia HL-60 cells, caused DNA fragmentation and inhibited proto-oncogene Bcl-2 expression in HL-60 cells by mediating reactive oxygen species such as hydrogen peroxide and the superoxide anion.

A number of mechanisms that may be involved in the chemopreventive effects of ginger and its components have been reported from the laboratory studies in a wide range of experimental models (Shukla and Singh, 2007). The cancer preventive activities of ginger are supposed to be mainly due to free radical scavenging, antioxidant pathways, alteration of gene expressions, and induction of apoptosis, all of which contribute towards decrease in tumour initiation, promotion, and progression (Baliga *et al.*, 2011).

Kim *et al.* (2005) observed that [6]-gingerol inhibited -12-O-tetradecanoyl-phorbol 13-acetate TPA-induced cyclooxygenase-2 (COX-2) expression in mouse skin *in vivo* by blocking the p38 Mitogen-activated protein kinases (MAP kinase)-NF-B signaling pathway. [6]-Gingerol was found to decrease the number of lung metastasis in mice implanted with B16F10 melanoma cells (Kim *et al.*, 2005). Jeong *et al.* (2009) reported that [6]-gingerol effectively suppressed *in vivo* tumour growth in HCT-116 cancer cell-bearing nude mice. Lee *et al.* (2008) found that 6-gingerol stimulated apoptosis through upregulation of NAG-1 and G(1) cell cycle arrest through downregulation of cyclin D1. The authors opine that multiple mechanisms must be involved in 6-gingerol action, including protein degradation as well as β-catenin, protein kinase C-epsilon (PKC-epsilon), and GSK-3β pathways.

On the other hand, Rhode *et al.* (2007) reported that 6-, 8-, and 10-gingerol had no effect and 6-shogaol could significantly inhibit the growth of A-2780 ovarian cancer cells. According to Sang *et al.* (2009) shogaols 6-, 8-, and 10 had much stronger growth inhibitory effects than gingerols (6-,8-, and 10-) on H-1299 human lung cancer cells and HCT-116 human colon cancer cells, especially when comparing 6-shogaol with 6-gingerol (IC50: ~8 μM vs. ~150 μM). In addition, they found that 6-shogaol had much stronger inhibitory effects on arachidonic acid release and nitric oxide (NO) synthesis than gingerol.

Liu and Zhu (2000) have observed that alcohol extract of *Zingiber officinale* can raise significantly the thymus index, spleen index and percentage of phagocytosis. Preclinical studies have also shown that ginger possesses chemo-preventive and antineoplastic properties. It is also reported to be effective in ameliorating the side effects of γ-radiation and of doxorubicin and cisplatin; to inhibit the efflux of anticancer drugs by P-glycoprotein and to possess cheosensitizing effects in certain neoplastic cells *in vitro* and *in vivo* (Pereira *et al.*, 2007).

Nausea that develops during the period that begins 24 hours after the administration of chemotherapy is called delayed nausea, and occurs in many patients with cancer. Meals high in protein decrease the nausea of motion sickness and pregnancy, possibly by reducing gastric dysrhythmias. As ginger has antinausea properties, Levine *et al.* (2008) investigated the combined effect of high protein and ginger and confirmed that the delayed nausea of chemotherapy could be reduced and in addition, the use of antiemetic medications could also be reduced. Thus, protein with ginger holds the potential of a novel, nutritional therapy for the delayed nausea of chemotherapy.

Ginger on *H. pylori*

The combinations of propolis extract + clarithromycin and *Z. officinale* extract + clarithromycin exhibited an improved inhibition of *H. pylori* with synergistic or additive activity. Interestingly, the susceptibility to combinations was significantly independent of the microbial clarithromycin susceptibility status. Only one *H. pylori* strain showed antagonism towards the *Z. officinale* extract + clarithromycin combination. The data demonstrated that combinations of propolis extract + clarithromycin and *Z. officinale* extract + clarithromycin have the potential to help control *H. pylori*-associated gastroduodenal disease (Nostro *et al.*, 2006).

The methanol extract of ginger rhizome inhibited the growth of all 19 strains *in vitro* with a minimum inhibitory concentration range of 6.25-50 micrograms/ml. One fraction of the crude extract, containing the gingerols, was active and inhibited the growth of all HP strains with an MIC range of 0.78 to 12.5 micrograms/ml and with significant activity against the CagA+ strains. These data demonstrated that ginger root extracts containing the gingerols inhibit the growth of *H. pylori* CagA+ strains *in vitro* and this activity may contribute to its chemo preventative effects (Mahady *et al.*, 2003).

Ginger is a strong antioxidant substance and may either mitigate or prevent generation of free radicals. It is considered a safe herbal medicine with only few and insignificant adverse/side effects. More studies are required in animals and humans on the kinetics of ginger and its constituents and on the effects of their consumption over a long period of time (Ali *et al.*, 2008).

Allergies

'Benifuuki', a tea (*Camellia Sinensis* L.) cultivar in Japan, is rich in anti-allergic epigallocatechin-3-O-(3-O-methyl) gallate (EGCG3"Me). 'Benifuuki' green tea and simultaneous addition of ginger extract remarkably suppressed cytokine (TNF-alpha and MIP-1alpha) secretion from mouse bone marrow-derived mast cells after antigen stimulation and, as expected, suppressed delay-type allergy. In the most severe cedar pollen scattering period, symptoms, *i.e.*, blowing the nose and itching eyes, were significantly relieved in the 'benifuuki' intake group compared with the placebo group, and blowing the nose, itching eyes and nasal symptom score, and at the 11th and 13th weeks, stuffy nose, throat pain and the nasal symptom medication score were significantly relieved in the 'benifuuki' containing ginger extract group compared to the placebo group (Maeda-Yamamoto *et al.*, 2007).

Ginger as an Analgesic

Sepahvand *et al.* (2010) showed that ginger extract elicited a significant anti nociceptive effect. In addition, in groups that received both morphine and ginger, the observed analgesia was higher than that in groups treated with either morphine or ginger extract. According to Ozgoli *et al.* (2009a) ginger was as effective as mefenamic acid and ibuprofen in relieving pain in women with primary dysmenorrhea. Further studies regarding the effects of ginger on other symptoms associated with dysmenorrhea and efficacy and safety of various doses and treatment durations of ginger are warranted.

Compared with placebo, ginger had no clinically meaningful or statistically significant effect on perceptions of muscle pain, Rated Perceived Exertion (RPE), work rate, HR, or VO2 during exercise. Recovery of VO2 and HR after the 30-min exercise bout followed a similar time course in the ginger and placebo conditions. Ginger consumption has also been shown to improve VO_2 recovery in an equine exercise model, but these results show that this is not the case in humans (Black and Oconnor, 2008). Darvishzadeh-Mahani *et al.* (2012) demonstrated that chronic morphine-injected rats displayed tolerance to the analgesic effect of morphine as well as morphine dependence. Ginger (50 and 100 mg/kg) completely prevented the development of morphine tolerance. In addition, concomitant treatment of morphine injected rats with Ginger (100 and 150 mg/kg) attenuated almost all of the naloxone-induced withdrawal signs which include weight loss, abdominal contraction, diarrhea, teeth chattering, and jumping. Moreover, morphine-induced L-type calcium channel over-expression in spinal cord was reversed by 100 mg/kg ginger indicating that ginger extract has a potential anti-tolerant/anti-dependence property against chronic usage of morphine.

Other Benefits

Osteo and Rheumatoid Arthritis

A highly purified and standardized ginger extract had a moderate but statistically significant effect on reducing symptoms of osteo-orthritis of the knee (Altman and Marcussen, 2001). Treatment with ginger extract (250 mg of Zingiberis Rhizoma per capsule) resulted in a highly statistically significant reduction in visual analog scale (VAS) of pain on movement and of handicap in a double blind, placebo controlled, crossover study of 6 months' duration. At the end of the study, the ginger extract group showed a significant superiority over the placebo group in the relief of gonarthritis (inflammation of the knee joint) (Wigle *et al.*, 2003).

Funk *et al.* (2009) observed a very significant joint-protective effect of ginger samples and suggested that nongingerol components are bioactive and can enhance the antiarthritic effects of gingerols. According to Srivastava and Mustafa (1989; 1992), one of the mechanisms by which ginger showed its ameliorative effects rheumatism and musculoskeletal disorders could be related to inhibition of prostaglandin and leukotriene biosynthesis, *i.e.*, it works as a dual inhibitor of eicosanoid biosynthesis.

Ginger on Cognition and Memory

Ginger extract and its active component, 6-gingerol, inhibited the cholinesterase activity which in turn increased acetylcholine, a neurotransmitter that plays an important role in learning and memory (Ghayur *et al.*, 2008). A recent study demonstrated that ginger extract enhanced the memory performance induced by cerebral ischemia by decreasing infarct volume in both cortical and subcortical areas (Wattanathorn *et al.*, 2011). The cognition enhancing effects of *Zingiber officinale* might be partly associated with the modulation effect of the extract on the alteration of both the monoamine system and the cholinergic system in various brain areas, including the prefrontal cortex and hippocampus. Recent accumulating lines of evidence showed that antioxidants could also improve cognitive performance in healthy elderly subjects (Perrig *et al.*, 1997;, Monteiro *et al.*, 2005). Therefore, the association between the antioxidant effects of *Zingiber officinale* and the cognitive enhancing effects still cannot be excluded (Wattanathorn *et al.*, 2011; Asnani and Verma, 2007). Saenghong *et al.* (2012) demonstrated that ginger extract enhances both attention and cognitive processing capabilities of healthy, middle-aged women, with no side effects reported. Therefore they suggested that that *Zingiber officinale* extract is a potential brain tonic to enhance cognitive function for middle-age women.

The coadminisration of monosodium glutamate and ginger root extract caused increase in monoamine content in most areas of the brain. This is may partly be attributable to an antagonistic action of ginger root extracts on monosodium glutamate effect thus was increasing the monoamine content. The ginger extract thus has a neuroprotective role against monosodium glutamate toxicity effect. (Waggas, 2009).

Ginger-Drug interaction

Few ginger-drug interactions have been reported in the literature. A series of synthetic gingerols and phenylalkanol analogues were found to inhibit arachidonic acid induced platelet serotonin release and aggregation based on an *in vitro* study in human blood (Koo *et al.*, 2001). Furthermore, ginger extracts have been reported to inhibit platelet aggregation induced by arachidonic acid, epinephrine, ADP or collagen based on *in vitro* studies (Srivastava, 1984a; 1984b; 1986; Suekawa *et al.*, 1986). However, *in vivo*, no significant effect on coagulation or on warfarin response was found in the rat following multiple 100 mg kg-1 doses of ginger extract (Weidner and Sigwart, 2000).

Phenprocoumon is used in Europe to slow blood. An objective causality assessment revealed that the adverse drug event as a result of the phenprocoumon and ginger interaction was probable (Krüth *et al.*, 2004).

Some medications that slow blood clotting include aspirin, clopidogrel (Plavix), diclofenac (Voltaren, Cataflam, others), ibuprofen (Advil, Motrin, others), naproxen (Anaprox, Naprosyn, others), dalteparin (Fragmin), enoxaparin (Lovenox), heparin, warfarin (Coumadin), and other medications for high blood pressure and heart disease include nifedipine (Adalat, Procardia), verapamil (Calan, Isoptin, Verelan), diltiazem (Cardizem), isradipine (Dyna Circ), felodipine (Plendil), amlodipine (Norvasc), and others. Because of the anti thrombic potential of ginger, it may interact with blood-thinning drugs and must be used carefully in patients with blood clotting disorders. Thus, Krüth *et al.* (2004) based on their investigations, also recommended to refrain from ingesting ginger and other herbals like garlic in situations where bleeding may be critical.

The water extracts of ginger has detoxifying and antioxidant effects. Therefore, Shati and Elsaid (2009) recommend the use of ginger to avoid alcohol toxicity.

Conclusions

Ginger has been used safely for thousands of years in cooking, and medicinally in folk and home remedies. Advanced technology enables the validation of these traditional experiences. In Hoffman's (2007) own words, "National Center for Complementary and Alternative Medicine has evaluated the results of the available studies, rating the reports from "suggestive" (for short-term use of Ginger for safe relief from pregnancy related nausea and vomiting), to "mixed" (when used for nausea caused by motion sickness, chemotherapy, or surgery), and to "unclear" for treating rheumatoid arthritis, osteoarthritis, or joint and muscle pain). Further work would clearly incorporate ginger in the mainstream therapeutic options, integrating east and west, old with new and render ginger as a true Universal Remedy".

References

Abdel-Aziz H, Windeck T, Ploch M, Verspohl EJ (2006). Mode of action of gingerols and shogaols on 5-HT3 receptors: binding studies, cation uptake by the receptor channel and contraction of isolated guinea-pig ileum. Eur. J. Pharmacol. 530 (1-2): 136–43.

Akhani SP, Vishwakarma SL, Goyal RK (2004). Antidiabetic activity of Zingiber officinale in streptozotocin-induced type I diabetic rats. J. Pharm. Pharmacol. 56 (1): 101–105.

Akoachere JF, Ndip RN, Chenwi EB, Ndip LM, Njock TE, Anong DN (2002). Antibacterial effect of Zingiber officinale and Garcinia kola on respiratory tract pathogens. East. Afr. Med. J. 79 (11): 588–92.

Al-Amin ZM, Thomson M, Al-Qattan KK, Peltonen-Shalaby R, Ali M (2006). Antidiabetic and hypolipidaemic properties of ginger (Zingiber officinale) in streptozotocin-induced diabetic rats. Br. J. Nutr. 96 (4): 660–66.

Ali BH, Blunden G, Tanira MO, Nemmar A (2008). Some phytochemical, pharmacological and toxicological properties of ginger (Zingiber officinale Roscoe): a review of recent research. Food Chem. Toxicol. 46 (2): 409–420.

Altman RD, Marcussen KC (2001). Effects of a ginger extract on knee pain in patients with osteoarthritis. Arthritis Rheum. 44 (11): 2531–38.

Apariman S, Ratchanon S, Wiriyasirivej B (2006). Effectiveness of ginger for prevention of nausea and vomiting after gynecological laparoscopy. *J. Med. Assoc. Thai.* 89 (12): 2003–2009. Article in Chinese.

Asnani V, Verma RJ (2007). Antioxidative effect of rhizome of Zingiber officinale on paraben induced lipid peroxidation: an *in vitro* study. Acta. Poloniae Pharmaceutica. 64 (1): 35–37.

Asnani VM, Verma RJ (2009). Ameliorative effects of ginger extract on paraben-induced lipid peroxidation in the liver of mice.Acta. Pol. Pharm. 66 (3): 225–28.

Backon J (1986). Ginger: Inhibition of thromboxane synthetase and stimulation of prostacyclin: Relevance for medicine and psychiatry. Medical Hypotheses. 20. (3): 271–78.

Baliga MS, Haniadka R, Pereira MM, D'Souza JJ, Pallaty PL, Bhat HP, Popuri S (2011). Update on the chemopreventive effects of ginger and its phytochemicals. Crit. Rev. Food Sci. Nutr. 51 (6): 499–523.

Bhandari U, Kanojia R and Pillai KK (2005). Effect of ethanolic extract of Zingiber officinale on dyslipidaemia in diabetic rats. J. Ethnopharmacol. 97: 227–30.

Bhandari U, Sharma JN, Zafar R (1998). The protective action of ethanolic ginger (Zingiber officinale) extract in cholesterol fed rabbits. J. Ethnopharm. 61 (2): 167–71.

Black CD, Oconnor PJ (2008). Acute effects of dietary ginger on quadriceps muscle pain during moderate-intensity cycling exercise Dept. of Kinesiology, Georgia

College and State University, Milledgeville, GA, USA. Int. J. Sport. Nutr. Exerc. Metab. 18 (6): 653–64.

Bliddal H, Rosetzsky A, Schlichting P, Weidner MS, Andersen LA, Ibfelt HH, Christensen K, Jensen ON,Barslev J (2000). A randomized, placebo-controlled, cross-over study of ginger extracts and ibuprofen in osteoarthritis. Osteoarthritis Cartilage. 8: 9–12.

Bone ME, Wilkinson DJ, Young JR, McNeil J, Charlton S (1990). Ginger root—a new antiemetic. The effect of ginger root on postoperative nausea and vomiting after major gynaecological surgery. Anaesthesia. 45 (8): 669–71.

Bordia A, Verma SK, Srivastava KC (1997). Effect of ginger (*Zingiber officinale* Rosc.) and fenugreek (*Trigonella foenum-graecum* L.) on blood lipids, blood sugar, and platelet aggregation ion patients with coronary heart disease. Prostaglandins. Leukot. Essent. Fatty Acids. 56 (5): 379–84.

Borrelli F, Capasso R, Aviello G, Pittler MH, Izzo AA (2005). Effectiveness and safety of ginger in the treatment of pregnancy-induced nausea and vomiting. Obstet. Gynecol. 105 (4): 849–56.

Bryer E (2005). A literature review of the effectiveness of ginger in alleviating mild-to-moderate nausea and vomiting of pregnancy. J Midwifery Women's Health. 50 (1): e1–3.

Cady RK, Schreiber CP, Beach ME and Hart CC (2005). Gelstat Migrainew (sublingually administered feverfew and ginger compound) for acute treatment of migraine when administered during the mild pain phase. Med. Sci. Monit. 11: 165–69.

Chaiyakunapruk N (2006). The efficacy of ginger for the prevention of postoperative nausea and vomiting: a meta-analysis. Am. J. Obstet. Gynecol. 194 (1): 95–99.

Chen JC, Huang LJ, Wu SL, Kuo SC, Ho TY, Hsiang CY (2007). Ginger and its bioactive component inhibit enterotoxigenic *Escherichia coli* heat-labile enterotoxin-induced diarrhea in mice. J. Agric. Food Chem. 55 (21): 8390–97.

Chevallier A (1996). The Encyclopedia of Medicinal Plants. London: Dorling Kindersley Ltd.

Connell DW, McLachlan R (1978) Natural pungent compounds: examination of gingerols, shogaols, paradols and related compounds by thin-layer and gas chromatography. J Chromatogr. 67: 29–35.

Darvishzadeh-Mahani F, Esmaeili-Mahani S, Komeili G, Sheibani V, Zare L (2012).Ginger (*Zingiber officinale* Roscoe) prevents the development of morphine analgesic tolerance and physical dependence in rats. J. Ethnopharmacol. 141 (3): 901–907.

Dugasani S, Pichika MR, Nadarajah VD, Balijepalli MK, Tandra S, Korlakunta JN (2010). Comparative antioxidant and anti-inflammatory effects of [6]-gingerol, [8]-gingerol, [10]-gingerol and [6]-shogaol. J. Ethnopharmacol. 127 (2): 515–20.

Duke JA (2002). Handbook of Medicinal Herbs. Boca Raton: CRC Press. 327–29.

Ensiyeh J, Sakineh MA (2009). Comparing ginger and vitamin B6 for the treatment of nausea and vomiting in pregnancy: a randomised controlled trial. Midwifery. 25 (6): 649–53.

Ernst E, Pittler MH (2000). Efficacy of ginger for nausea and vomiting: a systematic review of randomized clinical trials. B. J. Anaesth. 84 (3): 367–71.

Feng T, Su J, Ding ZH, Zheng YT, Li Y, Leng Y, Liu JK (2011). Chemical constituents and their bioactivities of "Tongling White Ginger" (*Zingiber officinale*). J. Agric. Food Chem. 59 (21): 11690–95.

Fischer-Rasmussen W, Kjaer SK, Dahl C, Asping U (1991). Ginger treatment of hyperemesis gravidarum. Eur. J. Obstet. Gynecol. Reprod. Biol. 38 (1): 19–24.

Fuhrman B, Rosenblat M, Hayek T, Coleman R, Aviram M (2000). Ginger extract consumption reduces plasma cholesterol, inhibits LDL oxidation, and attenuates development of atherosclerosis in atherosclerotic, apolipoprotein E-deficient mice. J. Nutr. 130 (5): 1124 -.31.

Funk JL, Frye JB, Oyarzo JN, Timmermann BN (2009). Comparative Effects of Two Gingerol-Containing *Zingiber officinale* Extracts on Experimental Rheumatoid Arthritis (perpendicular). J. Nat. Prod. 2009 Feb. 13.

Ghayur MN, Gilani AH (2005a). Pharmacological basis for the medicinal use of ginger in gastrointestinal disorders. Dig. Dis. Sci. 50 (10): 1889–97.

Ghayur MN, Gilani, AH (2005b). Ginger Lowers Blood Pressure Through Blockade of Voltage-Dependent Calcium Channels. J. Cardiovasc. Pharmacol. 45 (1): 74–80.

Ghasemzadeh A, Jaafar HZ, Rahmat A (2010). Antioxidant activities, total phenolics and flavonoids content in two varieties of Malaysia young ginger (*Zingiber officinale* Roscoe). Molecules.15 (6): 4324–33.

Gonlachanvit S, Chen YH, Hasler WL, Sun WM, Owyang C. (2003) Ginger reduces hyperglycemia-evoked gastric dysrhythmias in healthy humans: possible role of endogenous prostaglandins. J Pharmacol Exp Ther. 307 (3): 1098–1103.

Hoffman T (2007). Ginger: an ancient remedy and modern miracle drug. Hawaii Med J. 6 (12): 326–27.

Huang QR, Iwamoto M, Aoki S, Tanaka N, Tajima K, Yamahara J, Takaishi Y, Yoshida M, Tomimatsu T, Tamai Y (1991). Anti-5-hydroxytryptamine3 effect of galanolactone, diterpenoid isolated from ginger. Chem Pharm Bull (Tokyo). 39 (2): 397–99.

Jeong CH, Bode AM, Pugliese A, Cho YY, Kim HG, Shim JH, Jeon YJ, Li H, Jiang H, Dong Z (2009). [6]-Gingerol suppresses colon cancer growth by targeting leukotriene A4 hydrolase. Cancer Res. 69: 5584–91.

Jiang X, Williams KM, Liauw WS, Ammit AJ, Roufogalis BD, Duke CC, Day RO and McLachlan AJ (2005). Effect of ginkgo and ginger on the pharmacokinetics and pharmacodynamics of warfarin in healthy subjects. British Journal of Clinical Pharmacology. 59 (4): 4425–32.

Kim EC, Min JK, Kim TY, Lee SJ, Yang HO, Han S, Kim YM, Kwon YG (2005a). [6]-Gingerol, a pungent ingredient of ginger, inhibits angiogenesis *in vitro* and *in vivo*. Biochem. Biophys. Res. Commun. 335: 300–308.

Kim SO, Kundu JK, Shin YK, Park JH, Cho MH, Kim TY, Surh YJ (2005b). [6]-Gingerol inhibits COX-2 expression by blocking the activation of p38 MAP kinase and NF-kappaB in phorbol ester-stimulated mouse skin. Oncogene. 24: 2558–67.

Kiuchi F, Iwakami S, Shibuya M, Hanaoka F, Sankawa U (1992). Inhibition of prostaglandin and leukotriene biosynthesis by gingerols and diaryl heptanoids. Chem. Pharm. Bull. (Tokyo) 40: 387–91.

Koo KL, Ammit AJ, Tran VH, Duke CC, Roufogalis BD (2001). Gingerols and related analogues inhibit arachidonic acid-induced human platelet serotonin release and aggregation. Thromb. Res. 103: 387–97.

Krüth P, Brosi E, Fux R, Mörike K, Gleiter CH (2004). Ginger-associated overanticoagulation by phenprocoumon. Ann. Pharmacother. 38 (2): 257–60.

Kundu JK, Na HK, Surh YJ (2009). Ginger-derived phenolic substances with cancer preventive and therapeutic potential. Forum Nutr. 61: 182–92.

Langner E, Greifenberg S, Gruenwald J (1998). Ginger: history and use. Adv. Ther. 15: 25–44.

Lee SH, Cekanova M, Baek SJ (2008). Multiple mechanisms are involved in 6-gingerol-induced cell growth arrest and apoptosis in human colourectal cancer cells. *Mol. Carcinog.* 47 (3): 197–208.

Levine ME, Gillis MG, Koch SY, Voss AC, Stern RM, Koch KL (2008). Protein and ginger for the treatment of chemotherapy-induced delayed nausea. J. Altern. Complement. Med. 14 (5): 545–51.

Lin RJ, Chen CY, Lee JD, Lu CM, Chung LY, Yen CM (2010). Larvicidal constituents of *Zingiber officinale* (ginger) against Anisakis simplex. Planta. Med. 76 (16): 1852–58.

Liu H, Zhu Y (2002). Effect of alcohol extract of *Zingiber officinale* rose on immunologic function of mice with tumour]. Wei. Sheng. Yan. Jiu. 31 (3): 208–209.

Lu P, Lai BS, Liang P, Chen ZT, Shun SQ (2003). [Antioxidation activity and protective effection of ginger oil on DNA damage *in vitro*] Zhongguo Zhong Yao Za Zhi. 28 (9): 873–75. [Article in Chinese].

Maeda-Yamamoto M, Ema K, Shibuichi I (2007). *In vitro and in vivo* anti-allergic effects of 'benifuuki' green tea containing O-methylated catechin and ginger extract enhancement. Cytotechnology. 55 (2-3): 135–42.

Mahady GB, Pendland SL, Yun GS, Lu ZZ, Stoia A (2003). Ginger (*Zingiber officinale* Roscoe) and the gingerols inhibit the growth of Cag A+ strains of Helicobacter pylori. Anti-cancer Res. 23 (5A): 3699–702.

Mascolo N, Jain R, Jain SC, Capasso F (1989). Ethnopharmacologic investigation of ginger (*Zingiber officinale*) Journal of Ethnopharmacology. 27 (1-2): 129–40.

Monteiro SC, Matté C, Bavaresco CS, Netto CA, Wyse ATS (2005). Vitamins E and C pretreatment prevents ovariectomy-induced memory deficits in water maze. Neurobiology of Learning and Memory 84 (3): 192–99.

Mustafa T, Srivastava KC (1990). Ginger (*Zingiber officinale*) in migraine headache. J Ethnopharmacol 29: 267–73.

Nicoll R, Henein MY (2009). Ginger (*Zingiber officinale* Roscoe): a hot remedy for cardiovascular disease? Int. J. Cardiol. 131 (3): 408–409.

Nostro A, Cellini L, Di Bartolomeo S, Cannatelli MA, Di Campli E, Procopio F, Grande R, Marzio L, Alonzo V (2006). Effects of combining extracts (from propolis or *Zingiber officinale*) with clarithromycin on Helicobacter pylori.Phytother. Res. 20 (3): 187–90.

Nurtjahja-Tjendraputra E, Ammit AJ, Roufogalis BD, Tran VH, Duke CC (2003). Effective anti-platelet and COX-1 enzyme inhibitors from pungent constituents of ginger. *Thromb. Res.* 111 (4-5): 259–65.

Ozgoli G, Goli M, Moattar F (2009a). Comparison of Effects of Ginger, Mefenamic Acid, and Ibuprofen on Pain in Women with Primary Dysmenorrhea. J Altern Complement Med. 2009 Feb. 13.

Ozgoli G, Goli M, Simbar M (2009b). Effects of Ginger Capsules on Pregnancy, Nausea, and vomiting J Altern Complement Med. 2009 Feb 28. Epub ahead of print.

Park M, Bae J, Lee DS (2008). Antibacterial activity of [10]-gingerol and [12]-gingerol isolated from ginger rhizome against periodontal bacteria. Phytother. Res. 22 (11): 1446–49.

Park KK, Chun KS, Lee JM, Lee SS, Surh YJ (1998). Inhibitory effects of [6]-gingerol, a major pungent principle of ginger, on phorbol ester-induced inflammation, epidermal ornithine decarboxylase activity and skin tumour promotion in ICR mice. Cancer Lett. 129: 139–44.

Penna SC, Medeiros MV, Aimbire FS, Faria-Neto HC, Sertie JA, Lopes-Martins RA (2003). Anti-inflammatory effect of the hydralcoholic extract of *Zingiber officinale* rhizomes on rat paw and skin edema. Phytomed. 10: 381–85.

Pereira MM, Haniadka R, Chacko PP, Palatty PL, Baliga MS (2011). *Zingiber officinale* Roscoe (ginger) as an adjuvant in cancer treatment: a review. J. B.U.O.N. 16 (3): 414–24.

Perrig WJ, Perrig P, Stahelin HB (1997). The relation between antioxidants and memory performance in the old and very old. Journal of the American Geriatrics Society. 45 (6): 718–24.

Pertz HH, Lehmann J, Roth-Ehrang R, Elz S (2011). Effects of ginger constituents on the gastrointestinal tract: role of cholinergic M3 and serotonergic 5-HT3 and 5-HT4 receptors. Planta. Med. 77 (10): 973–78.

Phillips S, Ruggier R, Hutchinson SE (1993). *Zingiber officinale* (ginger)—an antiemetic for day case surgery. Anaesthesia. 48 (8): 715–17.

Platel K, Rao A, Saraswathi G, Srinivasan K (2002). Digestive stimulant action of three Indian spice mixes in experimental rats. Digestive stimulant action of three Indian spice mixes in experimental rats. Nahrung. 46 (6): 394–98.

Platel K, Srinivasan K (1996). Influence of dietary spices or their active principles on digestive enzymes of small intestinal mucosa in rats. Int. J. Food Sci. Nutr. 47 (1): 55–59.

Portnoi G, Chng LA, Karimi-Tabesh L Koren G, Tan MP, Einarson A (2003). Prospective comparative study of the safety and effectiveness of ginger for the treatment of nausea and vomiting in pregnancy. *Am. J. Obstet. Gynecol.* 189 (5): 1374–77.

Qidwai W, Alim SR, Dhanani RH, Jehangir S, Nasrullah A, Raza A (2003). Use of folk remedies among patients in Karachi Pakistan. J. Ayub. Med. Coll. Abbottabad. 15 (2): 31–33.

Ranganathan R, Vijayalakshmi R, Parameswari P (2012). Ethno medicinal plants and their utilization by villagers in Jawadhu hills of Thiruvannamalai district of Tamilnadu, India. I.J.P.R.D. 4 (04): 174–83.

Rhode J, Fogoros S, Zick S, Wahl H, Griffith KA, Huang J, Liu JR (2007). Ginger inhibits cell growth and modulates angiogenic factors in ovarian cancer cells. BMC Complement. Altern. Med. 7: 44.

Saenghong N, Wattanathorn J, Muchimapura S, Tongun T, Piyavhatkul N, Banchonglikitkul C, Kajsongkram T (2012). *Zingiber officinale* Improves Cognitive Function of the Middle-Aged Healthy Women. Evid. Based Complement. Alternat. Med. 2012: 383062.

Sang S, Hong J, Wu Hou, Liu J, Yang CS, Pan Min-Hsiung, Badmaev V, Ho Chi Tang (2009). Increased Growth Inhibitory Effects on Human Cancer Cells and Anti-Inflammatory Potency of Shogaols from *Zingiber officinale* Relative to Gingerols. Agric. Food Chem. 57 (22): 10645–50.

Sankaranarayanan S, Bama P, Ramachandran J, Kalaichelvan P.T, DeccaramanM, Vijayalakshimi M, Dhamotharan R, Dananjeyan B and Sathya Bama S (2010). Ethnobotanical study of medicinal plants used by traditional users in Villupuram district of Tamil Nadu, India. Journal of Medicinal Plants Research. 4 (12): 1089 -1101.

Semwal P, Pardha P, Kala CP, Sajwan BS (2010). Medicinal plants used by local Vaidyas in Ukhimath block, Uttarkhand, Indian Journal of Traditional Knowledge. 9 (3): 480–85.

Sepahvand R, Esmaeili-Mahani S, Arzi A, Rasoulian B, Abbasnejad M (2010). Ginger (*Zingiber officinale* Roscoe) elicits antinociceptive properties and potentiates morphine-induced analgesia in the rat radiant heat tail-flick test. J. Med. Food. 13 (6): 1397–401.

Shati AA, Elsaid FG (2009). Effects of water extracts of thyme (*Thymus vulgaris*) and ginger (*Zingiber officinale* Roscoe) on alcohol abuse. Food Chem. Toxicol. 47 (8): 1945–49.

Shukla Y, Singh M (2007). Cancer preventive properties of ginger: a brief review. Food Chem. Toxicol. 45 (5): 683–90.

Sripramote M, Lekhyananda N (2003). A randomized comparison of ginger and vitamin B6 in the treatment of nausea and vomiting of pregnancy. J. Med. Assoc. Thai. 86 (9): 846–53.

Srivastava KC (1986). Isolation and effects of some ginger components of platelet aggregation and eicosanoid biosynthesis. Prostaglandins Leukot. Med. 25: 187–98.

Srivastava KC (1984a). Aqueous extracts of onion, garlic and ginger inhibit platelet aggregation and alter arachidonic acid metabolism. Biomed. Biochim. Acta. 43: S335–46.

Srivastava KC. (1984b). Effects of aqueous extracts of onion, garlic and ginger on platelet aggregation and metabolism of arachidonic acid in the blood vascular system: *in vitro* study. Prostaglandins. Leukot. Med.13: 227–35.

Srivastava KC, Mustafa T (1989). Ginger (*Zingiber officinale*) and rheumatic disorders. Medical Hypotheses. 29: 25–28.

Srivastava KC, Mustafa T (1992). Ginger (*Zingiber officinale*) in rheumatism and musculoskeletal disorders. Medical Hypotheses. 39: 343–48.

Suekawa M, Aburada M, Hosoya E (1986a). Pharmacological studies on ginger. II.Pressor action of [6]-shogaol in anaesthetized rats, or hindquarters, tail and mesenteric beds of rats. J. Pharmacobiodyn. 9: 842–52.

Suekawa M, Ishige A, Yuasa K, Sudo K, Aburada M, Hosoya E (1984). Pharmacological studies on ginger.I. Pharmacological actions of pungent constituents, [6]-gingerol and [6]-shogaol. J. Pharmacobiodyn. 7: 836–48.

Suekawa M, Yuasa K, Isono M, Sone H, Ikeya Y, Sakakibara I, Aburada M, Hosoya E (1986b). Pharmacological studies on ginger. IV. Effect of (6)-shogaol on the arachidonic cascade. Nippon. Yakurigaku. Zasshi. 88: 263–269.

Surh YJ, Lee F, Lee MJ (1998). Chemo protective properties of some pungent ingredients present in red pepper and ginger. Mut. Res. 402: 259-267.

Surh YJ, Park KK, Chun KS, Lee LJ, Lee E, Lee SS (1999). Anti-tumour-promoting activities of selected pungent phenolic substances present in ginger. J. Environ. Pathol. Toxicol. Oncol. 18 (2): 131–39.

Thomson M, Al Qattan KK, Al Sawan SM, Alnaqeeb MA, Khan I, Ali M (2002). The use of ginger (*Zingiber officinale* Rosc.) as a potential anti-inflammatory and antithrombotic agent. Prostaglandins. Leukot. Essent. Fatty Acids. 67 (6): 475–78.

Ursell A (2000). The Complete Guide to Healing Foods, pp. 112–14. London: Dorling Kindersley Ltd.

USDA (2012). National Nutrient Database for Standard Reference, Release 25.

Varma KR, Jain TC, Bhattacharyya SC (1962). Structure and stereochemistry of zingiberol and juniper camphor. Tetrahedron. 18: 979.

Verma RJ, Asnani V (2007). Ginger extract ameliorates paraben induced biochemical changes in liver and kidney of mice. Acta. Pol. Pharm. 64 (3): 217–20.

Verma SK, Singh J, Khamesra R, Bordia A (1993). Effect of ginger on platelet aggregation in man. Indian J. Med. Res. 98: 240–42.

Vutyavanich T, Kraisarin T, Ruangsri R (2001). Ginger for nausea and vomiting in pregnancy: randomized, double-masked, placebo-controlled trial. Obstet. Gynecol. 97 (4): 577–82.

Waggas AM (2009). Neuroprotective evaluation of extract of ginger (*Zingiber officinale*) root in monosodium glutamate-induced toxicity in different brain areas male albino rats. Pakistan Journal of Biological Sciences. 12 (3): 201–12.

Wang CC, Chen LG, Lee LT, Yang LL (2003). Effects of 6-gingerol, an antioxidant from ginger, on inducing apoptosis in human leukemic HL-60 cells. *In vivo*. 17 (6): 641–45.

Wattanathorn J, Jittiwat J, Tongun T, Muchimapura S, Ingkaninan K (2011). *Zingiber officinale* mitigates brain damage and improves memory impairment in focal cerebral ischemic rat. Evidence-Based Complementary and Alternative Medicine. 2011: 8 pages. Article. ID 429505.

Weidner MS, Sigwart K (2000). The safety of a ginger extract in the rat. J. Ethnopharmacol. 73: 513–20.

Wigler I, Grotto I, Caspi D, Yaron M (2003). The effects of Zintona EC (a ginger extract) on symptomatic gonarthritis. Osteoarthritis Cartilage. 11 (11): 783–89.

Willetts KE, Ekangaki A, Eden JA (2003). Effect of a ginger extract on pregnancy-induced nausea: a randomised controlled trial. Aust. N. Z. J. Obstet. Gynaecol. 43 (2): 139–44.

Zainab M. Al-Amin, Martha Thomson, Khaled K. Al-Qattan, Riitta Peltonen-Shalaby and Muslim Ali (2006). Antidiabetic and hypolipidaemic properties of ginger (*Zingiber officinale*) in streptozotocin-induced diabetic rats. British Journal of Nutrition. 96: 660–66.

Zhou HL, Deng YM, Xie QM (2006). The modulatory effects of the volatile oil of ginger on the cellular immune response *in vitro* and *in vivo* in mice. J. Ethnopharmacol. 105 (1-2): 301–305.

Chapter 10

Mustard Seeds

(*Brassica nigra/B. juncea/B. alba*)

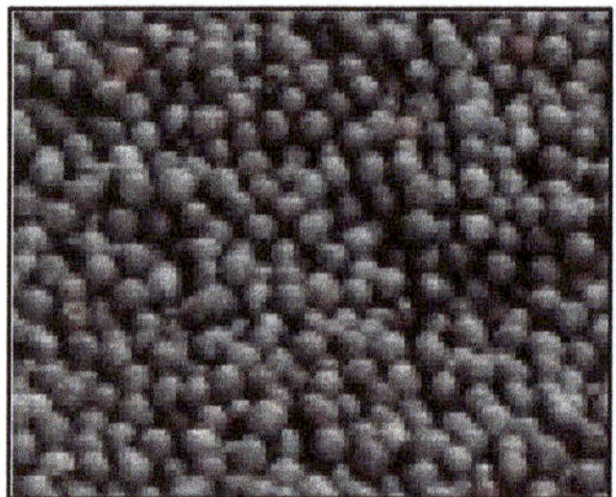

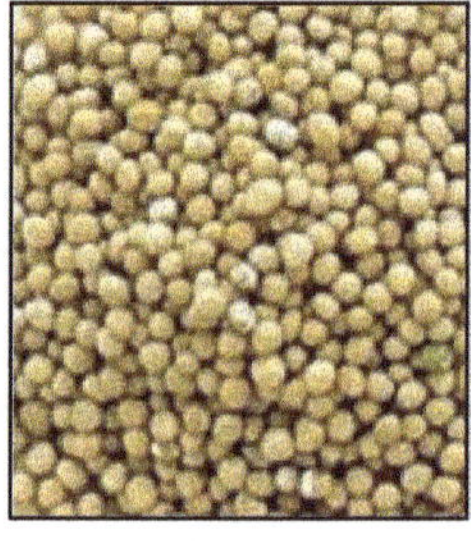

Mustard is a spice with a strong flavour. Ancient Sanskrit writings dating back approximately 5,000 years, mentioned mustard seeds. The origin of mustard seeds can be traced to different areas of Mediterranean region, Europe and Asia. Major producers of mustard seeds include Canada, Hungary, Great Britain, India, Pakistan and the United States. The plant reaches about 4-5 feet in height and bears golden yellow coloured flowers. Its tiny, round seeds measuring about 1 mm in diameter are encased inside a fruit pod in a similar fashion like green pea pod. Though mustard is a winter crop, it also grows well in temperate regions.

Varieties of Mustard seeds

Mustard (commonly called as Rai) comes from the cabbage family and can be found in forty different varieties. There are 3 main varieties of mustard seeds grown worldwide-the white (yellow), black and brown. Brown and black mustard seeds return higher yields than their yellow counterparts.

- ☆ **White Mustard (*Brassica alba*):** is a round hard seed, beige or straw yellow coloured, slightly larger than the other two varieties. The seeds are mildly pungent. Whole white mustard seed is used in pickling and in spice mixtures for cooking meats and seafood. Powdered mustard is usually made from white mustard seed and is often called mustard flour.

- ☆ **Black Mustard (*Brassica nigra*):** Commonly seen in South Asia, it is a round hard seed, varying in colour from dark brown to black, smaller and much more pungent than the other two varieties. Black mustard seed has the strongest flavour than the brown one.
- ☆ **Brown Mustard (*Brassica juncea*):** is native to sub-Himalayan plains of Northern India. Is similar in size to the black variety and varies in colour from light to dark brown. It is more pungent than the white, less than the black. The brown seed is pounded with other spices in the preparation of curry powders and pastes.

Nutritive Value of Mustard Seeds

Mustard seeds are a very good source of ω-3 fatty acids, dietary fiber, protein, as well as niacin, calcium, iron, manganese, magnesium, phosphorus, selenium and zinc.

Nutritional Value per 100 g

Nutrient	*Amount*	*Nutrient*	*Amount*
Energy (kcal)	508	Carbohydrates (g)	28.09
Dietary fiber (g)	12.2	Fat (g)	36.24
Fatty acids, total saturated	1.989	Protein (g)	26.08
Fatty acids, total monounsaturated	22.578	Fatty acids, total polyunsaturated	20.088
Calcium (mg)	266	Iron (mg)	9.21
Magnesium (mg)	370	Phosphorus (mg)	528
Potassium (mg)	738	Sodium (mg)	13
Zinc (mg)	6.08	Riboflavin (Vit.B2) mg)	0.261
Thiamine (Vit. B1) (mg)	0.805	Vitamin B6 (mg)	0.397
Niacin (Vit. B3) (mg)	4.733	Vitamin C (mg)	7.1
Folate (Vit. B9) (μg)	162	Vitamin K (mcg)	5.4
Vitamin A (IU)	31		

USDA (2012).

Phytochemical Constituents of Mustard Seeds

Seven phenolic acids; *viz.*, tannic, gallic, caffeic, cinnamic, chlorogenic, ferulic and vanillic acids were identified in black mustard. Maximum amount of tannic and gallic acids were observed in black mustard among many other spices (Singh *et al.*, 2004). Phenolics are known to significantly contribute to the flavour, taste, and medicinal properties of food. Nair *et al.* (1998) found flavonoid (a sum of quercetin, kaempferol, luteolin and pelargonidin) content to be high (> 100 mg/100 gm) in mustard seeds. The nutritional value of meal from low glucosinolate mustard was equal or superior to that of canola meal samples derived from *B. napus* and *B. rapa* cultivars (Newkirk *et al.*, 1997).

Therapeutic Uses of Mustard seeds

Early physicians, including Hippocrates used mustard seed in their medicines. And even today, in many parts of the world, mustard seeds are used medicinally. It was imported to US through Spanish missionaries and seen as a cure-all. Mustard is an age-old purgative. This can be necessary in cases of accidental poisoning.

These small seeds are rich in glucosinolates and also contain the enzyme myrosinase which can break glucosinolates into isothiocyanates. The selenium concentrated in these seeds adds on to the antioxidant benefits and helps in prevention of cancer, cardiovascular diseases, obesity etc. selenium is also known for its anti-inflammatory benefits that can reduce the incidence of asthma, rheumatoid arthritis, cataracts etc (Iyer *et al.*, 2009).

Antioxidant

Concentration of malondialdehyde showed a significant decrease, while hydroperoxides and conjugated dienes were significantly increased in liver and heart of both the experimental groups. SOD and catalase activity was found to be increased in liver and heart of both the spices administered groups. Glutathione levels in liver, heart and kidney were lowered in rats administered these spices. Glutathione reductase, glutathione peroxidase and glutathione S-transferase activity showed a sharp increase in the experimental groups compared to the controls (Khan *et al.*, 1996 b). Again the same authors (Khan *et al.*, 1997) have reported that this spice alters the peroxidation (thiobarbituric acid reactive substances) level to a beneficial extent. Histological studies also focused on modulation of hepatic functions to near normal level.

Antimicrobial

The use of mustard flour at levels of >5-10 per cent to eliminate *E. coli* O157:H7 from fresh ground beef was found to be a good method (Nadarajah *et al.*, 2005). Compounds generated by the enzymatic hydrolysis of glucosinolates naturally present in mustard powder are potently bactericidal against *Escherichia coli* O157:H7. Because *E. coli* O157:H7 can survive the dry fermented sausage manufacturing process, 2, 4, and 6 per cent (wt/wt) hot mustard powder or 6 per cent (wt/wt) cold mustard powder were added to dry sausage batter inoculated with *E. coli* O157:H7 at about 7 log CFU/g to evaluate the antimicrobial effectiveness of the powders. The 6 per cent dehydrated mustard powder treatment provided the most rapid reductions of *E. coli* O157:H7 (yielding <0.20 log CFU/g after 24 days) by an unknown mechanism and was the least detrimental ($P < 0.05$) to sausage texture (Graumann and Holley (2008).

Bacteria can degrade naturally occurring glucosinolates in mustard and form isothiocyanates with antimicrobial activity. Sausage batches containing hot mustard powder (active myrosinase), cold mustard powder (inactivated myrosinase), autoclaved mustard powder (inactivated myrosinase) and no mustard flour (control) were examined. Interestingly, both pairs of starter cultures yielded similar results. Elimination of *E. coli* O157:H7 (>5 log cfu/g) occurred after 31 days in the presence of hot flour and in 38 days when the cold flour was added but not in the control. The autoclaved powder caused more rapid bactericidal action against *E. coli* O157:H7, yielding a >5 log cfu/g reduction in 18 days. This may have been a result of the formation and/or release of antimicrobial substances by the autoclave treatment. Autoclaved mustard powder could potentially solve an important challenge facing the meat industry as it strives to manufacture safe dry fermented sausages (Luciano *et al.*, 2011). According to Nilson and Holley (2012) on hams treated with mustard powder for 21 days, *E. coli* O157:H7 was reduced by 3 log cfu /g compared to only a 1 log cfu/g reduction in the control. By 45 days, mustard powder caused a reduction of >5 log cfu/g *E. coli* O157:H7, whereas it took 80 d for numbers in control hams to be similarly reduced.

An antimicrobial edible film was developed from defatted mustard meal (*Sinapis alba*) (DMM), a byproduct from the bio-fuel industry, without incorporating external antimicrobials. The film-coating retarded the growth of *L. monocytogenes* in smoked salmon at 5, 10, and 15°C and the antimicrobial effect during storage was more noticeable when the coating was applied before inoculation than when it was applied after inoculation. The tensile strength, percentage elongation, solubility in water cxu, and water vapor permeability of the anti microbial film were 2.44 ± 0.19 MPa, 6.40 ± 1.13 per cent, 3.19 ± 0.90 per cent, and 3.18 ± 0.63 gmm/kPa hm(2), respectively. The antimicrobial DMM films have been shown to be suitable to be applied to foods as wraps or coatings to control the growth of *L. monocytogenes* (Lee *et al.*, 2012).

An antifungal protein (18.9 kDa) designated juncin was isolated from seeds of the Japanese takana (*Brassica juncea* var. *integrifolia*) by Ye and Ng (2009). The protein exhibited antifungal activity towards the phytopathogens *Fusarium oxysporum*, *Helminthosporium maydis*, and *Mycosphaerella arachidicola* with IC-50 values of 13.5, 27, and 10 μM, respectively. It inhibited the proliferation of hepatoma (HepG2) and breast cancer (MCF7) cells with IC-50 values of 5.6 and 6.4 μM, respecitvely, and the activity of HIV-1 reverse transcriptase with an IC(50) of 4.5 μM. Its N-terminal sequence differed from those of antifungal proteins of *Brassica campestris* and *Brassica alboglabra*.

Diabetes

Magnesium in mustard seeds helps to regulate blood glucose and help diabetics prevent sharp spikes in their blood glucose levels. A significant hypoglycaemic action of *Brassica juncea* has been reported by Khan *et al.* (1995b) in experimental animals. The metabolic alterations induced by *Brassica juncea* included an increase in the concentration of hepatic glycogen and glycogenesis due to increased activity of glycogen synthetase, and reduction in glycogenolysis and gluconeogenesis due to decreased activity of glycogen phosphorylase and gluconeogenic enzymes. Streptozotocin (STZ; 100mg/kg) induced diabetic rats were fed 10 per cent of *Brassica juncea* (BJ) seed powder for 60 days. Although feeding of the BJ showed a trend towards improvement in most of the parameters, (serum glucose levels, body weight, urine volume, serum creatinine, and urinary albumin), results were not statistically different from the Diabetic control except in serum creatinine values in BJ-fed rats on day 70. Thus, Grover *et al.* (2003) suggested that mustard plants can be best utilized by promoting them as preferable food adjuvants for diabetic patients.

Feeding of a fructose diet containing 10 per cent *Brassica juncea* seeds powder for 30 days significantly decreased fasting serum glucose, insulin and cholesterol levels but did not normalize them. Thus, Yadav *et al.* (2004) confirmed that BJ can play a role in the management of pre-diabetic state of insulin resistance and should be promoted for use in patients prone to diabetes. Considering all the available information from animal experimentation as well as clinical trials where spices, their extracts or their active principles were examined for treatment of diabetes, *Brassica nigra* seeds have been reported to be hypoglycaemic (Srinivasan, 2005).

Administration of 200 mg/kg body weight of aqueous extract of the seeds of *B. nigra*, to diabetic animals daily once for one month brought down fasting serum glucose (FSG) levels while in the untreated group FSG remained at a higher value. In the treated animals the increase in glycosylated hemoglobin (HbA1c) and serum lipids was much less when compared with the levels in untreated diabetic controls (Anand *et al.*, 2007).

Cancer:

Isothiocyanates are valuable for their anti-cancer and anti-inflammatory benefits (Bhattacharya, *et al.*, 2010). Allyl isothiocyanate (AITC), which occurs in many common cruciferous vegetables, was recently shown to be selectively delivered to bladder cancer tissues through urinary excretion and inhibit bladder cancer development in rats. Mustard seeds are source of sinigrin, which is a precursor of AITC and thus anticarcinogenic.

The chemo-preventive potential of mustard seed oil was investigated by Hashim *et al.* (1998) on 7,12-dimethylbenz[a]anthracene-induced transplacental and translactational carcinogenesis in Swiss albino mice at two doses (0.05 and 0.10 ml per day from days 13 to 19 of gestation). The percentage of tumour incidence in the F1 progeny was reduced significantly at both dose levels from 65 per cent in the control group to 29 per cent and 16 per cent, respectively, in the experimental groups. When lactating mothers were given the mustard oil at dose levels of 0.05 and 0.10 ml per day for the first 15 days of lactation, the multiple site tumour incidences was brought down significantly from a control value of 70 per cent to 32 per cent and 18 per cent, in lower and higher dose groups respectively. Mustard oil exerts its effect by inducing the enzymes of drug detoxification and also by changing the profile of the antioxidant defense system.

The chemo-preventive property of an ethanolic extract of the seeds of *Brassica compestris* var sarason (mustard seed) on DMBA (7,12 dimethylbenz(a)anthracene induced skin papillomagenesis in male Swiss albino mice was reported by Qiblawi and Kumar (1999). A significant reduction in the values of tumour incidence, tumour burden and the cumulative number of papillomas was observed in mice treated orally with the seed extract continuously at peri and post initiational stages of papillomagenesis compared with the control groups.

Dietary ,ustard seeds suppresses 1,2-dimethylhydrazine (DMH)-induced immuno-imbalance as well as colon carcinogenesis in rats (Zhu *et al.*, 2012). Morphological and histological studies revealed that the mean number of neoplasms in the colon and intestine were significantly low in the mustard fed group (Khan *et al.*, 1996 a).

Uhl *et al.* (2003) observed that mustard juice is highly protective against benzo(a)pyrene ([B(a)P] induced DNA damage in human derived cells and that induction of detoxifying enzymes may account for its chemo-protective properties. Furthermore, their findings showed that the effects of crude juice cannot be explained by its allyl isothiocyanate contents.

More recently, Yuan *et al.* (2011) found a suspension of extracted mustard seed to suppress oxidized-LDL-induced macrophage respiratory burst *in vitro*, to prevent growth, and to induce apoptotic death of SW480 cells (a human colon cancer cell line), while no such effects were found for normal 3T3 cells. A diet enriched with mustard seeds decreased plasma levels of the lipid peroxidation product malonaldehyde in mice exposed to the colon cancer-inducer azoxymethane (AOM). Such a diet also dose-dependently enhanced the activity of several antioxidant enzymes, such as superoxide dismutase (SOD), catalase, and GSH-peroxidase and, moreover, reduced AOM-mediated formation of colon adenomas by about 50 per cent.

Hypolipidemia

Mustard seeds are valuable sources of essential fatty acids. The feasibility of synthesizing the cardioprotective ω-3 fatty acids in mustard has been explored and confirmed by Wu *et al.* (2005) through genetic modification. Using a series of transformations with increasing numbers of transgenes, they demonstrated the incremental production of PUFA achieving Arachidonic acid (AA) levels of up to 25 per cent and Eicosapentaenoic acid (EPA) levels of up to 15 per cent of total seed fatty acids. Both fatty acids were almost exclusively found in triacylglycerols, with AA located preferentially at sn-2 and sn-3 positions and EPA distributed almost equally at all three positions. Moreover, the reconstituted Docosahexaenoic acid biosynthetic pathway in plant seeds, demonstrated the practical feasibility of large-scale production of this important ω-3 fatty acids from mustard seeds.

Five per cent yellow or white mustard mucilage significantly ($p<0.05$) decreased the number of total (approximately 21 per cent inhibition) and large (approximately 50 per cent inhibition) aberrant crypt foci (ACF) in the colons of Sprague-Dawley rats compared to that in untreated controls. In addition, 5 per cent mustard mucilage supplemented diet significantly lowered ($p<0.05$) the number of total (approximately 63 per cent inhibition) and large (approximately 60 per cent inhibition) colonic ACF in Zucker obese rats compared to untreated obese rats, and had no effect on fasting plasma cholesterol or triglyceride levels (Eskin *et al.*, 2007).

Upon feeding with mustard, bile acids and neutral sterols showed a sharp increase thus decreasing the cholesterol and phospholipid levels in experimental animals as compared to the control (Khan *et al.*, 1996a).

Other Uses

Magnesium helps to relax muscles, thus reducing restless leg syndrome and inducing better sleep in insomniacs.The severity and incidence of migraine headaches have also been proven to reduce due to magnesium consumption. Magnesium also reduces asthma and lowers blood pressure. Being a rich source of magnesium, the use of mustard seeds in these disorders could be exploited. The effects of mustard are currently being studied for menopausal women and on migraine attacks.

Omega-3-fatty acids, tryptophan and niacin present in mustard seeds are all mood enhancers and can help to prevent stress. Omega-3- fatty acids in mustard seeds can also help to keep the skin soft and supple. Mustard seed oil generates warmth and is great for skin health. The high iron and calcium present in mustard seeds, make it a 'must-have' spice during pregnancy and lactation (USDA, 2012).

Safety Issues

Khan *et al.* (1995 a) observed that mustard fed to rats at doses equal to normal human intake did not cause any adverse effect on food efficiency ratio, red blood cell count, white blood cells, total count, differential counts or on the levels of blood constituents, like serum electrolytes, blood urea, hemoglobin, total serum protein, albumin-globulin ratio, fibrin level, glycosylated hemoglobin and the activity of glutamic oxaloacetic transaminase, glutamic pyruvic transaminase and alkaline phosphatase in serum. No histopathological changes were observed in the liver of rats administered curry leaf and mustard thus confirming the safety of its consumption.

Conclusion

The tiny mustard seeds seem to be mighty in therapeutic properties. But the available research studies are few and there is a need for further confirmative as well as explorative studies.

References

Anand P, Murali KY, Tandon V, Chandra R, Murthy PS (2007). Preliminary studies on antihyperglycemic effect of aqueous extract of *Brassica nigra* (L.) Koch in streptozotocin induced diabetic rats. Indian J. Exp. Biol. 45 (8): 696–701.

Bhattacharya A, Li Y, Wade KL, Paonessa JD, Fahey JW, Zhang Y (2010). Allyl isothiocyanate-rich mustard seed powder inhibits bladder cancer growth and muscle invasion. Carcinogenesis. 31 (12): 2105–2110.

Eskin NA, Raju J, Bird RP (2007). Novel mucilage fraction of *Sinapis alba* L. (mustard) reduces azoxymethane-induced colonic aberrant crypt foci formation in F344 and Zucker obese rats. Phytomedicine. 14 (7-8): 479–85.

Graumann GH, Holley RA (2008). Inhibition of *Escherichia coli* O157:H7 in ripening dry fermented sausage by ground yellow mustard. J. Food Prot. 71 (3): 486–93.

Grover JK, Yadav SP, Vats V (2003). Effect of feeding Murraya koeingii and *Brassica juncea* diet on [correction] kidney functions and glucose levels in streptozotocin diabetic mice. J. Ethnopharmacol. 85 (1): 1–5.

Hashim S, Banerjee S, Madhubala R, Rao AR (1998). Chemoprevention of DMBA-induced transplacental and translactational carcinogenesis in mice by oil from mustard seeds (Brassica spp.). Cancer Lett. 134 (2): 217–26.

Iyer A, Panchal, S, Poudyal H, Brown L (2009). Potential Health Benefits of Indian Spices in the Symptoms of the Metabolic Syndrome: A Review, Indian Journal of Biochemistry and Biophysics. 46: 467–81.

Khan BA, Abraham A, Leelamma S (1995 a). Haematological and histological studies after curry leaf (*Murraya koenigii*) and mustard (*Brassica juncea*) feeding in rats. Indian J. Med. Res. 102: 184–86.

Khan BA, Abraham A, Leelamma S (1995 b). Hypoglycaemic action of *Murraya koenigii* (curry leaf) and *Brassica juncea* (mustard): mechanism of action. Indian J. Biochem. Biophys. 32 (2): 106–108.

Khan BA, Abraham A, Leelamma S (1996 a). *Murraya koenigii* and *Brassica juncea*—alterations on lipid profile in 1-2 dimethyl hydrazine induced colon carcinogenesis. Invest. New Drugs. 14 (4): 365–69.

Khan BA, Abraham A, Leelamma S (1996 b). Role of *Murraya koenigii* (curry leaf) and *Brassica juncea* (Mustard) in lipid peroxidation. Indian J. Physiol. Pharmacol. 40 (2): 155–58.

Khan BA, Abraham A, Leelamma S (1997). Antioxidant effects of curry leaf, *Murraya koenigii* and mustard seeds, *Brassica juncea* in rats fed with high fat diet. Indian J. Exp. Biol. 35 (2): 148–50.

Lee HB, Noh BS, Min SC (2012). *Listeria monocytogenes* inhibition by defatted mustard meal-based edible films. Int. J. Food Microbiol. 153 (1-2): 99–105.

Luciano FB, Belland J, Holley RA (2011). Microbial and chemical origins of the bactericidal activity of thermally treated yellow mustard powder toward *Escherichia coli* O157:H7 during dry sausage ripening. Int. J. Food Microbiol. 145 (1): 69–76.

Nadarajah D, Han JH, Holley RA (2005). Use of mustard flour to inactivate *Escherichia coli* O157:H7 in ground beef under nitrogen flushed packaging. Int. J. Food Microbiol. 99 (3): 257–67.

Nair S, Nagar R, Gupta R (1998). Antioxidant phenolics and flavonoids in common Indian foods. J. Assoc. Physicians India. 46 (8): 708–710.

Newkirk RW, Classen HL, Tyler RT (1997). Nutritional evaluation of low glucosinolate mustard meals (*Brassica juncea*) in broiler diets. Poult. Sci. 76 (9): 1272–77.

Nilson AM, Holley RA (2012). Use of deodorized yellow mustard powder to control *Escherichia coli* O157:H7 in dry cured Westphalian ham. Food Microbiol. 30 (2): 400–407.

Qiblawi S, Kumar A (1999). Chemopreventive action by an extract from *Brassica compestris* (var Sarason) on 7,12-dimethylbenz(a)anthracene induced skin papillomagenesis in mice. Phytother. Res. 13 (3): 261–63.

Singh UP, Singh DP, Maurya S, Maheshwari R, Singh M, Dubey RS, Singh RB (2004). Investigation on the phenolics of some spices having pharmacotherapeutic properties. J. Herb. Pharmacother. 4 (4): 27–42.

Srinivasan K (2005). Plant foods in the management of diabetes mellitus: spices as beneficial antidiabetic food adjuncts. Int. J. Food Sci. Nutr. 56 (6): 399–414.

Uhl M, Laky B, Lhoste E, Kassie F, Kundi M, Knasmüller S (2003). Effects of mustard sprouts and allylisothiocyanate on benzo(a)pyrene-induced DNA damage in human-derived cells: a model study with the single cell gel electrophoresis/Hep G2 assay. Teratog. Carcinog. Mutagen. Suppl. 1: 273–82.

USDA (2012). National Nutrient Database for Standard Reference, Release 25.

Wu G, Truksa M, Datla N, Vrinten P, Bauer J, Zank T, Cirpus P, Heinz E, Qiu X (2005). Stepwise engineering to produce high yields of very long-chain polyunsaturated fatty acids in plants. Nat. Biotechnol. 23 (8): 1013–17.

Yadav SP, Vats V, Ammini AC, Grover JK (2004). *Brassica juncea* (Rai) significantly prevented the development of insulin resistance in rats fed fructose-enriched diet. J. Ethnopharmacol. 93 (1): 113–16.

Ye X, Ng TB (2009). Isolation and characterization of juncin, an antifungal protein from seeds of Japanese Takana (*Brassica juncea* var. *integrifolia*). J. Agric. Food Chem. 57 (10): 4366–71.

Yuan H, Zhu M, Guo W, Jin L, Chen W, Brunk UT, Zhao M (2011). Mustard seeds (*Sinapis alba* Linn) attenuate azoxymethane-induced colon carcinogenesis. Redox. Rep. 16 (1): 38–44.

Zhu M, Yuan H, Guo W, Li X, Jin L, Brunk UT, Han J, Zhao M, Lu Y (2012). Dietary mustard seeds (*Sinapis alba* Linn) suppress 1,2-dimethylhydrazine-induced immuno-imbalance and colonic carcinogenesis in rats. Nutr. Cancer. 64 (3): 464–72.

Chapter 11

Sesame Seeds

(*Sesamum indicum* Linn.)

Sesame seed is a traditional healthy oil seed commonly used in Asian countries. Sesame seeds are believed to represent a symbol of immortality. These seeds were thought to have first originated in India and were mentioned in early Hindu legends. From India, sesame seeds were introduced throughout the Middle East, Africa and Asia. Currently, the largest commercial producers of sesame seeds include India, China and Mexico. The commonly known varieties of sesame seeds are–white, yellow, black and red.

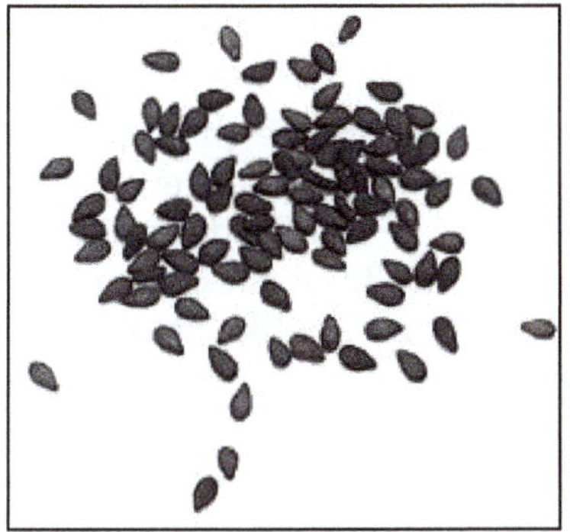

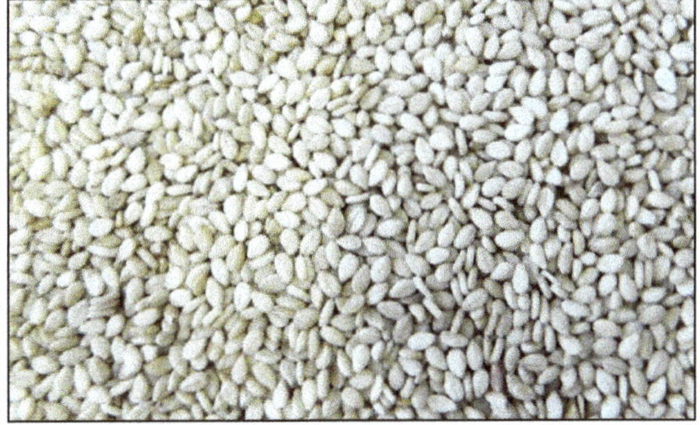

Nutritive Value

Sesame seeds contain up to 55 per cent oil and 20 per cent protein. Sesame proteins are limited in lysine but rich in tryptophan and methionine. Sesame oil is rich in linoleic and oleic acid (Martinchik, 2011). In addition, sesame seed oil contains

40 mg of vitamin E per 100 g of oil with the predominance of gamma-tocopherol over the other isomers of vitamin E (Martinchik, 2011). Sesame seeds are also a very good source of copper, magnesium and calcium.

Nutritive Value of Sesame Seeds

Nutrient	*Amount*	*Nutrient*	*Amount*
Energy (kcals)	515	Calcium (mg)	300
Carbohydrate (g)	17.1	Iron (mg)	56.7
Protein (g)	23.9	Phosphorus (mg)	224
Fat (g)	39	Thiamine (mg)	0.07
Riboflavin (mg)	0.97	Niacin (mg)	8.4

Gopalan *et al.*, 2010.

Phytochemical Composition

Sesame seeds contain large amounts of the plant lignans sesamin, sesamolin, and sesaminol glucosides (Fukuda *et al.*, 1985; Katsuzaki *et al.*, 1994), sesamolinol, pin (Namiki, 1995, Jiao *et al.*, 1998 and Shyu *et al.*, 2002). The three sesaminol glucosides isolated from sesame seed are sesaminol-22 -O-β-D-glucopyranosyl (1→2)-β-D-glucopyranoside; sesaminol-22-O-β-D-lucopyranoside and sesaminol-22-O-β-D-glucopyranosyl(1→2)-[β-D-glucopyranosyl(1→6)]-β-D-lucopyranoside (Katsuzaki *et al.*, 1994). Sesame seed contains large quantities of lignan glucosides (Ryu *et al.*, 1998), including pinoresinol glucosides (Katsuzaki *et al.*, 1992) and sesaminol glucosides (Katsuzaki *et al.*, 1994).

Eleven odor-active thiols, namely, 2-methyl-1-propene-1-thiol, (Z)-3-methyl-1-butene-1-thiol, (E)-3-methyl-1-butene-1-thiol, (Z)-2-methyl-1-butene-1-thiol, (E)-2-methyl-1-butene-1-thiol, 2-methyl-3-furanthiol, 3-mercapto-2-pentanone, 2-mercapto-3-pentanone, 4-mercapto-3-hexanone, 3-mercapto-3-methylbutyl formate, and 2-methyl-3-thiophenethiol, were recently identified in an extract of white sesame seeds and quantified using stable isotope dilution analyses (Tamura *et al.*, 2011).

Screening for aroma-active compounds in an aroma distillate obtained from freshly pan-roasted sesame seeds by aroma extract dilution analysis revealed 32 odorants in the FD factor range of 2-2048, of which 29 could be identified. The highest FD factors were found for the coffee-like smelling 2-furfurylthiol, the caramel-like smelling 4-hydroxy-2,5-dimethyl-3(2H)-furanone, the coffee-like smelling 2-thenylthiol (thiophen-2-yl-methylthiol), and the clove-like smelling 2-methoxy-4-vinylphenol. In addition, 9 odor-active thiols with sulfurous, meaty, and/or catty, black-currant-like odors were identified for the first time in roasted sesame seeds. Among them, 2-methyl-1-propene-1-thiol, (Z)-3-methyl-1-butene-1-thiol, (E)-3-methyl-1-butene-1-thiol, (Z)-2-methyl-1-butene-1-thiol, (E)-2-methyl-1-butene-1-thiol, and 4-mercapto-3-hexanone are new ones (Tamura *et al.*, 2010).

Processing of Sesame Seeds

Defatting of sesame seeds increases the crude protein, ash, crude fiber, carbohydrate and mineral contents. Defatted flour showed comparatively better foam capacity and stability, water absorption and emulsion capacities but diminished bulk density and oil absorption capacity (Egbekun and Ehieze, 1997). The emulsifying and foaming properties of enzymatically hydrolysed and dehydrated sesame seeds are improved in water (85 per cent) and at different pH levels (91-95 per cent), by the action of neutrase 0.5L and alcalase 0.6L (Saad *et al.*, 1984).

Processing of sesame seeds also influences the chemical constituents. Infra Red roasting of sesame seeds at 200° C for 30 min increased the efficiency of conversion of sesamolin to sesamol (51 per cent to 82 per cent) compared to conventional heating. The gamma-tocopherol content decreased by 17 per cent and 25 per cent in oils treated at 200°C and 220°C for 30 min, respectively. There were no significant differences in the tocopherol content and oxidative stability of the oil. Methionine and cysteine content of the flours remained unchanged due to roasting. The functional properties of defatted flours obtained from either Infra Red roasted or conventionally roasted sesame seeds remained the same. Sesame oil is stable to oxidation compared to other vegetable oils. This stability can be attributed to the presence of tocopherols and the formation of sesamol, the thermal degradation product of sesamolin (Kumar *et al.*, 2009a).

Sprouting was found to influence the composition of sesame seeds. Badifu and Akpagher (1996) boiled the seeds and allowed to sprout under ambient condition (30 ±2°C) with an objective to reduce or eliminate the bitter taste associated with them. There was slight increase (about 10 per cent) in protein content of sprouted seeds. The flour from the boiled seeds had the highest foam stability.

Germinated sesame seeds with noticeable reduction in fat content (23 per cent), were found to increase in linolenic acid, phosphorus and sodium from 0.38 per cent (w/w), 445 mg/100 g, and 7.6 mg/100 g before germination to 0.81 per cent (w/w), 472 mg/100 g, and 8.4 mg/100 g after germination, respectively. After germination the seeds contained considerable amount of calcium (462 mg/100 g), higher than that of soybean. Germinated seeds are excellent source of sesamol (475 mg/100 g) and alpha-tocopherol (32 mg/100 g) (Hahm *et al.*, 2009).

Therapeutic Value of Sesame Seeds/Oil

Sesame seeds or their products exhibit several health benefits in cardiovascular diseases, cancer, diabetes and other clinical conditions. They promotes growth due to the good quality protein. The health benefits of various fractions of sesame seed extract were found to be different *e.g.* decorticated sesame seed extracted with isopropanol showed body weight gain and food efficiency ratio in rats similar to those of the control groups fed diets prepared with casein and soybean meal. Hexane extract of decorticated sesame seed showed significant hypolidaemic antioxidant effect (Sen and Bhattacharya, 2001).

Sesame seed contains furfuran lignans with beneficial physiological activities, mainly sesamin, sesamolin, and sesaminol glucosides. Reported activities of sesame seed lignans include modulation of fatty acid metabolism, inhibition of cholesterol absorption and biosynthesis, antioxidant and vitamin E-sparing effects, hypotensive effects, improvement of liver functions in connection with alcohol metabolism, and antiaging effects (Kamal-Eldin *et al.*, 2011). Other functions include: specific inhibition of Δ5-desaturation of (n-6) fatty acids (Shimizu *et al.*, 1991; Chatrattanakunchai *et al.*, 2000) that interrupt the formation of proinflammatory 2-series prostaglandins (Utsunomiya *et al.*, 2000), hypocholesterolemic activity via inhibition of cholesterol synthesis and absorption (Hirata *et al.*, 1996). antihypertensive effect (Kita *et al.*, 1995; Nakano *et al.*, 2002; Matsumura *et al.*, 1995; 1998), protection against ethanol and carbon tetrachloride-induced liver damage (Akimoto *et al.*, 1993), synergy with α-tocopherol (Yamashita *et al.*, 2000), improvement of the bioavailability of γ-tocopherol (Kamal-Eldin *et al.*, 2000), and a suppressive effect against induced carcinogenesis in animals (Hirose *et al.*, 1992, Adlercreutz and Mazur, 1997; Thompson *et al.*, 2003 and Namiki 2007).

Antioxidant

The high antioxidative properties of sesame seed appear to be related to lignans, such as sesamin and sesamolin, sesamol (Budowski 1950), sesamolinol, pinoresinol, p1 (Fukuda *et al.*, 1985) and sesaminol (Kang *et al.*, 1998a; 1998b). Sesaminol, a phenolic lignan-type compound contained in sesame seed, is one of the most potent free radical scavengers (Kang *et al.*, 1998a). Pinoresinol glucosides and sesaminol glucosides possesses a lower peroxyl radical scavenging activity than the corresponding aglycone. However, these glucosides act as precursors of lipid-soluble antioxidative lignans (Osawa *et al.*, 1995).

Far-infrared irradiation of sesame seeds increased the antioxidant activity of methanolic extracts of defatted sesame seeds (Lee *et al.*, 2005). Ikeda *et al.* (2002) found sesame seed and its lignans to elevate gamma-tocopherol concentration due to the inhibition of cytochrome P(450) 3A-dependent metabolism of gamma-tocopherol. Further, Ikeda *et al.* (2003) observed that the dietary sesamin and sesaminol lowered the TBARS concentrations and decreased the red blood hemolysis. The dietary sesamin and sesaminol elevated the alpha-tocopherol concentrations in the plasma, liver, and brain of the rats fed a diet with or without DHA suggesting that dietary sesame lignans decrease lipid peroxidation as a result of elevating the alpha-tocopherol concentration in rats fed DHA. Later they (Ikeda *et al.*, 2007) reported that dietary sesame seed and its lignan stimulate ascorbic acid synthesis as a result of the induction of UDP-glucuronosyltransferase 1A and the 2B-mediated metabolism of sesame lignan in rats. The data also suggested that dietary sesame seed enhances antioxidative activity in the tissues by elevating the levels of two antioxidative vitamins, vitamin C and E.

The vitamin E concentrations were also significantly higher in supercritical carbondioxde extracts than in n-hexane extracts, and its concentrations in extracts corresponded with the antioxidant activity of extracts (Hu *et al.*, 2004). Yamashita *et al.* (2007) explains that sesame lignan sesaminol increases tocopherol concentrations in animals by suppressing the conversion of gamma-tocopherol to gamma-7-

hydroxymatairesinol. 7-hydroxymatairesinol, a structurally different plant lignan, does not have such properties.

Sesame seed oil (SO) is one of the most important edible oils in India as well as in Asian countries and has potent antioxidant properties. It showed a protective effect against the cypermethrin induced brain toxicity and this could be associated mainly with the attenuation of the oxidative stress and the preservation in antioxidant enzymes (Hussien *et al.*, 2011). The antioxidant in sesame oil, effectively protected DNA damage from lipid peroxidation induced by 4-Nitroquinoline-1-oxide (Arumugam and Ramesh, 2011). Hsu and Liu (2004a) showed that sesame oil could be used as a potent antioxidant to reduce oxidative stress after the onset of sepsis in rats. Sesame oil might attenuate hepatic lipid peroxidation by inhibiting superoxide anion and nitric oxide, at least partially, in experimental septic rats (Hsu *et al.*, 2008). The administration of sesame oil provided significant protection against cypermethrin-induced oxidative stress, biochemical changes, histopathological damage and genomic DNA fragmentation (Abdou *et al.*, 2012).

Sesame oil potently reduces renal oxidative stress by inhibiting the generation of ROS and nitric oxide in septic rats (Hsu *et al.*, 2002; 2004; 2005; Hsu and Liu, 2004a; Hsu and Liu, 2004b)). Further, sesame oil protects against gentamicin-induced renal injury by inhibiting renal oxidative stress in rats (Hsu *et al.*, 2010). Sesame oil significantly prevented the rise of serum blood urea nitrogen and creatinine levels. Furthermore, there was a parallel inhibition of the rise in levels of expression of renal lipid peroxidation, myeloperoxidase, hydroxyl radicals, superoxide anion, nitrite/nitrate, and inducible nitric oxide synthase in rats with gentamicin-plus-iodinated contrast-induced acute kidney injury. Hsu *et al.* (2011) concluded from these observations that sesame oil may attenuate aminoglycoside-plus-iodinated contrast-induced acute kidney injury by inhibiting renal oxidative stress in rats.

Anti-inflammatory

Sesame seed oil and Quil A (a saponin that emulsifies fat and potentiates immune response) when present in the diet exerted cumulative effects resulting in a decrease in the levels of dienoic eicosanoids with a reduction in IL-1beta and a concomitant elevation in the levels of IL-10 that were associated with a marked increase in survival of mice (Chavali *et al.*, 1997). Chavali *et al.* (2001) found sesamin, sesamol and other lignans in sesame seed oil to be responsible for an increase in survival after cecal ligation and puncture and also for an increase in the interleukin -10 levels in response to a nonlethal dose of endotoxin in mice. Sesame oil given 6 h after cecal ligation and puncture significantly increased survival rate (Hsu and Liu, 2004a).

Antimicrobial

A novel antimicrobial protein (SiAMP2) belonging to the 2S albumin family was isolated from Sesamum indicum kernels specifically inhibited *Klebsiella* sp. Specific regions in the molecule surface where cationic and hydrophobic residues are exposed and conserved, were proposed as being involved in antimicrobial activity (Maria-Neto *et al.*, 2011).

Sesame Seeds on CVD

Significant decreases in plasma total cholesterol, triglyceride, and VLDL and LDL cholesterol concentrations were observed by Sen and Bhattacharya (2001) in the rats fed diet containing decorticated sesame seed extracted with isopropanol than that of casein. Biswas *et al.* (2010) observed that sesame protein isolate decreases cholesterol concentration in plasma, increases HDL-cholesterol, and also decreases plasma and erythrocyte membrane lipid peroxidation with or without cholesterol fed diet in rats.

Sesamin, the major fat-soluble lignan in sesame seed, influences lipid metabolism (Hirata *et al.*, 1996; Ogawa *et al.*, 1995; Hirose *et al.*, 1991), and has an antihypertensive (Matsumura *et al.*, 1995; Kita *et al.*, 1995; Matsumura *et al.*, 1998; Nakano *et al.*, 2002), and anticancer activities (Hirose *et al.*, 1992; Miyahara *et al.*, 2000). Nakai *et al.* (2003) reported that sesamin undergoes cleavage of methylenedioxyphenyls to catechol or methoxy catechol structures in rat liver. A clear hypocholesterolemic effect elicited by sesamin (alone or in combination with vitamin E) was reported in studies conducted in rats (Sugano *et al.*, 1990; Hirose *et al.*, 1991; Nakabayashi *et al.*, 1995; Kamal-Eldin *et al.*, 2000).

Incubation with sesame oil increases the mycelial dihomo-gamma-linolenic acid content of an arachidonic acid-producing fungus, *Mortierella alpina*, but decreases its arachidonic acid content. Sesamin and related lignan compounds present in sesame seeds or its oil are specific inhibitors of delta 5 desaturase in polyunsaturated fatty acid biosynthesis in both microorganisms and animals (Shimizu *et al.*, 1991).

The mechanism of hypolipidaemic effect of sesame seeds was explained by Ashakumary *et al.* (1999) who observed dietary sesamin to decrease the hepatic activity and mRNA abundance of fatty acid synthase and pyruvate kinase, the lipogenic enzymes. However, this lignan increased the activity and gene expression of malic enzyme, another lipogenic enzyme. An alteration in hepatic fatty acid metabolism may therefore account for the serum lipid-lowering effect of sesamin in the rat.

Hirata *et al.* (1996) found a significant effect of dietary sesamin in the reduction of total cholesterol and LDL-cholesterol when it was administered together with vitamin E to human subjects. Nakabayashi *et al.* (1995) reported that the observed effect might be due to the synergism between these two dietary components. Sesame rich in lignans more profoundly affects hepatic fatty acid oxidation and serum triacylglycerol levels. Therefore, Sirato-Yasumoto (2001) confirmed that consumption of sesame rich in lignans results in alteration of lipid metabolism in a potentially beneficial manner. Peñalvo *et al.* (2006) analysed various studies on hypochleserolemic effect and concluded that sesamin does not seem to affect cholesterol biosynthesis or absorption in mice. Stanol ester alone or together with sesamin significantly attenuated the elevation of the cholesterol levels (Peñalvo *et al.*, 2006).

The hypercholesteraemic effect of sesame seed in rats appeared to be due to its fiber, sterol, polyphenol and flavonoid content that enhanced the fecal cholesterol excretion and bile acid production as well as increased the antioxidant enzyme activities (Visavadiya and Narasimhacharya, 2008). In contrast, feeding Defatted sesame flour to rabbits did not protect cholesterol-induced hypercholesterolemia as observed by Kang *et al.* (1999) but expected to have decreased susceptibility to oxidative stress in rabbits fed cholesterol, perhaps due to the antioxidative activity of sesaminol.

Diets containing 0.2 and 0.4 per cent sesamin lowered the amount of mature sterol regulatory element binding protein-1 to less than one-fifth of that in the animals fed a sesamin-free diet through a suppression of gene expression as well as the proteolysis of the membrane-bound precursor form of this transcriptional factor to generate the mature form (Ide *et al.*, 2001). The lignans modified the mRNA levels of not only many enzymes involved in hepatic fatty acid oxidation, but also proteins involved in the transportation of fatty acids into hepatocytes and their organelles, and in the regulation of hepatic concentrations of carnitine, CoA and malonyl-CoA. It is apparent that sesame lignans stimulate hepatic fatty acid oxidation by affecting the gene expression of various proteins regulating hepatic fatty acid metabolism (Ide *et al.*, 2009).

Alipoor *et al.* (2012) found that sesame seed supplementation decreased serum Total Cholesterol, LDL-cholesterol and lipid peroxidation, and increased antioxidant status in hyperlipidemic patients. Sesame lignans inhibited extreme changes of the n-6/n-3 ratio by reducing hepatic PUFA content. The reduction of hepatic PUFA content may have occurred because of the effects of sesame lignans on PUFA degradation (oxidation) and esterification (Umeda-Sawada *et al.*, 1998). Recently, the Scientific Advisory of the American Heart Association reported that high monounsaturated fatty acids diets tend to lower triglyceride concentrations (Kang *et al.*, 1998 b). Thus substitution of sesame oil with other edible oils lowers plasma triglyceride concentrations.

Sesame oil lowered blood pressure, decreased lipid peroxidation, and increased antioxidant status in hypertensive patients (Sankar *et al.*, 2006b). The lignans present in sesame oil are thought to be responsible for many of its unique chemical and physiological properties, including its antioxidant and antihypertensive properties. Sankar *et al.* (2006b) found significant elevations of vitamin C, vitamin E, ß-carotene, and reduced glutathione and the levels decreased once sesame oil substitution was stopped. Elevation of vitamin C upon the substitution of sesame oil could be due to its decreased utilization or due to increase in the levels of GSH, because vitamin C and GSH are synergistic antioxidants (Gerster, 1991). Epidemiological reports showed that carotenoids may play a preventive role in cardiovascular disease. Plasma levels of ß-carotene rose significantly upon the substitution of sesame oil, which could be due to the sparing action of vitamin E and sesame lignans. A significant reduction was noted in body weight and body mass index (BMI) upon sesame oil substitution. Significant reduction in TBARS and maintenance of the same even after withdrawal of sesame oil was also noted (Sankar *et al.*, 2006b). On the other hand, though supplementation with 25 g/d of sesame significantly increased the exposure to mammalian lignans there was no improvement in markers of cardiovascular disease risk in overweight or obese men and women (Wu *et al.*, 2009).

Wichitsranoi *et al.* (2011) observed that 4-week administration of black sesame meal significantly decreased systolic blood pressure and increased vitamin E level.

The change in Systolic pressure tended to be positively related to the change in plasma lipid, malondialdehyde, while the change in Diastolic pressure was negatively related to the change in vitamin E. Thus, Wichitsranoi *et al.* (2011) demonstrated the possible antihypertensive effects of black sesame meal on improving antioxidant status and decreasing oxidant stress; and thus, implying a beneficial effect of black sesame meal on prevention of CVD. Sesame oil reduced lipid peroxidation and hydroxyl radical, but failed to affect superoxide anion. Superoxide dismutase and catalase were increased, but glutathione was not affected, and the levels of nitrite were reduced. Further, sesame oil-treatment attenuated hepatic disorder in lipopolysaccharide-treated rats. Thus, parenteral sesame oil can be used to attenuate oxidative stress and relieve hepatic disorder after lipopolysaccharide intoxication in rats (Hsu *et al.*, 2004).

Sesame on Diabetes

Sesame oil consumption was shown to influence beneficially the blood glucose, glycosylated hemoglobin, lipid peroxidation, and antioxidant levels in diabetic rats (Ramesh *et al.*, 2005). Similarly, reduction of body weight, body mass index, girth of waist, girth of hip, and waist–hip ratio, plasma glucose, HbA1c, TC, LDL-C, and TG, TBARS level were observed by Sankar *et al.* (2006a). They also found the activities of enzymic and the levels of nonenzymic antioxidants increased upon substitution with sesame oil. Plasma sodium levels were reduced, while potassium levels were elevated indicating that substitution with sesame oil as the sole edible oil has an additive effect in further lowering BP and plasma glucose in hypertensive diabetics medicated with atenolol (beta-blocker) and glibenclamide (sulfonylurea). Sankar *et al.* (2011) also demonstrated the synergistic effect of sesame seed oil with glibenclamide that provides a safe and effective option for the drug combination useful in clinical practice for improvement of hyperglycemia.

Sesame lignans at 0.5 per cent level and alpha-tocopherol significantly ameliorated the alteration in lipid profile and the adverse free radical generative influence of DM induced by alloxan (Dhar *et al.*, 2007).

Sesame for Neuronal Health

Sesamin and sesamolin are the major lignans from sesame seeds. Previous reports (Hou *et al.*, 2003a; Lahaie-Collins *et al.*, 2008) showed that sesamin can protect against hypoxia-, H_2O_2-or 1-methyl-4-phenyl-pyridine (MPP^+)-induced brain and PC12 cells injuries. Sesamin also inhibits nitric oxide (NO) and cytokine production in lipopolysaccharide (LPS)-and oxidative-stressed BV-2 microglia (Hou *et al.*, 2003b; Hou *et al.*, 2004; Jeng *et al.*, 2005).

Sesame also benefits patients of neurodegenerative diseases. Hamada *et al.* (2009) reported that Sesamin may promote neuronal differentiation by tapping into the mitogen-activated protein kinase signaling pathway downstream from the TrkA receptor (a high-affinity nerve growth factor receptor) in pheochromocytoma cells. Sesamol could be used as an effective agent in the management of 3-nitropropionic acid-induced cognitive impairment and oxidative damage in striatal, cortex and hippocampal regions as well as neurotoxicity in animals (Kumar *et al.*, 2009b; 2010).

Hamada *et al.* (2011) also found that sesamin has the potential to reduce oxidative stress and ameliorate oxidative stress-related neurodegenerative diseases. Pre-treatment with Sesamol (SML) (5, 10, and 20 mg/kg) significantly improved body weight, locomotor activity, motor coordination, and attenuated oxidative damage in different regions of rat brain. Besides these, SML treatment also significantly improved mitochondrial enzymes in all regions of the brain as compared with the respective control (3-NP) group, thus suggesting that SML could be used as effective agents in the management of Huntington's disease.

Sesamin could protect Kainic acid (KA) induced status epilepticus (a period of continuous seizure activity/brain injury) through anti-inflammatory and partially antioxidative mechanisms. Hsieh *et al.* (2011) observed significant increase in plasma α-tocopherol level by 50 per cent and 55.8 per cent from rats without and with KA treatment, respectively with sesamin extract (30 mg/kg). It also decreased malondialdehyde (MDA) from 145 per cent to 117 per cent and preserved superoxide dismutase from 55 per cent of the vehicle control mice to 81 per cent of sesamin-treated mice, respectively to the normal levels ($p=0.013$). The treatment significantly decreased the mortality from 22 per cent to 0 per cent in rats as compared with the non-treated group. The decreased mortality in the sesamin-treated animals could also be confirmed by the sesamin effect *in vitro* that showed a decreased LDH release and Caspase-3 activation and increased cell viability in KA-stimulated PC12 cells (Hsieh *et al.*, 2011). The protective effect of sesamin and sesamolin on hypoxic neuronal and PC12 cells might be related to suppression of ROS generation and mitogen-activated protein kinases activation (Hou *et al.*, 2003b; 2004)) in hypoxia-stressed BV-2 cells.

A study with defatted sesame seeds extract (30, 100 and 300 mg/kg) given twice orally at 0 h and 2 h after onset of ischemia shows the reduction of brain infarct volume dose-dependently and improves sensory-motor function (Jamarkattel-Pandit *et al.*, 2010). The role of COX-2 mRNA and protein in KA-induced brain injury has been reported by Hashimoto *et al.* (1998); Sandhya *et al.* (1998) and Sanz *et al.* (1997). Sesame seed oil may inhibit activation of NADPH oxidase dependent inflammatory mechanism due to 6-Hydroxydopamine induced neurotoxicity in mice thus indicating its neuroprotective effect (Ahmad *et al.*, 2012).

Post-menopausal Syndrome

Sesame seed is a rich source of mammalian lignan precursors and sesamin is one of them. Enterolactone (EL) and enterodiol (ED) are produced from dietary plant lignans such as secoisolariciresinol diglucoside (SDG) or its aglycone secoisolariciresinol (SECO), matairesinol, 7-hydroxymatairesinol, lariciresinol, and pinoresinol (Heinonen *et al.*, 2001; Saarinen *et al.*, 2000) by the action of intestinal microbiota of humans and animals (Axelson *et al.*, 1982; Borriello *et al.*, 1985; Setchell *et al.*, 1980; Wang *et al.*, 2000; 2001). The transformation of furofuran lignans to mammalian lignans by intestinal microbiota involves the hydrolysis of glucoside, demethylenation of a methylene group, oxidation of dibenzylbutanediol to dibenzylbutyrolactone, and reductive cleavage of furofuran rings. Jan *et al.* (2009) demonstrated that STG could be converted to enterolactone and enterodiol by rat intestinal microflora. From intermediate metabolites of sesamin identified in rat urine by GC-MS, a tentative metabolic pathway of sesamin to mammalian lignans is suggested (Liu *et al.*, 2006). The mammalian lignans, enterolactone and enterodiol were shown to possess weak estrogenic and antiestrogenic activities that may protect against hormone-dependent diseases such as breast cancer. Sesaminol triglucoside (STG) is a furofuran lignan with methylenedioxyphenyls. The abundance of sesamin in sesame seeds indicates that they are a major food source of enterolactone precursors (Peñalvo *et al.*, 2005).

The effect of sesame on female reproductive hormones was well studied. Mammalian lignans were shown to be produced, for the first time, from precursors in food bars containing 25 g whole sesame seed or their combination (Flax seed Sesame seed–12.5 g each), in a randomized crossover study, healthy postmenopausal women were supplemented with the bars for 4 wk each separated by 4-wk washout periods by the bacterial flora in the colon. A significant increase in urinary mammalian lignan excretion similar to that after ingestion of flaxseed was detected after the ingestion of sesame seed (Coulman *et al.*, 2005).

In a recent study, Penalvo *et al.* (2005) demonstrated the conversion of sesamin to mammalian lignans enterodiol (ED) and enterolactone (EL) by *in vitro* fecal fermentation and the increased plasma EL and ED levels in healthy volunteers after sesame seed ingestion. In addition, Wu *et al.* (2006) demonstrated that ingestion of sesame seed benefits postmenopausal women by improving blood lipids, antioxidant status, and possibly sex hormone status.

Sesame Seeds in Cancer

Tanabe *et al.* (2011) revealed a novel function for Receptor tyrosine kinase EphA1 and EphB2 in the induction of autophagy, suggesting a tumour suppressor role for these proteins in colourectal cancer.

According to Harikumar *et al.* (2010) sesamin down regulated constitutive and inducible NF-kappaB activation induced by various inflammatory stimuli and carcinogens, and inhibited the degradation of I kappa Balpha (IKK), the inhibitor of NF-kappa B, through the suppression of phosphorylation of IKK and inhibition of activation of IKK protein kinase, thus resulting in the suppression of p65 phosphorylation and nuclear translocation, and NF-kappaB-mediated reporter gene transcription. The inhibition of IKK protein kinase activation was found to be mediated through the inhibition of TAK1 kinase. Sesamin may thus have potential against cancer and other chronic diseases through the suppression of a pathway linked to the NF-kappaB signaling.

Wound Healing

The Sesame seeds have been used traditionally for the treatment of wounds in Buldhana district of Maharashtra state. In the excision and burn wound models, the sesame treated animals showed significant reduction in period of epithelization and wound contraction (50 per cent). In the incision wound model a significant increase in the breaking strength was observed. Seeds and oil treatment (250 mg and 500 mg/kg; po) in dead space wound model, produced a significant increase in the breaking strength, dry weight and hydroxyproline content of the granulation tissue. The results suggest that S. indicum seeds and oil applied topically or administered orally possesses wound healing activity (Kiran and Asad, 2008).

Sesamol is the anti-oxidative constituent contained mainly in the processed sesame seed oil which has not been explored scientifically for its wound healing activity (Shenoy *et al.*, 2011). Sesamol could be a promising drug in normal as well as delayed wound healing processes as the tensile strength significantly increased with sesamol (SM) at 471.40±14.66g when compared to control at 300.60±9.16 g in normal and DM suppressed healing. SM treated rats showed a significant ($p<0.05$) rise in hydroxyproline levels at 6.45±0.45 mg when compared to control at 1.75±0.20 mg (Shenoy *et al.*, 2011).

Other Benefits of Sesame Seeds

Anti-aging

The anti-aging effect of sesame was elucidated to be due to the strong vitamin E activity caused by a novel synergistic effect of sesame lignans with tocopherols where in, the metabolic decomposition of tocopherols was inhibited by sesame lignans. In studies on the microbial production of polyunsaturated fatty acids, Namiki (2007) found the specific inhibitory action of sesame lignans on Delta5 desaturase in polyunsaturated fatty acid synthesis.

Conclusions

Most of the studies on the health benefits of sesame seeds have been on animal models. Studies on human subjects have been few. Anti-aging effects of the seeds would be of great value but there is just one study by Namiki *et al.* (2007) and thus future work needs to be focused on this aspect.

References

Abdou HM, Hussien HM, Yousef MI (2012). Deleterious effects of cypermethrin on rat liver and kidney: protective role of sesame oil. J. Environ. Sci. Health. B.47 (4): 306–314.

Adlercreutz H, Mazur W (1997). Phyto-oestrogens and Western diseases. Ann. Med. 29: 95–120.

Ahmad S, Khan MB, Hoda MN, Bhatia K, Haque R, Fazili IS, Jamal A, Khan JS, Katare DP (2012). Neuroprotective effect of sesame seed oil in 6-hydroxydopamine induced neurotoxicity in mice model: cellular, biochemical and neurochemical evidence. Neurochem. Res. 37 (3): 516–26.

Akimoto K, Kitagawa Y, Akamatsu T, Hirose N, Sugano, M, Shimizu S, Yamada H (1993). Protective effects of sesamin against liver damage caused by alcohol or carbon tetrachloride in rodents. Ann. Nutr. Metab. 37: 218–24.

Alipoor B, Haghighian MK, Sadat BE, Asghari M (2012). Effect of sesame seed on lipid profile and redox status in hyperlipidemic patients. Int. J. Food Sci. Nutr. Jan 23. [Epub ahead of print].

Arumugam P, Ramesh S (2011). Protective effects of sesame oil on 4-NQO-induced oxidative DNA damage and lipid peroxidation in rats. Drug Chem. Toxicol. 34 (2): 116–19.

Ashakumary L, Rouyer I, Takahashi Y, Ide T, Fukuda N, Aoyama T, Hashimoto T, Mizugaki M, Sugano M (1999). Sesamin, a sesame lignan, is a potent inducer of hepatic fatty acid oxidation in the rat. Metabolism. 48 (10): 1303–13.

Axelson M, Sjovall J, Gustafsson BE, Setchell KD (1982). Origin of lignans in mammals and identification of a precursor from plants. Nature. 298: 659–60.

Badifu GI, Akpagher EM (1996). Effects of debittering methods on the proximate composition, organoleptic and functional properties of sesame (*Sesamum indicum* L.) seed flour. Plant. Foods. Hum. Nutr. 49 (2): 119–26.

Biswas A, Dhar P, Ghosh S (2010). Antihyperlipidemic effect of sesame (*Sesamum indicum* L.) protein isolate in rats fed a normal and high cholesterol diet. J. Food Sci. 75 (9): H274–79.

Borriello SP, Setchell KD, Axelson M, Lawson AM (1985). Production and metabolism of lignans by the human faecal flora. J. Appl. Bacteriol. 58: 37–43.

Budowski P (1950). Sesame oil. III. Antioxidant properties of sesamol. J. Am. Oil Chem. Soc. 27: 264–67.

Chatrattanakunchai S, Fraser T, Stobart K (2000). Sesamin inhibits lysophosphatidylcholine acyltransferase in Mortierella alpina. Biochem. Soc. Trans. 28: 718–21.

Chavali SR, Utsunomiya T, Forse RA (2001). Increased survival after cecal ligation and puncture in mice consuming diets enriched with sesame seed oil. Crit. Care. Med. 29 (1): 140–43.

Chavali SR, Zhong WW, Utsunomiya T, Forse RA (1997). Decreased production of interleukin-1-beta, prostaglandin-E2 and thromboxane-B2, and elevated levels of interleukin-6 and -10 are associated with increased survival during endotoxic shock in mice consuming diets enriched with sesame seed oil supplemented with Quil-A saponin. Int. Arch. Allergy Immunol. 114 (2): 153–60.

Coulman KD, Liu Z, Hum WQ, Michaelides J, Thompson LU (2005). Whole sesame seed is as rich a source of mammalian lignan precursors as whole flaxseed. Nutr. Cancer. 52 (2): 156–65.

Dhar P, Chattopadhya K, Bhattacharyya D, Biswas A, Roy B, Ghosh S (2007). Ameliorative influence of sesame lignans on lipid profile and lipid peroxidation in induced diabetic rats. J. Agric. Food Chem. 55 (14): 5875–80.

Egbekun MK, Ehieze MU (1997). Proximate composition and functional properties of fullfat and defatted beniseed (*Sesamum indicum* L.) flour. Plant. Foods Hum. Nutr. 51 (1): 35–41.

Fukuda Y, Osawa T, Namiki M, Saki T (1985). Studies on antioxidative substances in sesame. Agric. Biol. Chem. 49: 301–306.

Gerster H. (1991). Potential role of ß-carotene in the prevention of cardiovascular disease. Int. J. Vit. Nutr. Res. 61: 277.

Gopalan C, Rama Sastri BV, Balasubramanian SC. (Revised and Updated by) Narasinga Rao BS, Deosthale, YG, Pant KC (2000). NIN, ICMR, Hyderabad, India.

Hahm TS, Park SJ, Martin Lo Y (2009). Effects of germination on chemical composition and functional properties of sesame (*Sesamum indicum* L.) seeds. Bioresour. Technol. 100 (4): 1643–47.

Hamada N, Fujita Y, Tanaka A, Naoi M, Nozawa Y, Ono Y, Kitagawa Y, Tomimori N, Kiso Y, Ito M (2009). Metabolites of sesamin, a major lignan in sesame seeds, induce neuronal differentiation in PC12 cells through activation of ERK1/2 signaling pathway. J. Neural. Transm. 116 (7): 841–52.

Hamada N, Tanaka A, Fujita Y, Itoh T, Ono Y, Kitagawa Y, Tomimori N, Kiso Y, Akao Y, Nozawa Y, Ito M (2011). Involvement of heme oxygenase-1 induction via Nrf2/ARE activation in protection against H2O2-induced PC12 cell death by a metabolite of sesamin contained in sesame seeds. Bioorg. Med. Chem. 19 (6): 1959–65.

Harikumar KB, Sung B, Tharakan ST, Pandey MK, Joy B, Guha S, Krishnan S, Aggarwal BB (2010). Sesamin manifests chemopreventive effects through the suppression of NF-kappa B-regulated cell survival, proliferation, invasion, and angiogenic gene products. Mol. Cancer. Res. 8 (5): 751–61.

Hashimoto K, Watanabe K, Nishimura T, Iyo M, Shirayama Y, Minabe Y (1998). Behavioral changes and expression of heat shock protein HSP-70 mRNA, brain-derived neurotrophic factor mRNA, and cyclooxygenase-2 mRNA in rat brain following seizures induced by systemic administration of kainic acid. Brain. Res. 804: 212–23.

Heinonen S, Nurmi T, Liukkonen K, Poutanen K, Wähälä K, Deyama T, Nishibe S, Adlercreutz H (2001). *In vitro* metabolism of lignans: new precursors of mammalian lignans enterolactone and enterodiol. J. Agric. Food Chem. 49: 3178–86.

Hirata F, Fujita K, Ishikura Y, Hosoda K, Ishikawa T, Nakamura H (1996). Hypocholesterolemic effect of sesame lignan in humans. Atherosclerosis. 122: 135–36.

Hirose N, Doi F, Ueki T, Akazawa K, Chijiiwa K, Sugano M, Akimoto K, Shimizu S, Yamada H (1992). Suppressive effect of sesamin against 7,12-dimethylbenz[a]-anthracene induced rat mammary carcinogenesis. Anticancer. Res. 12: 1259–65.

Hirose N, Inoue T, Nishihara K, Sugano M, Akimoto K, Shimizu S, Yamada H (1991). Inhibition of cholesterol absorption and synthesis in rats by sesamin. J. Lipid. Res. 32: 629–38.

Hou RC, Chen HL, Tzen JT, Jeng KC (2003a). Effect of sesame antioxidants on LPS-induced NO production by BV2 microglial cells. Neuroreport. 14 (14): 1815–19.

Hou RC, Huang HM, Tzen JT, Jeng KC (2003b). Protective effects of sesamin and sesamolin on hypoxic neuronal and PC12 cells. J. Neurosci. Res. 74 (1): 123–33.

Hou RC, Wu CC, Yang CH, Jeng KC (2004). Protective effects of sesamin and sesamolin on murine BV-2 microglia cell line under hypoxia. Neurosci. Lett. 367 (1): 10–13.

Hsieh PF, Hou CW, Yao PW, Wu SP, Peng YF, Shen ML, Lin CH, Chao YY, Chang MH, Jeng KC (2011). Sesamin ameliorates oxidative stress and mortality in kainic acid-induced status epilepticus by inhibition of MAPK and COX-2 activation. J. Neuroinflammation. 8: 57.

Hsu DZ, Chiang PJ, Chien SP, Huang BM, Liu MY (2004). Parenteral sesame oil attenuates oxidative stress after endotoxin intoxication in rats. Toxicology. 19 (1-2): 147–53.

Hsu DZ, Chien SP, Li YH, Chuang YC, Chang YC, Liu MY (2008). Sesame oil attenuates hepatic lipid peroxidation by inhibiting nitric oxide and superoxide anion generation in septic rats. J. Parenter. Enteral Nutr. 32 (2): 154–59.

Hsu DZ, Li YH, Chu PY, Periasamy S, Liu MY (2011). Sesame oil prevents acute kidney injury induced by the synergistic action of aminoglycoside and iodinated contrast in rats. Antimicrob. Agents. Chemother. 55 (6): 2532–36.

Hsu DZ, Liu MY (2002). Sesame oil attenuates multiple organ failure and increased survival rate during endotoxemia in rats. Crit. Care Med. 30: 1859–62.

Hsu DZ, Liu MY (2004a). Effects of sesame oil on oxidative stress after the onset of sepsis in rats. Shock. 22 (6): 582–85.

Hsu DZ, Liu MY (2004 b). Sesame oil protects against lipopolysaccharide-stimulated oxidative stress in rats. Crit. Care Med. 32: 227–31.

Hsu DZ, *et al.* (2005). Effect of sesame oil on oxidative-stress-associated renal injury in endotoxemic rats: involvement of nitric oxide and proinflammatory cytokines. Shock. 24: 276–80.

Hsu DZ, Liu CT, Li YH, Chu PY, Liu M (2010). Protective effect of daily sesame oil supplement on gentamicin-induced renal injury in rats. Shock. 33: 88–92.

Hu Q, Xu J, Chen S, Yang F (2004). Antioxidant activity of extracts of black sesame seed (*Sesamum indicum* L.) by supercritical carbon dioxide extraction. J. Agric. Food Chem. 52 (4): 943–47.

Hussien HM, Abdou HM, Yousef MI (2013). Cypermethrin induced damage in genomic DNA and histopathological changes in brain and haematotoxicity in rats: The protective effect of sesame oil. Brain Res. Bull. 92: 76-83.

Ide T, Ashakumary L, Takahashi Y, Kushiro M, Fukuda N, Sugano M (2001). Sesamin, a sesame lignan, decreases fatty acid synthesis in rat liver accompanying the down-regulation of sterol regulatory element binding protein-1. Biochim. Biophys. Acta. 1534 (1): 1–13.

Ide T, Nakashima Y, Iida H, Yasumoto S, Katsuta M (2009). Lipid metabolism and nutrigenomics–impact of sesame lignans on gene expression profiles and fatty acid oxidation in rat liver. Forum Nutr. 61: 10–24.

Ikeda S, Abe C, Uchida T, Ichikawa T, Horio F, Yamashita K (2007). Dietary sesame seed and its lignan increase both ascorbic acid concentration in some tissues and urinary excretion by stimulating biosynthesis in rats. J. Nutr. Sci. Vitaminol. (Tokyo). 53 (5): 383–92.

Ikeda S, Kagaya M, Kobayashi K, Tohyama T, Kiso Y, Higuchi N, Yamashita K (2003). Dietary sesame lignans decrease lipid peroxidation in rats fed docosahexaenoic acid. J. Nutr. Sci. Vitaminol. (Tokyo). 49 (4): 270–76.

Ikeda S, Tohyama T, Yamashita K (2002). Dietary sesame seed and its lignans inhibit 2,7,8-trimethyl- 2(2'-carboxyethyl)-6-hydroxychroman excretion into urine of rats fed gamma-tocopherol. J. Nutr. 132 (5): 961–66.

Jamarkattel-Pandit N, Pandit NR, Kim MY, Park SH, Kim KS, Choi H, Kim H, Bu Y (2010). Neuroprotective effect of defatted sesame seeds extract against *in vitro* and *in vivo* ischemic neuronal damage. Planta. Med. 76: 20–26.

Jan KC, Hwang LS, Ho CT (2009). Biotransformation of sesaminol triglucoside to mammalian lignans by intestinal microbiota. J. Agric. Food Chem. 57 (14): 6101–106.

Jeng KC, Hou RC, Wang JC, Ping LI (2005). Sesamin inhibits lipopolysaccharide-induced cytokine production by suppression of p38 mitogen-activated protein kinase and nuclear factor-kappaB. Immunol. Lett. 97: 101–106.

Jiao, Y., Davin, L. B. and Lewis, N. G (1998). Furanofuran lignan metabolism as a function of seed maturation in *Sesamum indicum*: Methylenedioxy bridge formation: In honour of Professor G. H. Neil Towers' 75th birthday. Phytochemistry. 49: 387–94.

Kamal-Eldin A, Frank J, Razdam A, Tengblad S, Basu S, Vessby B (2000). Effects of dietary phenolic compounds on tocopherol, cholesterol, and fatty acids in rats. Lipids. 35: 427–35.

Kamal-Eldin A, Moazzami A, Washi S (2011). Sesame seed lignans: potent physiological modulators and possible ingredients in functional foods and nutraceuticals. Recent Pat. Food Nutr. Agric. 3 (1): 17–29.

Kang MH, Kawai Y, Naito M, Osawa T (1999). Dietary defatted sesame flour decreases susceptibility to oxidative stress in hypercholesterolemic rabbits. J. Nutr. 129 (10): 1885–90.

Kang MH, Katsuzaki H, Osawa T (1998a). Inhibition of 2,22-azobis (2,4-dimethylvaleronitrile)-induced lipid peroxidation by sesaminols. Lipids 33: 1031–36.

Kang MH, Naito M, Tsujihara N, Osawa T (1998b). Sesamolin inhibits lipid peroxidation in rat liver and kidney. J. Nutr. 128: 1018–22.

Katsuzaki H, Kawakishi S, Osawa T (1994). Sesaminol glucosides in sesame seeds. Phytochemistry. 35: 773–76.

Katsuzaki, H., Kawasumi, M., Kawakishi, S. and Osawa, T. (1992) Structure of novel antioxidative lignan glucosides isolated from sesame seed. Biosci. Biotechnol. Biochem. 56: 2087–88.

Kiran K, Asad M (2008). Wound healing activity of *Sesamum indicum* L seed and oil in rats. Indian J. Exp. Biol. 46 (11): 77–82.

Kita S, Matsumura Y, Morimoto S, Akimoto K, Furuya M, Oka N, Tanaka T (1995). Antihypertensive effect of sesamin. II. protection against two-kidney, one-clip renal hypertension and cardiovascular hypertrophy. Biol. Pharm. Bull. 18: 1283–85.

Kumar CM, Appu Rao AG, Singh SA (2009 a). Effect of infrared heating on the formation of sesamol and quality of defatted flours from *Sesamum indicum* L. J. Food. Sci. 74 (4): H105–11.

Kumar P, Kalonia H, Kumar A (2009 b). Sesamol attenuate 3-nitropropionic acid-induced Huntington-like behavioral, biochemical, and cellular alterations in rats. J. Asian Nat. Prod Res. 11 (5): 439–50.

Kumar P, Kalonia H, Kumar A (2010). Protective effect of sesamol against 3-nitropropionic acid-induced cognitive dysfunction and altered glutathione redox balance in rats. Basic Clin. Pharmacol. Toxicol. 107 (1): 577–82.

Lahaie-Collins V, Bournival J, Plouffe M, Carange J, Martinoli MG (2008). Sesamin modulates tyrosine hydroxylase, superoxide dismutase, catalase, inducible NO synthase and interleukin-6 expression in dopaminergic cells under MPP-induced oxidative stress. Oxid. Med. Cell. Longev. 1: 54–62.

Lee SC, Jeong SM, Kim SY, Nam KC, Ahn DU (2005). Effect of far-Infra red irradiation on the antioxidant activity of defatted sesame meal extracts. J. Agric. Food Chem. 53 (5): 1495–98.

Liu Z, Saarinen NM, Thompson LU (2006). Sesamin is one of the major precursors of mammalian lignans in sesame seed (*Sesamum indicum*) as observed *in vitro* and in rats. J. Nutr. 136 (4): 906–912.

Martinchik AN (2011). [Nutritional value of sesame seeds]. Vopr. Pitan. 80 (3): 41–43. [Article in Russian].

Maria-Neto S, Honorato RV, Costa FT, Almeida RG, Amaro DS, Oliveira JT, Vasconcelos IM, Franco OL (2011). Bactericidal activity identified in 2S Albumin from sesame seeds and in silico studies of structure-function relations. Protein J. 30 (5): 340–50.

Matsumura Y, Kita S, Morimoto S, Akimoto K, Furuya M, Oka N, Tanaka T (1995). Antihypertensive effect of sesamin. I. protection against deoxycorticosterone acetate-salt-induced hypertension and cardiovascular hypertrophy. Biol. Pharm. Bull. 18: 1016–19.

Matsumura Y, Kita S, Tanida Y, Taguchi Y, Morimoto S, Akimoto K, Tanaka T (1998). Antihypertensive effect of sesamin. III. protection against development and maintenance of hypertension in stroke-prone spontaneously hypertensive rats. Biol. Pharm. Bull. 21: 469–73.

Miyahara Y, Komiya T, Katsuzaki H, Imai K, Nakagawa M, Ishi Y, Hibasami H (2000). Sesamin and episesamin induce apoptosis in human lymphoid leukemia Molt 4B cells. Int. J. Mol. Med. 6: 43–46.

Nakabayashi A, Kitagawa Y, Suwa Y, Akimoto K, Asami S, Shimizu S, Hirose N, Sugano M, Yamada Y (1995). Alfa-tocopherol enhances the hypocholesterolemic action of sesamin in rats. Int. J. Vit. Nutr. Res. 65: 162–68.

Nakai M, Harada M, Nakahara K, Akimoto K, Shibata H, Miki W, Kiso Y (2003). Novel antioxidative metabolites in rat liver with ingested sesamin. J. Agric. Food Chem. 51: 1666–70.

Nakano D, Itoh C, Takaoka M, Kiso Y, Tanaka T, Matsumura Y (2002). Antihypertensive effect of sesamin. IV. inhibition of vascular superoxide production by sesamin. Biol. Pharm. Bull. 25: 1247–49.

Namiki M (1995). The chemistry and physiological functions of sesame. Food Rev. Int. 11: 282–329.

Namiki M (2007). Nutraceutical functions of sesame: a review. Crit. Rev. Food Sci. Nutr. 47 (7): 651–73.

Ogawa H, Sasagawa S, Murakami T, Yoshizumi H (1995). Sesame lignans modulate cholesterol metabolism in the stroke-prone spontaneously hypertensive rat. Clin. Exp. Pharmacol. Physiol. Suppl. 22: S310–12.

Osawa T, Yoshida A, Kawakishi S, Yamashita K, Ochi H (1995). Protective role of dietary antioxidants in oxidative stress. Cutler, R. G. Packer, L. eds. Oxidative Stress and Aging Molecular and Cell. Biology. Basel, Switzerland. Updates: 367–77.

Penalvo JL, Heinonen SM, Aura AM, Adlercreutz H (2005). Dietary sesamin is converted to enterolactone in humans. J. Nutr. 135: 1056–62.

Peñalvo JL, Hopia A, Adlercreutz H (2006). Effect of sesamin on serum cholesterol and triglycerides levels in LDL receptor-deficient mice. Eur. J. Nutr. 45 (8): 439–44.

Ramesh B, Saravanan R, Pugalendi KV (2005). Influence of sesame oil on blood glucose, lipid peroxidation, and antioxidant status in streptozotocin diabetic rats. J. Med. Food. 8 (3): 377–81.

Ryu, S. N., Ho, C. T. and Osawa, T. (1998) High performance liquid chromatographic determination of antioxidant lignan glycosides in sesame varieties of sesame. J. Food Lipids 5: 17–28.

Saad R, Pérez C (1984). [Functional and nutritional properties of modified proteins of sesame (*Sesamum indicum*, L.)]. Arch. Latinoam. Nutr. 34 (4): 749–62. [Article in Spanish].

Saarinen NM, Warri A, Mäkelä SI, Eckerman C, Reunanen M, Ahotupa M, Salmi SM, Franke AA, Kangas L, Santti R (2000). Hydroxymatairesinol, a novel enterolactone precursor with antitumour properties from coniferous tree (Picea abies). Nutr. Cancer. 36: 207–16.

Sandhya TL, Ong WY, Horrocks LA, Farooqui AA (1998). A light and electron microscopic study of cytoplasmic phospholipase A2 and cyclooxygenase-2 in the hippocampus after kainite lesions. Brain Res. 788: 223–31.

Sankar D, Ali A, Sambandam G, Rao R (2011). Sesame oil exhibits synergistic effect with antidiabetic medication in patients with type 2 diabetes mellitus. Clin. Nutr. 30 (3): 351–58.

Sankar D, Rao MR, Sambandam G, Pugalendi KV (2006 a). A pilot study of open label sesame oil in hypertensive diabetics. J. Med. Food. 9 (3): 408–412.

Sankar D, Rao MR, Sambandam G, Pugalendi KV (2006 b). Effect of sesame oil on diuretics or Beta-blockers in the modulation of blood pressure, anthropometry, lipid profile, and redox status. Yale J. Biol. Med. 79 (1): 19–26.

Sanz O, Estrada A, Ferrer I, Planas AM (1997). Differential cellular distribution and dynamics of HSP70, cyclooxygenase-2, and c-Fos in the rat brain after transient focal ischemia or kainic acid. Neurosci. 80: 221–32.

Sen M, Bhattacharyya DK (2001). Nutritional quality of sesame seed protein fraction extracted with isopropanol. J. Agric. Food Chem. 49 (5): 2641–46.

Setchell KD, Lawson AM, Mitchell FL, Adlercreutz H, Kirk DN, Axelson M (1980). Lignans in man and in animal species. Nature. 287: 740–42.

Shenoy RR, Sudheendra AT, Nayak PG, Paul P, Kutty NG, Rao CM (2011). Normal and delayed wound healing is improved by sesamol, an active constituent of *Sesamum indicum* (L.) in albino rats. J. Ethnopharmacol. 133 (2): 608–612.

Shimizu, S., Akimoto, K., Shinmen, Y., Sugano, M. and Yamada, H (1991). Sesamin is a potent and specific inhibitor of D5 desaturase in polyunsaturated fatty acid biosynthesis. Lipids. 26: 512–16.

Shyu YS, Hwang LS (2002). Antioxidative activity of the crude extract of lignan glycosides from unroasted Burma black sesame meal. Food. Res. Int. 35: 357–65.

Sirato-Yasumoto S, Katsuta M, Okuyama Y, Takahashi Y, Ide T (2001). Effect of sesame seeds rich in sesamin and sesamolin on fatty acid oxidation in rat liver. J. Agric. Food. Chem. 49 (5): 2647–51.

Sugano M, Inoue T, Koba K, Yoshida K, Hirose N, Shinmen Y, Akimoto K, Amachi T (1990). Influence of sesame lignans on various lipid parameters in rats. Agric. Biol. Chem. 54:2669–73.

Tamura H, Fujita A, Steinhaus M, Takahisa E, Watanabe H, Schieberle P (2010). Identification of novel aroma-active thiols in pan-roasted white sesame seeds. J. Agric. Food Chem. 58 (12): 7368–75.

Tamura H, Fujita A, Steinhaus M, Takahisa E, Watanabe H, Schieberle P (2011). Assessment of the aroma impact of major odor-active thiols in pan-roasted white sesame seeds by calculation of odor activity values. J. Agric. Food Chem. 59 (18): 10211–18.

Tanabe H, Kuribayashi K, Tsuji N, Tanaka M, Kobayashi D, Watanabe N (2011). Sesamin induces autophagy in colon cancer cells by reducing tyrosine phosphorylation of EphA1 and EphB2. Int. J. Oncol. 39 (1): 33–40.

Thompson LU (2003). Flaxseed, lignans, and cancer. In: Thompson LU, Cunnane SC, editors. Flaxseed in human nutrition, 2nd ed. Champaign (IL): AOCS Press; 194–222.

Umeda-Sawada R, Ogawa M, Igarashi O (1998). The metabolism and n-6/n-3 ratio of essential fatty acids in rats: effect of dietary arachidonic acid and a mixture of sesame lignans (sesamin and episesamin). Lipids. 33 (6): 567–72.

Utsunomiya T, Chavali SR, Zhong WW, Forse, RA (2000). Effects of sesamin-supplemented dietary fat emulsions on the ex vivo production of lipopolysaccharide-induced prostanoids and tumour necrosis factor {alpha} in rats. Am. J. Clin. Nutr. 72: 804–808.

Visavadiya NP, Narasimhacharya AV (2008). Sesame as a hypocholesteraemic and antioxidant dietary component. Food Chem. Toxicol. 46 (6): 1889–95.

Wang LQ, Meselhy MR, Li Y, Nakamura N, Min BS, Qin GW, Hattori M (2001). The heterocyclic ring fission and dehydroxylation of catechins and related compounds by Eubacterium sp. strain SDG-2, a human intestinal bacterium. Chem. Pharm. Bull. (Tokyo). 49: 1640–43.

Wang LQ, Meselhy MR, Li Y, Qin GW, Hattori M (2000). Human intestinal bacteria capable of transforming secoisolariciresinol diglucoside to mammalian lignans, enterodiol and enterolactone. Chem Pharm Bull (Tokyo). 48: 1606–610.

Wichitsranoi J, Weerapreeyakul N, Boonsiri P, Settasatian C, Settasatian N, Komanasin N, Sirijaichingkul S, Teerajetgul Y, Rangkadilok N, Leelayuwat N (2011). Antihypertensive and antioxidant effects of dietary black sesame meal in pre-hypertensive humans. Nutr. J. 10: 82.

Wu JH, Hodgson JM, Puddey IB, Belski R, Burke V, Croft KD (2009). Sesame supplementation does not improve cardiovascular disease risk markers in overweight men and women. Nutr. Metab. Cardiovasc. Dis. 19 (11): 774–80.

Wu WH, Kang YP, Wang NH, Jou HJ, Wang TA (2006). Sesame ingestion affects sex hormones, antioxidant status, and blood lipids in postmenopausal women. J. Nutr. 136 (5): 1270–75.

Yamashita, K., Kagaya, M., Higuti, N. and Kiso, Y (2000). Sesamin and α-tocopherol synergistically suppress lipid-peroxide in rats fed with a high docosahexaenoic acid diet. Biofactors. 11: 11–13.

Yamashita K, Yamada Y, Kitou S, Ikeda S, Abe C, Saarinen NM, Santti R (2007). Hydroxymatairesinol and sesaminol act differently on tocopherol concentrations in rats. J. Nutr. Sci. Vitaminol. (Tokyo). 53 (5): 393–99.

Chapter 12

Turmeric

(*Curcuma longa* Linn.)

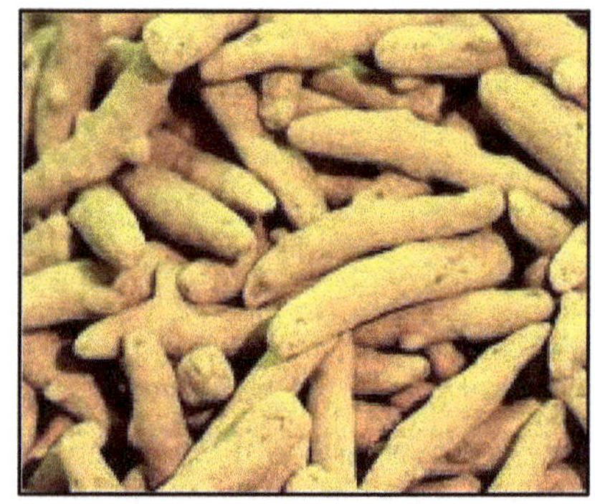

Turmeric was traditionally called Indian saffron. It is a dried rhizome from the family of Zangiberaceae and has been used in Indian and Chinese systems of medicine for a long time. It is available fresh as well as dry rhizomes and also as powder. It was listed in an Assyrian (now Northern Iraq) herbal dating from about 600 BC. Both the East and the West have held its medicinal property in high regard through the ages.

Use of turmeric dates back nearly 4000 years to the Vedic culture in India. It is extensively used in Ayurveda, Unani and Siddha medicine as a home remedy for various diseases (Chattopadhyay *et al.*, 2004; Abas *et al.*, 2005).

Turmeric was mentioned in the writings of Marco Polo concerning his 1280 journey to China and India; and it was first introduced to Europe in the 13th century by Arab traders. Vasco da Gama, a Portuguese sailor during 15th century, after his visit to India, truly introduced spices including turmeric to the West (Akram *et al.*, 2010).

Interestingly, Turmeric is known and being used in other parts of the world. The use of turmeric dates back nearly 4000 years to the ancient Vedic culture of India. Since then, it has been used an important spice, beauty product and in religious ceremonies. Turmeric was traditionally called Indian saffron because of its deep yellow-orange colour and has been used throughout history as a condiment, healing remedy and textile dye.

The plant is a native of Southern Asia and is cultivated throughout the warmer parts of the world. It is grown on a large scale in India, China, Java and East Indies. Rhizome may be 2 to 6 cm long and 1 to 1.7 cm thick. Leaves are very large, in tufts up to 1.2 ft. Flowers in autumnal spikes 10 to 15 cm long (Raghunathan and Mitra 1982). It has a peculiar fragrant/odor and a slightly bitter, acrid taste, like ginger.

Principal Constituents

Turmeric contains an acrid volatile oil, brown colouring matter, gum, starch, calcium chloride, woody fiber and a yellowish colouring matter named curcumin also known as diferuloylmethane. The chemical compounds diaryl heptanoids are responsible for the colouring matter in turmeric. Curcumin containing turmeric powder is obtained by digesting turmeric in boiling alcohol, filtering and evaporating the solution to dryness, the residue being digested in ether, filtered and evaporated.

Turmeric contains two major classes of secondary metabolites, the phenolic curcuminoids and the hydrophobic essential oil (Lantz *et al.,* 2005). The rhizome contains curcuminoids, curcumin, demethoxy curcumin, bis- demethoxycurcumin, 5'- methoxycurcumin and dihydrocurcumin which are found to be natural antioxidants. The fresh rhizomes also contain two new natural phenolics which possess antioxidant and anti-inflammatory activities and also two new pigments. Several sesquiterpenes, germacrone, turmerone, ar-(+)-, a-, ß- turmerones, ß- bisabolene, a-curcumene; zingiberene, ß- sesquiphellandene, bisacurone, curcumenone, dehydrocurdione, procurcumadiol, bis-acumol, curcumenol, isoprocurcumenol epiprocurcumenol, procurcumenol, zedoaronediol, curlone, and turmeronol A and turmeronol B have been found to be present in the rhizomes. The relative proportions of these terpenoids vary depending on the rhizome's geographic origin and method of extraction (Negi *et al.,* 1999, Jain *et al.,* 2007, Joshi *et al.,* 2003).

The rhizomes are also reported to contain four new polysaccharidesukonans– having activity on the Reticuloendothelial system, along with stigmasterol, ß-sitosterol, cholesterol and 2-hydroxymethyl anthraquinone (Toda *et al.,* 1985; Kiso *et al.,* 1983).

Kiuchi et al. (1993) isolated a new curcuminoid, cyclocurcumin (IV), from the nematocidally active fraction of turmeric, the rhizome of *Curcma longa,* together with three known curcuminoids, curcumin (I), demethoxycurcumin (II) and bisdemethoxycurcumin (III). Although the above curcuminoids were ineffective when they were applied independently, the nematocidal activity increased remarkably when they were mixed, suggesting a synergistic action between them.

The essential oil (6 per cent) from the rhizome contains d-a-phellandrene, d-sabinene, cineol, borneol, zingiberene, sesquiterpenes (turmerones). Pure turmeric powder has the highest curcumin concentration, averaging 3.14 per cent by weight (Tayyem *et al.,* 2006). The crystalline colouring matter, curcumin, is diferuloyl methane. It dissolves in concentrated sulphuric acid giving a yellow-red colouration. The yellow pigmented fraction, isolated from the rhizomes, contains the curcumins belonging to the dicinnamoyl- methane group. Aromatic oil, turmeric oil, composed of terpene-hydrocarbon-derivatives and sesquiterpenic ketones has also been isolated (The Wealth of India). Major constituents of the essential oil are l-curcamene (65.5 per cent), squiterpene (22 per cent), camphor (2.5 per cent), camphene (0.8 per cent). Other components include curcumin, curzerenone, curzenene, furanodienone, furanodiene, zederone, curculone, curcumol, procurcumenol, curcumadiol, curdione.

Funk *et al.* (2006 a, b) demonstrated potent and physiologically important effects of the curcuminoids (Chainani 2003). For example, they have elucidated a profound anti-arthritic effect of curcuminoid-containing turmeric extracts due to their ability to inhibit nuclear factor-êB (NF-êB) activation in experimental rheumatoid arthritis, thus blocking multiple downstream signaling pathways critical to joint inflammation, including cyclo-oxygenase (COX)-stimulated prostaglandin-E_2 (PGE_2) production (Funk *et al.*, 2006 a). Far less studied, and indeed, often discarded in the preparation of turmeric dietary supplements (AR), are turmeric's essential oils.

The biological properties of the multi-component essential oils of turmeric include antifungal (Apisariyakul, 1995), mosquitocidal (Roth *et al.*, 1998), antivenom (Ferreira *et al.*, 1992), antibacterial and antioxidant properties (Negi *et al.*, 1999, Jayaprakasha *et al.*, 2002).

Nutritional Value

Turmeric is an excellent source of both iron and manganese. It is also a good source of vitamin B6, dietary fiber and potassium.

Nutritional Value per 100 g

Nutrient	*Amount*	*Nutrient*	*Amount*
Energy (kcal)	354	Carbohydrates (g)	64.93
Dietary fiber (g)	21.1	Fat (g)	9.88
Protein (g)	7.83	Calcium (mg)	183
Iron (mg)	41.42	Magnesium (mg)	193
Phosphorus (mg)	268	Potassium (mg)	2525
Sodium (mg)	38	Zinc (mg)	4.35
Thiamine (Vit. B1) (mg)	0.152	Riboflavin (Vit.B2) (mg)	0.233
Niacin (Vit. B3) (mg)	5.140	Vitamin B6 (mg)	1.800
Folate (Vit. B9) (µg)	39	Vitamin C (mg)	25.9
Vitamin K (mcg)	13.4		

USDA (2012).

Therapeutic Uses of Turmeric

Besides flavouring food, turmeric, (affectionately called as "Kitchen Queen"), has been used in traditional medicine as a household remedy for various diseases. It is pungent, bitter and astringent. In Ayurveda, the traditional Indian system of herbal medicine, turmeric is believed to relieve gas, dispel worms, improve digestion, regulate menstruation, dissolve gallstones, relieve arthritis, subside phlegm, remove the impurities of blood and strengthen the overall energy of the body among other uses. In addition to its use as a spice and pigment, turmeric and its constituents mainly curcumin and essential oils showed a wide spectrum of biological actions. These include its anti-inflammatory, antioxidant, anticarcinogenic, antimutagenic, anticoagulant, antifertility, antidiabetic, antibacterial, antifungal, anti-protozoal, antiviral, anti-fibrotic, anti-venom, antiulcer, hypotensive and hypocholesterolemic activities (Rathaur *et al.*, 2012).

It is also believed to be appetizing and carminative. It is used for curing eczema, chronic sinusitis, anorexia, cough, anemia and fever. Further, it is used to remove phlegm and the impurities of blood. It is also believed to improve the complexion of the skin, purify breast milk and act against urinary disorders. Thus the traditional belief that turmeric is a multipurpose preventive and curative agent instigates the scientists to probe into these effects for scientific explanations.

Turmeric powder is used in auspicious ceremonies as it is found to be germicidal in effect aside of the psychological effect of the colour. Turmeric is used for bruises, leech bites, festering eye infection, and inflammation of the oral mucosa, inflammatory skin conditions and infected wounds. In folk medicine, turmeric is used for diarrheas, intermittent fever, dropsy, bronchitis, cold, worms, leprosy, kidney inflammation and cystitis.

Curcumin, a spice once relegated to the kitchen shelf, has moved into the clinic and may prove to be "Curecumin". Relevantly, several molecular targets have been identified for therapeutic/preventive effects of turmeric. Modern interest in turmeric began in 1971 when Indian researchers found evidence that whole turmeric possesses anti-inflammatory properties. Much of this observed activity seems to be due to the presence of a constituent curcumin (Ammon and Wahl, 1991).

Turmeric as an Antioxidant

Curcumin is a powerful antioxidant and protects the body against free radical damage (Sreejayan and Rao, 1996).

Aboul *et al.* (2011) demonstrated the promising anticonvulsant and potent antioxidant effects of curcumin in reducing oxidative stress, excitability and the induction of seizures in epileptic animals and improving some of the adverse effects of antiepileptic drugs.

Curcumin inhibited ovariectomy-induced bone loss, at least in part by reducing osteoclastogenesis as a result of increased antioxidant activity and impaired receptor activator of nuclear factor-êB ligand signaling. Kim *et al.* (2011) thus suggested that bone loss associated with estrogen deficiency could be attenuated by curcumin administration.

Antimicrobial Activity

Most exacerbations of asthma can be proven to be associated with bacterial infections and there is scientific evidence that frequent respiratory infections particularly bacterial infections provoke asthma attack. Turmeric extracts exhibited a moderate antibacterial activity against human pathogens causing upper respiratory infection namely *H. influenzae, S. pneumoniae, S. pyrogene* and *S. aureus*, by taking Gentamycin, Optochin, Bacitracin and Amoxicillin as reference standards (Nilani *et al.*, 2010).

Methicillin-resistant Staphylococcus aureus (MRSA) has been emerging worldwide as one of the most important hospital and community pathogens. Kim *et al.* (2005) demonstrated the ethyl acetate extract of turmeric to lower the MICs of ampicillin and oxacillin markedly against MRSA. In the bacterial invasion assay, MRSA intracellular invasion was significantly decreased in the presence of 0.125-2 mg/mL of turmeric extract compared with the control group. Thus the turmeric was shown to have the potential to restore the effectiveness of beta-lactams against MRSA, and inhibit the MRSA invasion of HMFs.

Waghmare *et al.* (2011) compared the efficacy of turmeric mouthwash and chlorhexidine gluconate mouthwash in prevention of gingivitis and plaque formation and stated that turmeric is definitely a good adjunct to mechanical plaque control. Further studies are required on turmeric based mouthwash to establish it as a low cost plaque control measure.

Application of turmeric powder over septic as well as aseptic wounds in rats and rabbits accelerated the process of healing to the extent of 23-24 per cent in both type of wounds (Gujral *et al.*, 1953).

Curcumin inhibits HIV *in vitro*, though human trials are needed to determine if it has any usefulness for treating humans with this condition (Barthelemy *et al.*, 1998). Some anti-HIV activity in human clinical studies; inhibits HIV long terminal repeat.

Anti-inflammatory Activity

Turmeric possesses anti-inflammatory property. With its vast array of molecular targets it has shown great potential as a therapeutic agent for various cancer types and for inflammatory conditions (Rajasekaran, 2011). Petroleum ether extracts of the rhizome showed significant anti-inflammatory activity in experimental animals without producing any toxicity or side effects. The anti-inflammatory activity of turmeric extracts has been attributed to curcumin and its analogues (Arora *et al.*, 1971; Ammon and Wahl, 1991; Rao *et al.*, 1982; Srimal and Dhawan, 1973). Arora *et al.* (1971) explained that the anti inflammatory effect of turmeric includes lowering of histamine levels, possibly by increasing production of natural cortisone by the adrenal glands.

Water extract of turmeric showed significant anti- inflammatory activity in acute carrageenin-induced oedema. Anti-inflammatory activity of the active principle curcumin was similar to cortisone and phenyl-butazone in carrageenin-induced edema in rats with an equivalent dose (Srimal and Dhawan 1973). Stabilizing effect on lysosomal membranes also has also been reported.

The volatile oil (1.6ml/kg) from the turmeric leaves showed as much anti-inflammatory activity as that of 100mg/kg Phenylbutazone upon oral administration on the exudative and proliferative phases of the inflammatory reaction in male albino rats with carrageenin-induced edema.

It has been shown that curcumin intake may also potently inhibit proinflammatory molecule expression. These effects are related, in part, to inhibition of the activities of the cyclooxygenase, lipoxygenase etc. In conjunctivitis, the eyes are washed with turmeric water. Its decoction is efficacious eyewash in catarrhal and purulent ophthalmia. Curcumin is also sometimes recommended for cataracts, chronic anterior uveitis (an inflammation of the iris of the eye) (Lal, 1999).

Turmeric has been used for centuries in Ayurvedic medicine as a treatment for inflammatory disorders including arthritis. On the basis of this traditional usage, dietary supplements containing turmeric rhizome and turmeric extracts are also being used in the western world for arthritis treatment and prevention. A preliminary trial in people with rheumatoid arthritis has indicated curcumin to be somewhat useful in reducing inflammation and symptoms such as pain and stiffness (Deodhar *et al.*, 1980). In a separate double-blind trial curcumin was found to be superior to placebo or phenylbutazone, a non steroidal anti inflammatory drug (NSAID) for alleviating post-surgical inflammation (Satoskar *et al.*, 1986).

Crude or refined essential oil extracts dramatically inhibited joint swelling (90-100 per cent inhibition) in female rats with streptococcal cell wall–induced arthritis when extracts were administered via intra peritoneal injection to maximize uniform delivery. However, Janet *et al.* (2010) observed that this antiarthritic effect was accompanied by significant morbidity and mortality. But though the oral administration of a 20-fold higher dose of the oil was non-toxic, it was only mildly joint-protective (20 per cent inhibition) (Funk *et al.*, 2010).

Curcumin also has been suggested for osteoarthritis. Thus turmeric is suggested in the management of rheumatoid and osteoarthritis because of its powerful anti-inflammatory properties as it helps to alleviate pain and stiffness associated with inflammation. It can be taken internally or topically. Funk *et al.* (2006a, b) found the essential oil-depleted turmeric fraction containing 41 per cent of the three major curcuminoids profoundly inhibited joint inflammation and periarticular joint destruction in a dose-dependent manner when treatment was started before, but not after, the onset of joint inflammation. A commercial sample containing 94 per cent of the three major curcuminoids was more potent in preventing arthritis than the essential oil-depleted turmeric fraction when compared by total curcuminoid dose per body weight. They concluded that three major curcuminoids are responsible for this antiarthritic effect, while the remaining compounds in the crude turmeric extract may inhibit this protective effect.

Based on the available pharmacological data obtained from *in vitro* and *in vivo* research, as well as clinical trials, Shehzad *et al.* (2012) foresee an opportunity to translate curcumin into clinics for the prevention of inflammatory diseases in the near future.

Gastrointestinal Disorders

Turmeric is an antacid, and, in small doses, acts as a carminative, stomachic, appetizer and tonic. In large doses, however, it appears to act as an antispasmodic inhibiting excessive peristaltic movement of the intestines. For ulcer curcumin is taken with meals to avoid possible stomach and intestinal ulcerations. Groups of 10 albino Porter strain rats received oral doses of 50 or 100 mg/kg of curcumin administered as a 2 per cent suspension in gum arabic daily for 6 days. At the high dose, gastric erosion was reported. Changes in the mucin content were reported to be the cause of the ulceration. Pretreatment with adrenergic, cholinergic, tryptaminergic and histaminergic receptor antagonists provided partial protection while metiamide pretreatment completely prevented the development of the lesions (Gupta *et al.*, 1980). Unlike standard anti-inflammatories, curcumin does not appear to cause stomach ulcers when taken in normal doses (Srimal and Dhawan, 1973). However, high doses might increase risk of ulcers (Gupta *et al.*, 1980).

An oral dose of 500mg/kg of the ethanol extract of turmeric produced significant antiulcerogenic activity in rats subjected to hypothermic-restraint stress and pyloric ligation. It also showed marked antiulcerogenic effect in indomethacin and reserpine, induced-gastric ulcers in rats. The extract had a highly significant protective effect against cytodestructive agents. Turmeric extract not only increased the gastric wall mucus significantly but also restored the non-protein sulfhydryl (NP-SH) content in the glandular stomachs of the rats (Rafatullah, *et al.*, 1990).

A double-blind placebo-controlled study including 106 people compared the effects of 500 mg curcumin 4 times daily against placebo (as well as against a locally popular over the counter treatment). After 7 days, 87 per cent of the curcumin group experienced full or partial relief of symptoms from dyspepsia as compared to 53 per cent of the placebo group (Thamlikitkul *et al.*, 1989). While a double-blind trial has found turmeric helpful for people with indigestion.

Contrary to these reports, turmeric does not appear to be effective for treating ulcers (Van Dau *et al.*, 1998; Kositchaiwat *et al.*, 1993). But there is some evidence that turmeric might be effective in its traditional role as an antiflatulent (Ammon and Wahl 1991; Thamlikitkul *et al.*, 1989).

Curcumin appears to stimulate gallbladder contractions, which may explain its traditional use for gallstones (Rasyid and Lelo 1999). However, such contractions could cause pain or serious complications. For this reason, individuals with gallbladder disease should only use curcumin on the advice of a physician. Because of its ability to stimulate the gall bladder, turmeric has also been suggested as a treatment for dyspepsia or indigestion (Thamlikitkul *et al.*, 1989). In Europe, gallbladder dysfunction or a lack of bile is thought to be the main cause of dyspepsia, however there is no evidence. Curcumin is especially recommended for hepatitis C patients.

In a randomized, multicenter, double-blind, placebo-controlled trial to assess the efficacy of curcumin as maintenance therapy in patients with quiescent ulcerative colitis, recurrence rates in curcumin-treated patients were significantly lower than in the placebo group (Hanai *et al.*, 2006). The mice receiving curcumin not only lost much less weight than the control animals, but when researchers checked their intestinal cell function, all the signs typical of colitis (mucosal ulceration, thickening of the intestinal wall, and the infiltration of inflammatory cells) were all much reduced. While the researchers are not yet sure exactly how curcumin achieves its protective effects, they think its benefits are the result of not only antioxidant activity, but also inhibition of a major cellular inflammatory agent called NF kappa-B. Although curcumin has been shown to be safe up to levels as high as 10 percent (100,000 ppm), the researchers showed effectiveness at a concentration as low as 0.25 per cent. This dose was well tolerated with no reduction in dietary intake. Thus curcumin is proved to be a cheap, well-tolerated, and effective therapy for inflammatory bowel disease. This food ingredient has for generations been regarded as a potent anti-inflammatory within many eastern civilizations.

In multidrug resistance gene deficient mice that spontaneously develop intestinal inflammation predominantly in the colon, addition of curcumin to the diet significantly reduced the histological signs of colonic inflammation (Nones *et al.*, 2009).

Diabetes

Medicinal effects of the essential oil in vertebrates have also been reported for stroke and diabetes. A single acute dose of 250-500 mg/kg oral or intraperitonial administration was neuroprotective in rats subjected to occlusive or embolic strokes (Rathore *et al.*, 2008; Dohare *et al.*, 2008a,b), while chronic dietary supplementation of essential oil (620 mg/kg/d) normalized serum glucose in diabetic mice (Nishiyama *et al.*, 2005, Honda *et al.*, 2006). Curcumin may ameliorate the damaging effects of long-term diabetes (Arun and Nalini, 2002) and is also recommended as a topical treatment to speed diabetic wound healing (Phan *et al.*, 2001).

Curcuma longa rhizome extract showed blood glucose lowering activity in experimentally induced–diabetic rats. After 3 and 6 hrs of curcuma injection (10 mg), there was a reduction by 37.2 percent and 54.5 percent respectively in the glucose levels (Tank *et al.*, 1990). Suryanarayana *et al.* (2007) observed that curcumin and turmeric controlled oxidative stress by inhibiting the increase in TBARS and protein carbonyls and reversing altered antioxidant enzyme activities without altering the hyperglycemic state in most of the tissues in STZ-induced hyperglycemic rats.

Lekshmi *et al.* (2012a) found the volatile oil of turmeric to inhibit glucosidase enzymes more effectively than the reference standard drug acarbose. Drying of rhizomes was found to enhance α-glucosidase and α-amylase inhibitory capacities of volatile oils. Ar-Turmerone, the major volatile component in the rhizome also showed potent α-glucosidase and α-amylase inhibition. Lekshmi and her colleagues (2012b) have also found turmerin to showgood DPPH and superoxide and moderate ABTS radical scavenging and Fe (II) chelation capacities. These results rationalise the traditional usage of turmeric rhizome preparations against diabetes.

Many of these therapeutic actions can be attributed to its potent antioxidant and anti-inflammatory activities. In view of the oxidative stress and inflammatory mechanisms of DM, curcumin can be considered suitable for the prevention and amelioration of diabetes (Meng *et al.*, 2012).

Obesity and type II diabetes mellitus are often associated with hyperleptinemia and commonly accompanied by nonalcoholic steatohepatitis, which could cause hepatic fibrosis. Tang and Chen (2010) found curcumin to eliminate stimulatory effects of leptin on hepatic stellate cells (HSC) activation and increased AMPK activity, leading to inducing expression of genes relevant to lipid accumulation and elevating the level of intracellular lipids.

Lin and colleagues (2011; 2012a,b) reported that curcumin inhibited the activation of hepatic stellate cells *in vitro*, a hallmark of non-alcoholic steatohepatitis and hepatic fibrogenesis associated with type 2 diabetes mellitus. They demonstrated that curcumin suppresses the advanced glycation end-products (AGEs)-mediated induction of the receptor for AGEs (RAGE) gene expression by increasing PPARγ activity and stimulating de novo synthesis of glutathione. As a result, downstream elements of RAGE-activated pathways are inhibited, which prevents oxidative stress, inflammation and hepatic stellate cell activation. On the basis of this report Stefanska (2012) suggested that curcumin may be a potential anti-fibrotic agent in type 2 diabetes and in liver conditions of different aetiology and in other disorders linked to the impairment of PPARγ activity, such as obesity and atherosclerosis.

Turmeric and Cancer

More recently, curcumin's therapeutic potential for preventing and treating various cancers is being recognized. As curcumin's therapeutic promise is being explored more systematically in various diseases, it has become clear that, due to its increased bioavailability in the gastrointestinal tract, curcumin may be particularly suited to treat gastrointestinal diseases.

Turmeric has been shown to inhibit chemical carcinogenesis. Curcumin inhibits colon cancer cell proliferation *in vitro* mainly by accumulating cells in the G2/M phase and that this effect is independent of its ability to inhibit prostaglandin synthesis. Curcumin is a strong inhibitor of arachidonic acid-induced edema of mouse ears *in vivo* and epidermal cyclooxygenase and lipoxygenase activities *in vitro*. (Huang *et al.*, 1997). Its mechanism of action is unknown but according to Hanif *et al.* (1997) curcumin may act by inhibiting arachidonic acid metabolism.

Curcumin has shown some promise in the prevention of oral carcinogenesis. In the 7, 12-dimethylbenz[a]anthracene (DMBA) hamster buccal pouch model of carcinogenesis, curcumin alone (Krishnaswamy *et al.*, 1998), or when administered together with piperine significantly reduced the formation of oral carcinoma, probably due to its anti-lipid peroxidative and antioxidant potential together with its effect on modulating carcinogen detoxification. Furthermore, its role in the attenuation of colonic cancer in animal models has also been established.

Li *et al.* (2002) observed that tea alone and in combination with curcumin significantly increased the apoptotic index in dysplasia and squamous cell carcinoma (SCC). Curcumin, alone and in combination with tea, significantly inhibited the angiogenesis in papilloma and SCC. The results suggested that green tea and curcumin had inhibitory effects against oral carcinogenesis at the post-initiation stage and such inhibition may be related to the suppression of cell proliferation, induction of apoptosis and inhibition of angiogenesis.

In the invasive oral squamous carcinoma cell line, curcumin exhibited anti-motility activity which was mediated by the inhibition of MAPK/ERK and NF-êB signaling and consequently down-regulation of proteolytic enzymes such as urokinase-type plasminogen activator and matrix metalloproteinases (Shin *et al.*, 2010). In the esophageal squamous cell carcinoma cell line HKESC-1, curcumin partially reversed the mitogenic effect of prostaglandin E2 (PGE2) that has been implicated in its growth. The chemopreventive effect in esophageal cancer has also been studied in rats with N-nitrosomethylbenzylamine (NMBA)-induced esophageal carcinogenesis, curcumin inhibited incidence and multiplicity of preneoplastic lesions when given during the post initiation phase and the initiation phase (Ushida *et al.*, 2000).

To prevent certain cancers curcumin acts like a "hypnotist" with cancer cells, tricking them into programming their own destruction. This process is called apoptosis. Curcumin induces cancer cell apoptosis. Cancer researchers are focusing on agents that induce apoptosis as the next generation of cancer drugs. One of the most effective nutrients available to induce apoptosis may be curcumin. Cancer patients should be taking 2000 mg to 4000 mg a day of curcumin extract with a heavy meal. In a wide range of cancer cells, curcumin has been shown to induce cell shrinkage, chromatin condensation, DNA fragmentation and block cellular signal transduction, all of which are characteristics of apoptosis. Curcumin inhibits tumourigenesis during both initiation and promotion (post-initiation) periods in several experimental animal models. Topical application of curcumin inhibits TPA-induced increases in the percent of epidermal cells in synthetic (S) phase of the cell cycle. In isolation, these compounds have demonstrated bioactivity *in vitro*, including cytotoxic and apoptotic effects in various cells (Aratanechemuge *et al.*, 2002, Ji *et al.*, 2004).

Nagabhushan and his colleagues (1987, 1988 and 1992) have shown that the curcumin in turmeric can inhibit the mutagenicity of polycyclic aromatic hydrocarbons (PAHs) (carcinogenic chemicals created by the burning of carbon based fuels including cigarette smoke), inhibit radiation-induced chromosome damage, prevent the formation of harmful heterocyclic amines and nitroso compounds, which may enter the body through certain processed foods, such as processed meat products that contain nitrosamines and irreversibly inhibit the multiplication of leukemia cells.

Curcumin present at micromolar concentration is able to inhibit the growth of estrogen-positive human breast MCF-7 cells induced individually or by a mixture of the pesticides endosulfane, DDT and chlordane or 17-beta estradiol. When curcumin and genistein were added together to MCF-7 cells, a synergistic effect resulting in a total inhibition of the induction of MCF-7 cells by the highly estrogenic activity of endosulfane/chlordane/DDT mixtures was noted. Thus it is evident that the combination of curcumin and genistein in the diet has the potential to reduce the proliferation of estrogen positive cells by mixtures of pesticides or 17-beta estradiol. Since it is difficult to remove pesticides completely from the environment or the diet, and since both turmeric and soybeans are not toxic to humans, their inclusion in the diet in order to prevent hormone related cancers deserves consideration (Duncan *et al.*, 1999). Curcumin acts upon oxidative stress in human breast epithelial cells transformed by the effect of radiation in the presence of estrogen (Calaf *et al.*, 2011).

The chemopreventive efficacy of an aqueous turmeric extract and its constituents, curcumin-free aqueous turmeric extract and curcumin given 2 weeks before, during and after the carcinogen treatment to female Swiss mice was demonstrated by Azuine *et al.* (1992) by significant inhibiton of the incidence and multiplicity of forestomach tumours. Menon *et al.* (1999) found that curcumin effectively inhibited metastasis (uncontrolled spread) of melanoma (skin cancer) cells. This may be due to its antioxidant activity in the body.

Contrary to the many remarkably encouraging reports on curcumin's anti-cancer benefits, there are sporadic reports that curcumin interfered with, rather than potentiated, the effects of anti-cancer chemotherapy (Somasundaram *et al.*, 2002). Another study found no significant therapeutic effect against prostate cancer (Imaida *et al.*, 2001) a finding that stands in stark contrast to numerous other studies that have noted significant anti-prostate cancer activity by curcumin (Nakamura *et al.*, 2002; Dorai *et al.*, 2001). This contradiction has led some experts to caution against taking curcumin during chemotherapy, except under an oncologist's supervision.

Turmeric on Heart Health

Researchers in Egypt noted that curcumin protected rats from oxidative stress injury following experimentally induced stroke (Ghoneim, 2002). But rats fed a diet causing high blood sugar, when received high doses of curcumin actually developed cataracts somewhat faster, (Suryanarayana *et al.*, 2003) possibly due to increased oxidative stress. Srivastava *et al.* (1985) have shown turmeric to be able to reduce platelets from clumping together, which in turn improves circulation and may help protect against atherosclerosis. In laboratory tests on animals and *in vitro*, scientists have shown that curcumin prevents lipid peroxidation and the oxidation of cellular and subcellular membranes that are associated with atherosclerosis (Sreejayan and Rao, 1994; Quiles *et al.*, 1998; 2002; Ramirez-Tortosa 1999; Mesa *et al.*, 2003).

Moreover, curcumin acts to lower total cholesterol levels. Perhaps even more important, it prevents peroxidation of LDL cholesterol. Since curcumin is an antioxidant it is capable of destroying the free radicals that lead to lipid peroxidation. It raises HDL cholesterol levels, even as it reduces LDL levels. In a small study of human volunteers, Mesa *et al.* (2003) reported a highly significant 29 per cent increase in HDL among subjects who consumed 500 mg of curcumin per day for seven days. Subjects also experienced a decrease in total serum cholesterol of more than 11 per cent, and a decrease in serum lipid peroxides of 33 per cent (Soni and Kuttan, 1992). Though further human studies are needed, these findings are promising. Mesa *et al.* (2003) also noted that curcumin may prevent the effects caused by a high fat diet on cholesterol during development of atherosclerosis.

Very recently it has been found that curcumin pretreatment attenuates the I/R injury as evidenced by (a) loss of cardiac mechanical work, (b) oxidant stress (increase in lipid peroxidation and decrease in reduced glutathione content) and (c) decrease in the activity of the antioxidant enzymes superoxide dismutase and glutathione reductase in both cardiac tissue and isolated mitochondria, and (d) decrease in mitochondrial respiratory capacity (González-Salazar *et al.*, 2011).

The volatile oil is significantly active in removing sputum, relieving cough and preventing asthma (Li *et al.*, 1998).

Turmeric as an Antifertility Agent

The petroleum ether, alcoholic and aqueous extracts of rhizomes of *Curcuma longa* inhibited fertility when administered on days 1-7 of pregnancy at doses of 100 or 200 mg/kg to female albino rats. Studies on rabbits on the contrary did not produce anti-ovulatory effects (Garg *et al.*, 1978, Garg, 1974).

Other Benefits of Turmeric

Curcumin has been shown to be a potential treatment for multiple sclerosis (Natarajan and Bright, 2002, Arun and Nalini, 2002). Curcuminoids are shown to possess significant antihepatotoxic action. An extract of the crude drug "ukon", the rhizomes of turmeric, exhibited intense preventive activity against carbon tetrachloride-induced liver injury *in vivo* and *in vitro* (Kiso *et al.*, 1983).

Some studies have noted a link between turmeric consumption and a decreased incidence of Alzheimer's disease, an effect that may well be related to curcumin's ability to block signaling pathways that lead to inflammation (Lim *et al.*, 2001, Kim *et al.*, 2001). In animal models of AD, curcumin reduced levels of amyloid and oxidized proteins and prevented cognitive deficits. The interaction of curcumin with Cu and Fe suggested another potential mechanism by which it could mediate its effects against AD animal models (Baum and Ng, 2004). The doctors at the All India Institute of Medical Sciences have found that turmeric can cure epilepsy, too. They have also found it effective in boosting memory and reducing stress as turmeric, when administered orally with phenytoin, significantly prevented cognitive impairment and oxidative stress. Ezz *et al.* (2011) and Du *et al.* (2012) have shown the anticonvulsant activity of curcumin in the pilocarpine rat model of seizures, and that modulation of free radicals and nitric oxide synthase may be involved in this effect.

Curcumin and valproate (standard drug) ameliorated most of the changes in amino acid concentrations and reduced the histopathological abnormalities including seizures, in the pilocarpine-induced epileptic rats suggesting that the antiepileptic effect of curcumin can find its use as an anticonvulsant (Noor *et al.*, 2012).

Xu *et al.* (2011) explained the neuroprotection and modulation of neuroplasticity exhibited in his study by curcumin against corticosterone and its relation to 5-hydroxy tryptamine (5-HT) receptors might be mediated, at least in part, via the 5-HT receptor-cAMP-PKA-CREB signal pathway.

Safety Issues

Because it has been consumed safely by millions of people literally for millennia, turmeric is a safe food ingredient. Turmeric is not a commonly allergenic food and is not known to contain measurable amounts of goitrogens, oxalates, or purines.

Turmeric is on the FDA's GRAS (generally recognized as safe) list, and curcumin, too, is believed to be extremely nontoxic (Ammon and Wahl, 1991; Shankar *et al.*, 1980). Side effects are rare and if at all, are generally limited to the usual mild stomach distress. However, safety on those with severe liver or kidney disease has not been established. Due to curcumin's effects on the gallbladder, individuals with gallbladder disease should use curcumin only on the advice of a physician. It has been used in large quantities as a condiment with no adverse reactions. However, curcumin is poorly absorbed by the gut. But its absorption and bioavailability are significantly enhanced by the addition of piperine, a natural alkaloid derived from black pepper. Interestingly, this again is a traditional practice in India, as the recipes usually have both these ingredients. LD (50) has been said to be 4.7mg/kg body weight. In the sub acute models LD (50), was 10 to 20 mg/kg body weight.

Interestingly, Sharma *et al.* (2009) demonstrated that curcumin exerts a protective effect against aluminium-induced elevation of ageing-related changes by modulating the extent of oxidative stress (by upregulating the activities of antioxidant enzymes) and by regulating the activities of Na(+), K(+) ATPase, PKC and AChE, suggesting that curcumin counters aluminium-induced enhancement in ageing-related processes. Bala *et al.* (2006) also demonstrated the antioxidative, antilipofusinogenesic and anti-ageing effects of curcumin in the brain.

Conclusions

Although the pharmacological safety of curcumin promises a great potential for treatment and prevention of various diseases, the relatively low bioavailability of curcumin is a major hurdle for clinical development. The nanotechnology-based approaches to increase curcumin delivery *in vivo* are evolving and are very promising in overcoming the problem of bioavailability of curcumin. It is a high potential drug for gastrointestinal cancers and inflammatory diseases as well as liver fibrosis. Curcumin appears to prevent certain cancers, inhibit cardiovascular disease, and quell inflammation, and may even offer protection against Alzheimer's disease.

References

Abas F, Lajis NH, Shaari K, Israf DA, Stanslas J, Yusuf UK, and Raof SM (2005). A labdane diterpene glucoside from the rhizomes of Curcuma longa. J. Nat. Prod. 68: 1090–93.

Aboul Ezz HS, Khadrawy YA, Noor NA (2011). The Neuroprotective Effect of Curcumin and Nigella sativa Oil Against Oxidative Stress in the Pilocarpine Model of Epilepsy: A Comparison with Valproate. Neurochem Res. 2011 Jul 13. [Epub ahead of print].

Akram M, Shahab-Uddin, Khan AA, Chani U, Hanan A, Mohiuddin E and Asif M (2010). Curcuma longa and Curcumin- A review article. Rom. J. Plant. Biol. 55: 65–72.

Ammon HPT, Wahl MA (1991). Pharmacology of Curcuma longa. Planta. Med. 57: 1–7.

Apisariyakul A, Vanittanakom N, Buddhasukh D (1995). Antifungal activity of turmeric oil extracted from Curcuma longa (Zingiberaceae) *J. Ethnopharmacol.* 49: 163–69.

Aratanechemuge Y, Komiya T, Moteki H, Katsuzaki H, Imai K, Hibasami H (2002). Selective induction of apoptosis by ar-turmerone isolated from turmeric (Curcuma longa L) in two human leukemia cell lines, but not in human stomach cancer cell line. *Int. J. Mol. Med.* 9: 481–84.

Arora RB, Basu N, Kapoor V, Jain AP (1971). Anti-inflammatory studies on *Curcuma longa* (turmeric). *Ind. J. Med. Res.* 59: 1289–95.

Arun N, Nalini N (2002). Efficacy of turmeric on blood sugar and polyol pathway in diabetic albino rats. Plant Foods Hum. Nutr. 57 (1): 41–52.

Azuine MA, Kayal JJ, Bhide SV (1992). Protective role of aqueous turmeric extract against mutagenicity of direct-acting carcinogens as well as benzo [alpha] pyrene-induced genotoxicity and carcinogenicity. J. Cancer Res. Clin. Oncol. 118 (6): 447–52.

Bala K, Tripathy BC, Sharma D (2006). Neuroprotective and anti-ageing effects of curcumin in aged rat brain regions. Biogerontology. 7 (2): 81–89.

Barthelemy S, Vergnes L, Moynier M, *et al.* (1998). Curcumin and curcumin derivatives inhibit Tat-mediated transactivation of type 1 human immunodeficiency virus long terminal repeat. *Res. Virol.* 149: 43–52.

Baum L, Ng A (2004). Curcumin interaction with copper and iron suggests one possible mechanism of action in Alzheimer's disease animal models. J. Alzheimers. Dis. 6: 367–77; discussion 443–49.

Calaf GM, Echiburú-Chau C, Roy D, Chai Y, Wen G, Balajee AS (2011). Protective role of curcumin in oxidative stress of breast cells. Oncol. Rep. 26 (4): 1029–35.

Chainani-Wu N (2003). Safety and anti-inflammatory activity of curcumin: a component of tumeric (Curcuma longa) *J. Altern. Complement. Med.* 9: 161-168.

Chattopadhyay I, Biswas K, Bandyopadhyay U, and Banerjee RK (2004). Turmeric and curcumin: Biological actions and medicinal applications. Curr. Sci. 87: 44–50.

Deodhar SD, Sethi R, Srimal RC. (1980). Preliminary study on antirheumatic activity of curcumin (diferuloyl methane). Indian J. Med. Res. 71: 632–34.

Dohare P, Garg P, Sharma U, Jagannathan NR, Ray M (2008a). Neuroprotective efficacy and therapeutic window of curcuma oil: in rat embolic stroke model. *BMC Complem. Altern. Med.* 8: 55.

Dohare P, Varma S, Ray M (2008b). Curcuma oil modulates the nitric oxide system response to cerebral ischemia/reperfusion injury. *Nitric Oxide.* 19: 1 -11.

Dorai T, Cao YC, Dorai B, Buttyan R, Katz AE (2001).Therapeutic potential of curcumin in human prostate cancer. III. Curcumin inhibits proliferation, induces apoptosis, and inhibits angiogenesis of LNCaP prostate cancer cells *in vivo*. Prostate. 47 (4): 293–303.

DU P, Tang HY, Li X, Lin HJ, Peng WF, Ma Y, Fan W, Wang X (2012). Anticonvulsive and antioxidant effects of curcumin on pilocarpine-induced seizures in rats. Chin. Med. J. (Engl).125 (11): 1975–79.

Duncan AM, Merz BE, Xu X, Nagel TC, Phipps WR, Kurzer MS (1999). Soy isoflavones exert modest hormonal effects in premenopausal women. J. Clin. Endocrinol. Metab. 84 (1): 192–97.

Ezz HS, Khadrawy YA, Noor NA (2011). The neuroprotective effect of curcumin and Nigella sativa oil against oxidative stress in the pilocarpine model ofepilepsy: a comparison with valproate. Neurochem. Res. 36 (11): 2195–204.

Ferreira LA, Henriques OB, Andreoni AA, Vital GR, Campos MM, Habermehl GG, de Moraes VL. (1992) Antivenom and biological effects of ar-turmerone isolated from Curcuma longa (Zingiberaceae)[erratum appears in Toxicon. 30 (12): 1637] *Toxicon.* 30: 1211–18.

Funk JL, Frye JB, Oyarzo JN, Kuscuoglu N, Wilson J, McCaffrey G, Stafford G, Chen G, Lantz RC, Jolad SD, Solyom AM, Kiela PR, Timmermann BN (2006a). Efficacy and mechanism of action of turmeric supplements in the treatment of experimental arthritis. *Arthritis Rheum.* 54 (11): 3452–64.

Funk JL, Frye JB, Oyarzo JN, Zhang H, Barbara N, Timmermann BN (2010). Antiarthritic Effects and Toxicity of the Essential Oils of Turmeric (Curcuma longa L.) J. Agric. Food Chem. 58 (2): 842–49.

Funk JL, Oyarzo JN, Frye JB, Chen G, Lantz RC, Jolad SD, Solyom AM, Timmermann BN (2006b). Turmeric extracts containing curcuminoids prevent experimental rheumatoid arthritis. *J. Nat. Prod.* 69 (3): 351–55.

Garg SK (1974). Effect of Curcuma longa (rhizomes) on fertility in experimental animals. Planta. Med. 26 (3): 225–27.

Garg SK, Mathur VS, Chaudhury RR (1978). Screening of Indian plants for antifertility activity. Indian J. Exp. Biol. 16 (10):1077–79.

Ghoneim AI, Abdel-Naim AB, Khalifa AE, El-Denshary ES (2002). Protective effects of cur cumin against ischaemis-reperfusion insult in rat forebrain. Pharmacol Res. 46 (3): 273–79.

González-Salazar A, Molina-Jijón E, Correa F, Zarco-Márquez G, Calderón-Oliver M, Tapia E, Zazueta C, Pedraza-Chaverri J (2011). Curcumin Protects from Cardiac Reperfusion Damage by Attenuation of Oxidant Stress and Mitochondrial Dysfunction. Cardiovasc. Toxicol. 2011 Jul 19. [Epub ahead of print].

Gujral ML, Choudhury NK, Saxena PN (1953). The effect of certain indigenous remedies on the healing of wounds and ulcers. J Indian Med Assoc. 22 (7):273–76.

Gupta B, Kulshrestha VK, Srivastava RK *et al.* (1980). Mechanisms of curcumin induced gastric ulcer in rats. Indian J. Med. Res. 71: 806–14.

Hanai H, Iida T, Takeuchi K, Watanabe F, Maruyama Y, Andoh A, Tsujikawa T, Fujiyama Y, Mitsuyama K, Sata M, *et al.* (2006). Curcumin maintenance therapy for ulcerative colitis: randomized, multicenter, double-blind, placebo-controlled trial. Clin Gastroenterol Hepatol. 4: 1502–506.

Hanif R, Qiao L, Shiff SJ, Rigas B (1997). Curcumin, a natural plant phenolic food additive, inhibits cell proliferation and induces cell cycle changes in colon adenocarcinoma cell lines by a prostaglandin-independent pathway. Lab. Clin. Med. 130 (6): 576–84.

Honda S, Aoki F, Tanaka H, Kishida H, Nishiyama T, Okada S, Matsumoto I, Abe K, Mae T (2006). Effects of ingested turmeric oleoresin on glucose and lipid metabolisms in obese diabetic mice: a DNA microarray study. *J. Agric. Food Chem.* 54: 9055–62.

Huang AC, Lin SY, Su CC, Lin SS, Ho CC, Hsia TC, Chiu TH, Yu CS, Ip SW, Lin TP, Chung JG (2008). Effects of curcumin on N-bis(2-hydroxypropyl) nitrosamine (DHPN)-induced lung and liver tumourigenesis in BALB/c mice *in vivo*. *In vivo*. 22 (6): 781–85.

Imaida K, Tamano S, Kato K, Ikeda Y, Asamoto M, Takahashi S, Nir Z, Murakoshi M, Nishino H, Shirai T (2001). Lack of chemopreventive effects of lycopene and curcumin on experimental rat prostate carcinogenesis. Carcinogenesis. 22 (3): 467–72.

Jain V, Prasad V, Pal R, Singh S (2007). Standardization and stability studies of neuroprotective lipid soluble fraction obtained from Curcuma longa. *J. Pharm. Biomed. Anal.* 44: 1079–86.

Janet L. Funk, Jennifer B. Frye, Janice N. Oyarzo, Huaping Zhang and Barbara N. Timmermann (2010). Anti-Arthritic Effects and Toxicity of the Essential Oils of Turmeric (Curcuma longa L.). J. Agric. Food Chem. 58 (2): 842–49.

Jayaprakasha GK, Jena BS, Negi PS, Sakariah KK. (2002) Evaluation of antioxidant activities and antimutagenicity of turmeric oil: a byproduct from curcumin production. *Z. Naturforsch. [C]* 57: 828–35.

Ji M, Choi J, Lee J, Lee Y (2004). Induction of apoptosis by ar-turmerone on various cell lines. *Int. J. Mol. Med.* 14: 253–56.

Joshi J, Ghaisas S, Vaidya A, Vaidya R, Kamat DV, Bhagwat AN, Bhide S (2003). Early human safety study of turmeric oil (Curcuma longa oil) administered orally in healthy volunteers. *J. Assoc. Physicians India.* 51:1055–60.

Kim DS, Park SY, Kim JK (2001). Curcuminoids from Curcuma longa L. (Zingiberaceae) that protect PC12 rat pheochromocytoma and normal human umbilical vein endothe- lial cells from beta (1-42) insult. Neurosci. Lett. 303 (1): 57–61.

Kim KJ, Yu HH, Cha JD, Seo SJ, Choi NY, You YO (2005). Antibacterial activity of Curcuma longa L. against methicillin-resistant Staphylococcus aureus. Phytother. Res. 19 (7): 599–604.

Kim WK, Ke K, Sul OJ, Kim HJ, Kim SH, Lee MH, Kim HJ, Kim SY, Chung HT, Choi HS (2011). Curcumin protects against ovariectomy-induced bone loss and decreases osteoclastogenesis. J. Cell. Biochem. 2011 Jul 5. [Epub ahead of print].

Kiso Y, Suzuki Y, Watanabe N, Oshima Y, Hikino H (1983). Antihepatotoxic Principles of Curcuma longa Rhizomes1. Planta. Med. 49 (11): 185–87.

Kiuchi F, Goto Y, Sugimoto N, Akao N, Kondo K, Tsuda Y (1993). Nematocidal activity of turmeric: synergistic action of curcuminoids. Chem. Pharm. Bull. (Tokyo). 41 (9): 1640–43.

Kositchaiwat C, Kositchaiwat S, Havanondha J (1993). *Curcuma longa* Linn. in the treatment of gastric ulcer comparison to liquid antacid: a controlled clinical trial. J. Med. Assoc. Thai. 76: 601–605.

Krishnaswamy K, Goud VK, Sesikeran B, Mukundan MA, Krishna TP. (1998) Retardation of experimental tumourigenesis and reduction in DNA adducts by turmeric and curcumin. Nutr. Cancer. 30: 163–66.

Lal B, Kapoor AK, Asthana OP, *et al.* (1999). Efficacy of curcumin in the management of chronic anterior uveitis. Phytother. Res. 13: 318–13.

Lantz RC, Chen GJ, Solyom AM, Jolad SD, Timmermann BN (2005). The effect of turmeric extracts on inflammatory mediator production. *Phytomedicine.* 12: 445–52.

Lekshmi PC, Arimboor R, Indulekha PS, Menon AN (2012a). Turmeric (*Curcuma longa* L.) volatile oil inhibits key enzymes linked to type 2 diabetes. Int. J. Food Sci. Nutr. 63 (7): 832–34.

Lekshmi PC, Arimboor R, Raghu KG, Menon AN (2012b). Turmerin, the antioxidant protein from turmeric (*Curcuma longa*) exhibits antihyperglycaemic effects. Nat. Prod. Res. 26 (17): 1654–58.

Li C, Li L, Luo J, Huang N (1998). Effect of turmeric volatile oil on the respiratory tract. China Journal of Chinese Materia Medica. 23 (10): 624–25.

Li N, Chen X, Liao J, Yang G, Wang S, Josephson Y, Han C, Chen J, Huang MT, Yang CS (2002). Inhibition of 7,12-dimethylbenz[a]anthracene (DMBA)-induced oral carcinogenesis in hamsters by tea and curcumin. Carcinogenesis. 23: 1307–313.

Lim GP, Chu T, Yang F, Beech W, Frautschy SA, Cole GM (2001). The curry spice curcumin reduces oxidative damage and amyloid pathology in an Alzheimer transgenic mouse. J. Neurosci. 21 (21): 8370–77.

Lin J, Chen A (2011). Curcumin diminishes the impacts of hyperglycemia on the activation of hepatic stellate cells by suppressing membrane translocation and gene expression of glucose transporter-2. Mol. Cell. Endocrinol. 333 (2): 160–71.

Lin J, Tang Y, Kang Q, Chen A (2012b). Curcumin eliminates the inhibitory effect of advanced glycation end-products (AGEs) on gene expression of AGE receptor-1 in hepatic stellate cells *in vitro*. Lab. Invest. 92 (6): 827–41.

Lin J, Tang Y, Kang Q, Feng Y, Chen A (2012a). Curcumin inhibits gene expression of receptor for advanced glycation end-products (RAGE) in hepatic stellate cells *in vitro* by elevating PPARγ activity and attenuating oxidative stress. Br. J. Pharmacol. 166 (8): 2212–27.

Meng B, Li J, Cao H (2012). Antioxidant and anti-inflammatory activities of curcumin on diabetes mellitus and its complications. Curr. Pharm. Des. 2012 Oct 23. [Epub ahead of print].

Menon LG, Kuttan R, Kuttan G (1999). Anti-metastatic activity of curcumin and catechin. *Cancer Lett.* 141:159–65.

Mesa MD, Aguilera CM, Ramirez-Tortosa CL (2003). Oral administration of a turmeric extract inhibits erythrocyte and liver micro- some membrane oxidation in rabbits fed with an atherogenic diet. Nutrition. 19 (9): 800–804.

Nagabhushan M, Amonkar AJ, Bhide SV (1987). *In vitro* antimutagenicity of curcumin against environmental mutagens. Food Chem. Toxicol. 25 (7): 545–47.

Nagabhushan M, Bhide SV. (1992) Curcumin as an inhibitor of cancer. J. Am. Coll. Nutr. 11 (2): 192–98.

Nagabhushan M, Nair UJ, Amonkar AJ, D'Souza AV, Bhide SV (1988). Curcumins as inhibitors of nitrosation *in vitro*. Mutat. Res. 202 (1):163–69.

Nakamura K, Yasunaga Y, Segawa T, (2002) Curcumin down-regulates AR gene expres- sion and activation in prostate cancer cell lines. Int J Oncol. 21 (4):825-30.

Natarajan C, Bright JJ (2002). Curcumin inhibits experimental allergic encephalomyelitis by blocking signaling through janus kinase- STAT pathway in T lymphocytes IL-12. J. Immunol. 168 (12): 6506–513.

Negi PS, Jayaprakasha GK, Jagan Mohan Rao L, Sakariah KK (1999). Antibacterial activity of turmeric oil: a byproduct from curcumin manufacture. *J. Agric. Food Chem.* 47: 4297–300.

Nilani P, Duraisamy B, Dhamodaran P, Ravichandran P, Elango K (2010). Effect of Selected Antiasthmatic Plant Constituents Against Micro Organism Causing Upper Respiratory Tract Infection. Anc. Sci.Life. 29 (3): 30–32.

Nishiyama T, Mae T, Kishida H, Tsukagawa M, Mimaki Y, Kuroda M, Sashida Y, Takahashi K, Kawada T, Nakagawa K, Kitahara M (2005). Curcuminoids and sesquiterpenoids in turmeric (*Curcuma longa* L.) suppress an increase in blood glucose level in type 2 diabetic KK-Ay mice. *J. Agric. Food Chem.* 53: 959–63.

Nones K, Dommels YE, Martell S, Butts C, McNabb WC, Park ZA, Zhu S, Hedderley D, Barnett MP, Roy NC (2009). The effects of dietary curcumin and rutin on colonic inflammation and gene expression in multidrug resistance gene-deficient (mdr1a-/-) mice, a model of inflammatory bowel diseases. Br. J. Nutr. 101: 169–81.

Noor NA, Aboul Ezz HS, Faraag AR, Khadrawy YA (2012). Evaluation of the antiepileptic effect of curcumin and *Nigella sativa* oil in the pilocarpine model of epilepsy in comparison with valproate. Epilepsy. Behav. 24 (2): 199–206.

Phan TT, See P, Lee ST, Chan SY (2001). Protective effects of curcumin against oxidative damage on skin cells *in vitro*: its implication for wound healing. J Trauma. 51 (5): 927–31.

Quiles JL, Aguilera C, Mesa MD, Ramirez- Tortosa MC, Baro L, Gil A (1998). An ethanolic- aqueous extract of *Curcuma longa* decreases the susceptibility of liver microsomes and mitochondria to lipid peroxidation in atherosclerotic rabbits. Biofactors. 8 (1- 2): 51–57.

Quiles JL, Mesa MD, Ramirez-Tortosa CL (2002). *Curcuma longa* extract supplementation reduces oxidative stress and attenuates aortic fatty acid streak development in rabbits. Arterioscler. Thromb. Vasc. Biol. 22 (7): 1225–31.

Rafatullah S, Tariq M, Al-Yahya MA, Mossa JS, Ageel AM (1990). Evaluation of turmeric (*Curcuma longa*) for gastric and duodenal antiulcer activity in rats. J. Ethnopharmacol. 29 (1): 25–34.

Raghunathan K, Mittra R (1982). Pharmacognosy of Indigenous Drugs. Central Council for Research in Ayurveda and Siddha. New Delhi.

Rajasekaran SA (2011). Therapeutic potential of curcumin in gastrointestinal diseases. World J Gastrointest. Pathophysiol. 2 (1): 1–14.

Ramirez-Tortosa MC, Mesa MD, Aguilera MC (1999). Oral administration of a turmeric extract inhibits LDL oxidation and has hypocholesterolemic effects in rabbits with experimental atherosclerosis. Atherosclerosis. 147(2): 371–78.

Rao DS, Sekhara NC, Satyanarayana MN, Srinivasan (1970). Effect of curcumin on serum and liver cholesterol levels in the rat. J. Nutr. 100: 1307–15.

Rao TS, Basu N, Siddiqui HH (1982). Anti-inflammatory activity of curcumin analogues. Indian J. Med. Res.75: 574–78.

Rasyid A, Lelo A (1999). The effect of curcumin and placebo on human gall-bladder function: an ultrasound study. Aliment. Pharmacol. Ther. 13 (2): 245–49.

Rasyid A, Rahman AR, Jaalam K, Lelo A (2002). Effect of different curcumin dosages on human gall bladder. Asia Pac. J. Clin. Nutr. 11 (4): 314–18.

Rathaur P, Waseem Raja, PW. Ramteke and Suchit A John. (2012). Turmeric: The Golden Spice of Life. IJPSR. 3 (7): 1987–94.

Rathore P, Dohare P, Varma S, Ray A, Sharma U, Jagannathan NR, Ray M (2008). Curcuma oil: reduces early accumulation of oxidative product and is anti-apoptogenic in transient focal ischemia in rat brain. Neurochem. Res. 33 (9): 1672–82.

Roth GN, Chandra A, Nair MG (1998). Novel bioactivities of *Curcuma longa* constituents. J. Nat. Prod. 61: 542–45.

Satoskar RR, Shah SJ, Shenoy SG. (1986). Evaluation of anti-inflammatory property of curcumin (diferuloyl methane) in patients with postoperative inflammation. Int. J. Clin. Pharmacol. Ther. Toxicol. 24: 651–54.

Shankar TNB, Shantha NV, Ramesh HP, *et al.* (1980). Toxicity studies on turmeric (*Cucurma longa*): acute toxicity studies in rats, guinea pigs and monkeys. Indian J. Exp. Biol. 18: 73–75.

Sharma D, Sethi P, Hussain E, Singh R (2009). Curcumin counteracts the aluminium-induced ageing-related alterations in oxidative stress, Na+, K+ ATPase and protein kinase C in adult and old rat brain regions. Biogerontology. 10 (4): 489–502.

Shehzad A, Rehman G, Lee YS (2012). Curcumin in inflammatory diseases. Biofactors. 2012 Dec 22. doi: 10.1002/biof.1066. [Epub ahead of print].

Shin HK, Kim J, Lee EJ, Kim SH. (2010) Inhibitory effect of curcumin on motility of human oral squamous carcinoma YD-10B cells via suppression of ERK and NF-kappaB activations. Phytother Res. 24(4):577-82.

Somasundaram S, Edmund NA, Moore DT, Small GW, Shi YY, Orlowski RZ (2002). Dietary curcumin inhibits chemotherapy-induced apoptosis in models of human breast cancer. Cancer Res. 62 (13): 3868–75.

Soni KB, Kuttan R. (1992) Effect of oral curcumin administration on serum peroxides and cholesterol levels in human volunteers. Indian J. Physiol. Pharmacol. 36 (4): 273–75.

Sreejayan N, Rao MNA. (1996) Free radical scavenging activity of curcuminoids. Arzneimittelforschung. 46: 169–71.

Sreejayan, N. Rao MN (1994). Curcuminoids as potent inhibitors of lipid peroxidation. J Indian Physiol. Pharmacol. 46 (12): 1013–16.

Srimal RC, Dhawan BN (1973) Pharmacology of diferuloyl methane (curcumin), a non-steroidal anti-inflammatory agent. J. Pharm. Pharmacol. 25: 447–52.

Srivastava R, Dikshit M, Srimal RC, Dhawan BN (1985). Antithrombotic effect of curcumin. Thromb. Res. 40 (3): 413–17.

Stefanska B (2012). Curcumin ameliorates hepatic fibrosis in type 2 diabetes mellitus–insights into its mechanisms of action. Br. J. Pharmacol. 166 (8): 2209–211.

Suryanarayana P, Krishnaswamy K, Reddy GB (2003). Effects of curcumin on galactose-induced cataractogenesis in rats. Mol. Vis. 9: 223–30.

Suryanarayana P, Satyanarayana A, Balakrishna N, Kumar PU, Reddy GB (2007). Effect of turmeric and curcumin on oxidative stress and antioxidant enzymes in streptozotocin-induced diabetic rat. Med. Sci. Monit. 13 (12): BR 286–92.

Tank R, Sharma N and Dixit VP. (1990), curcuma longa. Indian Drugs., 27, 11, 587-589.

Tang Y, Chen A (2010). Curcumin protects hepatic stellate cells against leptin-induced activation *in vitro* by accumulating intracellular lipids. Endocrinology. 151 (9): 4168–77.

Tayyem RF, Heath DD, Al-Delaimy WK, Rock CL (2006).Curcumin content of turmeric and curry powders. Nutr. Cancer. 55 (2): 126–31.

Thamlikitkul V, Bunyapraphatsara N, Dechatiwongse T (1989). Randomized double blind study of *Curcuma domestica* Val. for dyspepsia. J. Med. Assoc. Thai. 72: 613–20.

The Wealth of India: Raw Materials (1953). Council for Scientific and Industrial Research. New Delhi. Vol. II: 402.

Toda S, Miyase T, Arichi H, Tanizawa H, Takino Y (1985). Natural antioxidants. III. Antioxidative components isolated from rhizome of *Curcuma longa* L. Chem. Pharm. Bull. (Tokyo). 33 (4): 1725–28.

USDA (2012). National Nutrient Database for Standard Reference, Release 25.

Ushida J, Sugie S, Kawabata K, Pham QV, Tanaka T, Fujii K, Takeuchi H, Ito Y, Mori H (2000). Chemopreventive effect of curcumin on N-nitrosomethylbenzylamine-induced esophageal carcinogenesis in rats. Jpn. J. Cancer Res. 91: 893–98.

Van Dau N, Ngoc Ham N, Huy Khac D *et al.* (1998). The effects of a traditional drug, turmeric (*Curcuma longa*), and placebo on the healing of duodenal ulcer. Phytomedicine. 5: 29–34.

Waghmare PF, Chaudhari AU, Karhadkar VM, Jamkhande AS (2011). Comparative evaluation of turmeric and chlorhexidine gluconate mouthwash in prevention of plaque formation and gingivitis: a clinical and microbiological study. J. Contemp. Dent. Pract. 12 (4): 221–24.

Xu Y, Li S, Vernon MM, Pan J, Chen L, Barish PA, Zhang Y, Acharya AP, Yu J, Govindarajan SS, Boykin E, Pan X, O'Donnell JM, Ogle WO (2011). Curcumin prevents corticosterone-induced neurotoxicity and abnormalities of neuroplasticity via 5-HT receptor pathway. J Neurochem. 2011 Jun 20. [Epub ahead of print].

Chapter 13

Barley

(*Hordeum vulgare* L.)

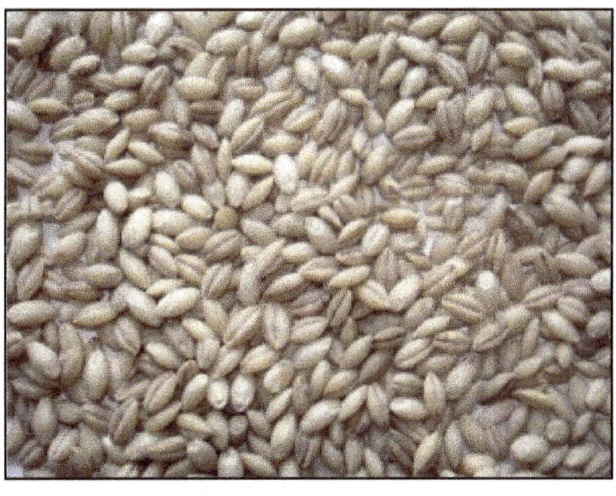

Barley is the oldest grain in the world. Traced back to 18.000 B.C, and valued in all cultures. This was considered as the holy gift of Gods 5.000 years ago in Egypt. In British Isles, Barley dates back to 3000 BC and in Scandinavia Norway: 2000–1700 B.C. This grain preceded oats in Scotland. In Eastern Europe Barley is the best crop for the high altitudes. *Barley* was cultivated in the East as food for horses and asses, and also as a staple food for the poor and for the people at large in times of distress.

Dehulled barley contains bran and germ, making it a nutritious and popular health food. It is polished through steaming, known as "pearling" to remove bran and later processed into a variety of products, including flour, flakes (similar to oatmeal), and grits.The flour made from pearl barley is known as the patent barley (Simon, 1963).

Historical Global Use of Barley

Barley seems to have been the principal bread cereal among the Hebrews, Greeks, and Romans. The Jews especially held the grain in high esteem. In Korea barley was used as a Rice extender as well as in beverages and condiments. In Tibet "tsampastsampas" a mixture of barley flour, tea and butter was a popular dish. In early 17th century, US used barley mostly for making malt and beer. It was also said to soothe and calm the bowels. Many people associate barley with making beer, but in other parts of the world it is a primary grain for food. In Asia, barley seeds are fermented and added to soybeans, salt and seaweed as a flavouring food.

Barley Fiber

β-glucan is a soluble dietary fibre fraction of barley, the levels of which range from 3 to 7.5 per cent for whole-grain and pearled products; and from 2.7 to 23 per cent for various types of barley flour products (Ames *et al.*, 2006; Dudgeon-Bollinger *et al.*, 1997; Andersson *et al.*, 2000; Kiryluk J *et al.*, 2000; Marconi *et al.*, 2000; Newman *et al.*, 1990). Variation in β-glucan among flour samples is also dependent on the method of flour extraction or sieving and particle size (Ames *et al.*, 2006; Dudgeon-Bollinger *et al.*, 1997; Kiryluk J *et al.*, 2000; Marconi *et al.*, 2000; Edney *et al.*, 1991). Many studies have reported the efficacy of β-glucan in terms of the lipid lowering effect, blood sugar reduction, weight reduction, immune-modulation, and anticarcinogenic effect). Kalra and Jood (2000) compared cultivars of barley differing in β-glucan content and showed that quantity and solubility of barley β-glucan were strong predictors of its cholesterol-lowering ability in rats. However, Wilson *et al.* (2004) showed that both high-molecular-weight and low-molecular-weight β-glucan concentrates from barley lowered cholesterol to similar levels and through similar mechanisms in hamsters.

Properties of β-glucan such as molecular weight, extractability or solubility, and viscosity potentially influence its physiological effect in the body (Bhatty, 1997; Bhatty *et al.*, 1991; Wood *et al.*, 1994; 2000; 2007; Storsley, 2001; Lazaridou and Biliaderis, 2007; Aman and Hesselman, 1984). However, the various processing techniques of barley could affect its β-glucan functionality by altering the molecular structure and viscosity without affecting the content (Wood *et al.*, 2000; Wood, 2002; Tosh 2007; Jones *et al.*, 2008).

Nutritional Value of Raw Barley

Barley is a low calorie, high fiber and micronutrient rich food. Especially it is a good source of B vitamins. Barley is not as rich a source of vitamin E.

Therapeutic Value of Barley

For many centuries man has been using barley seeds and leaves as food and medicine. Barley seeds are ground into flour for baking or processed for use as a cereal. Malt sugar, another common derivative of barley, is used as a natural laxative. In Asia, barley seeds are fermented and added to soybeans, salt, and seaweed for flavouring food. The First clinical research trial was conducted in Denmark. Barley is

Nutritional Value of Raw Barley (per 100 g)

Nutrient	*Amount*	*Nutrient*	*Amount*
Thiamine (mg)	0.19	Riboflavin (mg)	0.1
Niacin (mg)	4.6	Pantothenic acid (mg)	0.3
Pyridoxine (mg)	0.3	Folate (μg)	23.0
VitaminA (IU)	22	Energy (Cal)	352
Carbohydrate (g)	77.7	Fat (g)	1.0
Protein (g)	10	Fibre (g)	15.6
Calcium (mg)	29.0	Iron (mg)	2.5
Magnesium (mg)	79.0	Potassium (mg)	280.0
Zinc (mg)	2.1		

USDA (2012).

Nutritional Value of Cooked Pearl Barley/Cup

Nutrient	*Amount*	*Nutrient*	*Amount*
Calories (kcal)	193	Protein (g)	4
Fat (gm)	1	Carbohydrate (g)	44
Total dietary fiber (g)	6	Calcium (mg)	17
Iron (mg)	2.1	Magnesium (mg)	35
Phosphorus (mg)	85	Potassium (mg)	146
Sodium (mg)	5	Zinc (mg)	1.2
Copper (mg)	0.16	Manganese (mg)	0.4
Selenium (mcg)	13.5	Thiamin (mg)	0.13
Riboflavin (mg)	0.10	Niacin (mg)	3.23
Pantothenic acid (mg)	0.21	Vitamin B6 (mg)	0.18
Vitamin A (IU)	11	Vitamin E (mg)	0.01
Vitamin K (mcg)	1.25	Folate (mg)	25

USDA (2012).

highly valued for its dietary fiber especially, the β-glucans. The fermentability of β-glucans and their ability to form highly viscous solutions in the human gut may constitute the basis of their health benefits. Consequently, the applicability of β-glucan as a food ingredient is being widely considered with the dual purposes of increasing the fiber content of food products and enhancing their health properties (El Khoury *et al.*, 2012). Malt sugar, a common derivative of barley, is used as a natural laxative. In India Barley was used in the form of barley tea and barley water for treating type 2 diabetes. Some of the therapeutic benefits of barley are discussed below.

Diabetes

Soluble fiber from barley and oats lower the acute glucose and insulin response to a meal. Whole grain barley which has a similar glycemic index as whole wheat can reduce blood glucose response to a meal for up to 10 hours after consumption (Nilsson, *et al.*, 2006). The Glycemic Index (GI) of barley beta glucan (BB) spaghetti decreased with increasing BB concentrations. In particular, the GI of 10 per cent BB spaghetti was 54 per cent lower (P d"0.02; GI = 29) than that of the control (GI = 64). The spaghetti showed incremental areas under the curve (IAUC) values lower than that of the spaghetti without β-glucan (Chillo *et al.*, 2011). The effect was attributed to colonic fermentation of indigestible carbohydrates. Jose-Cunilleras (2004) also reported that in horses, ingestion of oat groats, corn, and barley result in similar plasma glucose area under curve and had a glycemic index of approximately 60. GI values were 78, 81, 49 and 34 for whole-wheat crackers, whole-wheat cookies, barley crackers and barley cookies respectively (Casiraghi *et al.*, 2006).

Several factors can affect glycemic and insulinemic responses from cereal foods. Some suggested factors lowering the responses are: intact botanical structure, high amylose/high ss-glucan cereal varieties, organic acid produced during fermentation and food processes inducing retrogradation of starch. Alminger and Eklund-Jonsson (2008) suggest that cereal products with beneficial influence on postprandial plasma glucose and insulin responses can be tailored by fermentation.

Comparing oat and barley, Behall *et al.* (2005) found the particle size had little effect on the glycemic responses. Both oat and barley meals reduced glycemic responses; the high soluble fiber content of barley appeared to be a factor in the greater reduction observed.

Liljeberg *et al.* (2005) observed that barley porridges produce postprandial glucose and insulin responses similar to the white wheat bread reference, suggesting that the naturally occurring dietary fiber in these whole-meal flours has no impact on the glucose tolerance. In contrast, all high fiber barley products induced significantly lower responses than did the reference product, with the glycemic and insulin indices ranging from 57 to 72 or 42 to 72 per cent, respectively. It is concluded that "lente" products of high sensory quality can be prepared from a barley genotype with an elevated content of soluble dietary fiber.

Naismith *et al.* (1991) found in the diabetic rats fed barley the blood glucose concentration, water consumption and weight loss was significant. They assume that a factor other than the fiber content of the cereals may be responsible for the difference in response. Again in adult diabetic rats, a diet containing barley had a modulating effect on the symptoms of diabetes (blood glucose concentration and water consumption) when compared with a starch or sucrose-based diet. Supplementation of the sucrose-based diet with an amount of trivalent inorganic chromium calculated to be equivalent to the available chromium in the barley-based diet abolished the differences in response to the diabetic state. Mahdi and Naismith (1991) and Mahdi *et al.* (1994) postulate that the beneficial effect of barley might be explained by its very high content of chromium (5.69 mcg/g).

On feeding horses with whole, finely ground, steamed, steam-flaked and popped barley in order to ascertain if any changes in pre-caecal starch digestibility caused by barley processing would affect metabolic responses. Thus, Vervuert *et al.* (2007) confirmed the post-prandial changes in plasma glucose and insulin after intake of the different barley products, but also showed that there was no association of the highest degree of gelatinization in the different barley diets with the most pronounced glycemic or insulinaemic response. Again Vervuert *et al.* (2008) observed the highest peak serum glucose and serum insulin concentrations after feeding the extruded barley, lower concentrations after feeding the micronised barley and the lowest concentrations after feeding the rolled barley.

Poppitt *et al.* (2007) investigated the postprandial effect of a highly enriched barley beta-glucan product on blood glucose, insulin and lipids when given with a high-CHO food and a high-CHO drink. Healthy men were fed 10g dose of barley beta-glucan fibre supplement (Cerogen) having 6.31 g beta-glucan was added to food and drink controls. They concluded that a high dose barley beta-glucan supplement can improve glucose control when added to a high-CHO starchy food, probably due to increased gastrointestinal viscosity, but not when added to a high-CHO beverage where rapid absorption combined with decreased beta-glucan concentration and viscosity obviated this mechanism.

Gao *et al.* (2012) demonstrated that the intake of Tea Polyphenols (TP) + Barley Beta Glucan (BBG) has beneficial effects on glucose tolerance, lipid metabolism, and serum antioxidant status. They also reported that TP + BBG is better than TP or BBG alone in improving glucose metabolism and antioxidant status in diabetic rats suggesting that polyphenol-rich cereal foods are helpful in type 2 diabetes.

The research findings of Bays *et al.* (2011) suggested that 6 g/d BBG consumed in a beverage over 12 weeks may improve insulin sensitivity among hyperglycemic individuals with no prior diagnosis of diabetes mellitus, and experience no change in body weight.

CVD

The consumption of dietary fiber, especially water-soluble fiber (5-10 g per day), has been shown to be inversely associated with coronary heart disease (Pereira *et al.*, 2004). The cholesterol-lowering activities of oats and barley are commonly attributed to the beta-glucan fractions. As beta-glucan is present in both grains and appears to be chemically similar, Judd and Truswell (1981), Ikegami *et al.* (1996), Lupton *et al.* (1994), McIntosh *et al.* (1991), Newman *et al.* (1989a, 1989b) and Delaney *et al.* (2003) demonstrated that the cholesterol-lowering potency of beta-glucan is approximately identical whether its origin was oats or barley.

Barley and β-glucan isolated from barley lowered total and low-density lipoprotein cholesterol by 0.30 mmol/l and 0.27 mmol/l respectively, compared with control (AbuMweis, 2010; German *et al.*, 1996; Oakenfull *et al.*, 1991). But Biörklund *et al.* (2005) compared barley beta glucan with oat beta glucan and found that a daily consumption of 5 g of barley beta-glucans in a beverage did not improve the lipid and glucose metabolism, but the oat beta-glucans did. Martinez *et al.* (1992) observed that the high soluble fiber content of barley exerts a hypocholesterolemic effect in chicks regardless of dietary fat source, possibly mediated through lowered fat absorption.

Aller *et al.* (2004) showed that an increase in soluble fiber intake of 4 g as part of a normal diet reduced LDL cholesterol levels by 12.8 per cent in healthy humans. But Tiwari and Cummins (2011) reported that consumption of 3 g/d of oat or barley β-glucan is sufficient to decrease blood cholesterol, and the FDA concluded that daily consumption of 3 g of soluble β-glucan from whole-grain barley or certain dry milled barley products would produce the same cholesterol-lowering effect as oat products (lowering plasma total cholesterol by 5–8 per cent). The required dosage for a single food is 0.75 g in a single serving (FDA, 2006). The ability of barley β-glucan soluble fiber to lower serum cholesterol is thought to occur through a combination of factors and mechanisms. Fermentation of β-glucan in the colon, results in the production of short-chain fatty acids, which impede cholesterol biosynthesis (Wilson *et al.*, 2004).

Similar results have been reported in hamsters fed hyper-cholesterolemic diets (Kahlon *et al.*, 1993; Zhang *et al.*, 1994; Chen *et al.*, 1981; De Groot *et al.*, 1963). According to Talati *et al.* (2009) barley-derived beta-glucan beneficially affected total cholesterol, LDL-cholesterol, and triglycerides, but not HDL-cholesterol. On the other hand, Beer *et al.* (1995) observed that though oat bran beta-glucan did not alter significantly the serum total cholesterol, LDL cholesterol and triglyceride concentrations, HDL cholesterol was significantly higher ($P < 0.05$) during the test period. So, according to these authors, the effect of oat bran preparations on serum cholesterol levels cannot be estimated by the beta-glucan content but by the measurement of solubility and viscosity of the beta-glucan.

There are various mechanisms by which cholesterol is reduced by dietary fiber: increased production of short chain fatty delayed intestinal absorption of glucose and lipids and inhibition of absorption and re-absorption of cholesterol and bile acids accompanied by increased excretion of bile acids (Beer *et al.*, 1995; Bridges *et al.*, 1992; Lia *et al.*, 1995; 1997; Bourdon *et al.*, 1995; Anderson and Bridges, 1993; Pins *et al.*, 2006; 2007; Wilson *et al.*, 2004). The reduced absorption may be caused by the high viscosity of β-glucan solutions, which increases the viscosity of the intestinal contents (Wursch and Pi-Sunyer, 1997; Lairon, 2001; Jenkins *et al.*, 2002; Wood *et al.*, 2002).

According to Wilson *et al.* (2003; 2004) barley beta-glucan possesses cholesterol-lowering and antiatherogenic activities that occur at both lower and higher molecular weight. Pins *et al.* (2005) and and Keenan *et al.* (2007) in their randomized, controlled, human studies observed a dose response of 9–15 per cent reduction in LDL cholesterol, but molecular weight did not significantly influence cholesterol lowering effect.

Burger *et al.* (1982) substituted 5-20 per cent high-protein barley flour for corn in a corn-based diet and observed a significant weight gain (p less than 0.01) of 10 to 20 per cent in 2-week-old chickens, inhibition of cholesterol biosynthesis by 45-65 per cent and a 3-fold increase in fatty acid synthetase thus opined that high-protein barley flour contains inhibitor(s) of cholesterol biosynthesis and growth factor(s) when compared to a corn-based diet. On the contrary, Drozdowski *et al.* (2009) observed the expression of genes involved in fatty acid synthesis and down regulation of cholesterol metabolism with the high viscosity beta-glucan extracts which also reduced intestinal fatty-acid-binding protein and fatty acid transport protein 4 mRNA.

Addition of barley bran flour or barley oil was found to enhance the cholesterol-lowering effect of the NCEP step 1 diet in individuals with hypercholesterolemia (Lupton *et al.*, 1994). Yu *et al.* (2004) observed that supplementation with 15 g of barley Leaf extract for 4 weeks decreased plasma lipids and inhibited LDL oxidation in hyperlipidemic smokers and/or non-smokers. Oda *et al.* (1994) also reported barley gums to suppress the elevation of serum and liver triglyceride concentrations in diet induced hyperglyceridemic rats.

Barley diet (25 per cent) lowered serum total cholesterol by 16.4 per cent but it was not dose dependent as higher percent barley diet did not show further lowering of cholesterol (Ranhotra *et al.*, 1998). Abd El-Mageed (2011) on the basis of his observations recommended that dietary intake of plant mixture of celery; chicory, and barley at 15 per cent (5 per cent of each) concentration can be beneficial to patients suffering from hypercholesterolemia and liver diseases.

McIntosh *et al.* (1991) showed that a 4-wk diet enriched with barley foods containing 8 g β-glucan per day reduced total and LDL cholesterol in moderately hypercholesterolemic men by 6.0 and 6.8 per cent, respectively, compared with wheat foods containing 1.5 per cent β-glucan and whole-grain barley flour products containing 9.6 per cent β-glucan per day for 4 wk, which showed 12 and 14 per cent reduction in total and LDL cholesterol in cholesterolemic men.

Madhujith and Shahidi (2007) proved that phenolic extracts from whole barley kernel possess high antioxidant, antiradical, and antiproliferative potentials. Specifically, antioxidants slow down the rate of oxidative damage by scavenging the free radicals that form when body cells use oxygen. An *in vivo* study conducted by Hoang *et al.* (2011) suggested that the hypocholesterolemic effects of barley are primarily the result of reduced dietary cholesterol uptake and bile acid resorption. Reduced expression of intestinal apical sodium dependent bile acid transporter and intestinal Niemann-Pick C1-like 1 may play a key role in the regulation of dietary cholesterol and bile acid metabolism in mice consuming a diet containing barley.

Both the barley protein- and casein-enriched breads, showed no differences in their effects on serum LDL cholesterol or C-reactive protein which are measures of oxidative stress or blood pressure. Nevertheless, because no adverse effects were observed on cardiovascular risk factors, Jenkins *et al.* (2010) suggested barley protein as an additional option for raising the protein content of the diet. Lahouar *et al.* (2011) indicated that the diet enriched with dietary fiber of barley variety "Rihane" could be effective in decreasing the atherogenic risk factors in rats.

Barley oil extracted with hexane from the grain of a high oil waxy hull-less barley was found to contain more than threefold polyunsaturated fatty than that of margarine. According to Wang *et al.* (1993) alpha-tocotrienol and polyunsaturated fatty acids are hypocholesterolemic components in barley oil.

Addition of refined beta-glucan or waxy barley to the diet resulted in greater bile acid excretions ($p < 0.05$) compared to the control group. The activity of cholesterol

7a-hydroxylase (CYP7A1).waxy barley diet was up-regulated by 2 to 3 times and the beta-glucan diet by 1.5 times. Hepatic CYP7A1 mRNA level paralleled the increases in enzyme activity. The results of this study suggest that the hypocholesterolemic effects of both beta-glucan and a waxy barley diet may be due to the enhancement of CYP7A1 expression resulting from increased fecal excretion of bile acids (Yang *et al.*, 2003).

The U.S. FDA allowed a claim for β-glucan soluble fiber from whole-grain barley and certain barley milling fractions for reducing plasma cholesterol levels and reducing the risk of heart disease (FDA, 2006). But Ames and Rhymer, (2008) feel that more research is needed to fully understand the mechanism of cholesterol reduction and the role of beta-glucan molecular weight, viscosity, and solubility

Cancer

Insoluble fiber is the type of fiber that helps the body to maintain regular bowel function. Studies show that insoluble fiber may be beneficial in lowering the risk for certain cancers such as colon cancer. Kanauchi (2008) showed the promising antineoplastic effects of prebiotic treatment. Modulation of intestinal environment by prebiotic germinated barley foodstuff prevents chemo-induced colonic carcinogenesis in rats. Germinated Barley showed anti-tumourigenicity in the rat model. Changes in the colonic environment featured through the increase of butyrate production were found. Although a more detailed observation is required, this study showed the promising antineoplastic effects of prebiotic treatment.

Spent barley grain is a good source of proteins, polyphenolics, fatty acids (including alpha-linolenic), vitamin E, and minerals. The insoluble dietary fiber-rich source from barley, spent barley grain was significantly more effective at preventing induced tumours than soluble fiber rich commercial barley bran. Pure cellulose and outer layer barley bran were, by comparison, only moderately effective in cancer prevention (McIntosh *et al.*, 1993).

Germinated Barley (GBF) has been shown to reduce both clinical activity and mucosal damage in ulcerative colitis (UC) with mild to moderate activity. The cumulative recurrence rate in the GBF group with steroid tapering treatment was significantly lower compared to the control group. No side effects related to GBF were observed. GBF appeared to be effective and safe as a maintenance therapy to taper steroid dose and prolong remission in patients with UC (Hanai, 2003).

According to Faghfoori *et al.* (2011) consumption of 30 g of GBF daily during two months of the study along with standard drug therapy reduced the level of serum TNF-α, IL- 6 and–8 in patients with ulcerative colitis. GBF group showed a significant decrease in clinical activity index (especially, the degree of visible blood in stools and the presence of nocturnal diarrhea) compared with the control group ($p<0.05$). No side effects related to GBF were observed. In conclusion, GBF can reduce the clinical activity of UC over long term as well as short term administration.

McIntosh *et al.* (1996) reported that commercially available barley bran to significantly reduce tumour incidence and burden influencing both the initiatory as well as promotional stages of chemically induced carcinogenesis.

Obesity

Lupton *et al.* (1993) found barley bran flour to accelerate gastrointestinal transit time and increase fecal weight. Son *et al.* (2008) also reported the gut transit time to be shortened in the barley group which showed significantly lower triglycerides, total cholesterol and LDL-C, and higher HDL-C than the other groups of rats fed different grains, thus improving several cardiovascular risk factors induced by obesity. Molecular weight of the barley fiber was found to alter the effects on body weight in human subjects with the high-MW fiber significantly decreasing body weight (Smith *et al.*, 2008).

The energy intake recorded in females at the lunch test showed that the energy intake of the participants fed with barley beta glucan supplemented biscuits was significantly lower than that of the control group (3048 kJ vs. 3890 kJ), suggesting that Beta glucan enriched biscuit was able to influence appetite ratings, but did not modify food intake in a short time period (Vitaglione *et al.* (2010).

Inflammatory Bowel Disorder

Barley-derived beta-glucan has been proved to decrease the bloating and abdominal pain score after the 30th day of the intervention (Day 30-37) as compared to placebo in the poly pectomized patients (Turunen, 2011).

Germinated barley foodstuff (GBF) is a prebiotic product and reduces colonic mucosal inflammation and the clinical symptoms observed in ulcerative colitis. The preliminary study demonstrated that, GBF effectively prevented the colitis-related dysplasia and inflammatory change in a chronic and sub-acute colitis model by modulating the intestinal environment as a prebiotic. This prebiotic may contribute to prevention of mucosal damage, proliferative effects on epithelium in regeneration stage and steady state (Kanauchi *et al.*, 2004).

In addition, certain other studies have suggested that dietary fiber exerts a therapeutic effect on inflammatory bowel disease patients. GBF suppressed the infiltration of the mucosal mast cells, and prevented the distraction of both collagen and elastic fibers. These effects may be closely associated with its inhibitory effects on mucosal mast cells, and the destruction of the mucosal connective tissues (Araki *et al.*, 2007).

Barley Beer

A large part of the barley crop is used for malting, for which barley is the best suited grain. It is a key ingredient in beer and whisky production. Two-row barley is traditionally used in German and English beers. Six-row barley was traditionally used in US beers, but both varieties are in common usage now. Distilled from green beer whisky has been made primarily from barley in Ireland and Scotland, while other countries have utilized more diverse sources of alcohol; such as the more common corn, rye and wheat in the USA. Barley wine was an alcoholic drink in the 18th century. It was prepared by boiling barley in water, then mixing the barley water with white wine and other ingredients like borage, lemon and sugar. In the 19th century a different barley wine was made prepared from recipes of ancient Greek origin (Ayto,

1990). Non-alcoholic drinks such as barley water (Ayto, 1990) and barley tea (called mugicha in Japan) have been made by boiling barley in water.

Other Benefits

Zhang *et al.* (1990) determined the frequency of gallstones, concentration of bile acids and cholesterol in bile, concentration of cholesterol in serum, and structure of the small intestinal mucosa in male Syrian Golden hamsters fed a stone provoking fibre-free diet with or without supplementation of brewer's spent grain (BSG), a concentrated barley fibre source from the by-product of brewing. A significantly lower frequency of gallstones was found in the animals with 10 per cent BSG dietary supplementation. Addition of 30 per cent BSG after an initial 6-week period with a fibre-free, stone provoking diet seemed to dissolve previously formed gallstones. Total bile acid concentration was higher in bile from animals given a diet supplemented with 10 per cent BSG. In addition, the cholesterol concentration in both serum and bile was lower in the 30 per cent BSG supplemented group. Thus even the spent barley grain has been found to possess preventive and curative property with regard to gallstones.

Storage of Barley Bread

Increasing viscous dietary fiber in snacks may have several nutritional advantages, Moriartey *et al.* (2011) demonstrated that solubility and thus viscosity of β-glucan can be impacted by different storage conditions applied to some bakery products, like muffins (Moriartey *et al.*, 2011). Therefore, they recommended that β-glucan-fortified bread be consumed fresh for greatest β-glucan solubility and viscosity, though β-glucan solubility of approximately 40 per cent is still achievable upon frozen storage of the bread for up to 2 weeks (Moriartey *et al.*, 2011).

Conclusions

New barley cultivars have been generated specifically for food use, possessing increased beta-glucan, desirable starch composition profiles, and improved milling/processing traits (Bird *et al.*, 2004; Coles *et al.*, 2007; Shimizu *et al.*, 2008). These advances in barley production, coupled with the establishment of a government-regulated health claim for barley beta-glucan, will stimulate new processing opportunities for barley foods and provide consumers with reliable, healthy food choices.

References

Abd El-Mageed NM (2011). Hepatoprotective effect of feeding celery leaves mixed with chicory leaves and barley grains to hypercholesterolemic rats. Pharmacogn. Mag. 7 (26):151–56.

AbuMweis SS, Jew S, Ames NP (2010). β-glucan from barley and its lipid-lowering capacity: a meta-analysis of randomized, controlled trials. Eur. J. Clin. Nutr. 64 (12): 1472–80.

Aller R, de Luis DA, Izaola O, La Calle F, del Olmo L, Fernandez L, Arranz T, Hernandez JMG (2004). Effect of soluble fiber intake in lipid and glucose levels in healthy subjects: a randomized clinical trial. Diabetes Res. Clin. Pract. 65: 7–11.

Alminger M, Eklund-Jonsson C (2008). Whole-grain cereal products based on a high-fibre barley or oat genotype lower post-prandial glucose and insulin responses in healthy humans. Eur. J. Nutr. 47 (6): 294–300.

Aman P, Hesselman K (1984). Analysis of starch and other main constituents of cereal grains. Swed. J. Agric. Res. 14: 135–40.

Ames N, Rhymer C, Rossnagel B, Therrien M, Ryland D, Dua S, Ross K (2006). Utilization of diverse hulless barley properties to maximize food product quality. Cereal Foods World. 41: 23–28.

Ames NP, Rhymer CR (2008). Issues surrounding health claims for barley. J. Nutr. 138 (6): 1237S-4.

Andersson AA, Andersson R, Aman P (2000). Air classification of barley flours. Cereal Chem. 77: 463–67.

Anderson JW, Bridges SR (1993). Hypo-cholesterolemic effects of oat bran in humans. In: Wood PJ, editor. Oat bran. St. Paul: American Association of Cereal Chemists. pp.139–57.

Araki Y, Kanauchi O, Sugihara H, Fujiyama Y, Hattori T (2007). Germinated barley foodstuff suppresses dextran sulfate experimental colitis in rats: the role of mast cells. Int. J. Mol. Med. 19 (2): 257–62.

Ayto J (1990). The glutton's glossary: a dictionary of food and drink terms. London: Routledge. pp. 16–17. ISBN 0415026474.

Bays H, Frestedt JL, Bell M, Williams C, Kolberg L, Schmelzer W, Anderson JW (2011). Reduced viscosity Barley β-Glucan versus placebo: a randomized controlled trial of the effects on insulin sensitivity for individuals at risk for diabetes mellitus. Nutr. Metab. (Lond). 8: 58.

Beer MU, Arrigoni E, Amado R (1995). Effects of oat gum on blood cholesterol levels in healthy young men. Eur. J. Clin. Nutr. 49: 517–22.

Behall KM, Scholfield DJ, Hallfrisch J (2005). Comparison of hormone and glucose responses of overweight women to barley and oats. J. Am. Coll. Nutr. 24 (3): 182–88.

Bhatty RS (1997). Milling of regular and waxy starch hull-less barleys for the production of bran and flour. Cereal Chem. 74: 693–99.

Bhatty RS, MacGregor AW, Rossnagel BG (1991). Total and acid-soluble beta-glucan content of hullless barley and its relationship to acid-extract viscosity. Cereal Chem. 68: 221–27.

Biörklund M, van Rees A, Mensink RP, Onning G (2005). Changes in serum lipids and postprandial glucose and insulin concentrations after consumption of beverages with beta-glucans from oats or barley: a randomised dose-controlled trial. Eur. J. Clin. Nutr. 59 (11): 1272–81.

Bird AR, Jackson M, King RA, Davies DA, Usher S, Topping DL (2004). A novel high-amylose barley cultivar (Hordeum vulgare var. Himalaya 292) lowers plasma cholesterol and alters indices of large-bowel fermentation in pigs. Br. J. Nutr. 92: 607–15.

Bourdon I, Yokoyama W, Davis P, Hudson C, Backus R, Richter D, Knuckles B, Schneeman BO. (1999).Postprandial lipid, glucose, insulin, and cholecystokinin responses in men fed barley pasta enriched with beta-glucan. Am. J. Clin. Nutr. 69: 55–63.

Bridges SR, Anderson JW, Deakins DA, Dillon DW, Wood CL. (1992). Oat bran increases serum acetate of hypercholesterolemic men. Am. J. Clin. Nutr. 56: 455-59.

Burger WC, Qureshi AA, Prentice N, Elson CE (1982). Effects of different fractions of the barley kernel on the hepatic lipid metabolism of chickens. Lipids. 17 (12): 956–63.

Casiraghi MC, Garsetti M, Testolin G, Brighenti F (2006). Post-prandial responses to cereal products enriched with barley beta-glucan. J. Am. Coll. Nutr. 25 (4): 313–20.

Chen WJL, Anderson JW, Gould MR (1981). Effects of oat bran, oat gum and pectin on lipid metabolism of cholesterol-fed rats. Nutr. Rep. Int. 24: 1093–98.

Chillo S, Ranawana DV, Pratt M, Henry CJ (2011). Glycemic response and glycemic index of semolina spaghetti enriched with barley β-glucan. Nutrition. 27 (6): 653–58.

Coles GD, Roberts SJ, Butler RC, Morrell MK, Rowarth JS (2007). The role of beta-glucan in barley. In: Salovaara H, Gates F, Tenkanen M, editors. Dietary fibre components and functions. Wageningen: Academic Publishers. pp. 65–74.

Davidson MH, Dugan LD, Burns JH, Bova J, Story K, Drennan KB (1991). The hypocholesterolemic effects of β-glucan in oatmeal and oat bran. J. Am. Med. Assoc. 265: 1833–39.

De Groot AP, Luyken R, Pikaar NA (1963). Cholesterol lowering effect of rolled oats. Lancet. 2: 303–304.

Delaney B, Nicolosi RJ, Wilson TA, Carlson T, Frazer S, Zheng GH, Hess R, Ostergren K, Haworth J, Knutson N (2003). Beta-glucan fractions from barley and oats are similarly anti-atherogenic in hyper-cholesterolemic Syrian golden hamsters. J. Nutr. 133 (2): 468–75.

De Vries, A (1976). Dictionary of Symbols and Imagery. Amsterdam: North-Holland Publishing Company. pp. 34–35.

Drozdowski LA, Reimer RA, Temelli F, Bell RC, Vasanthan T, Thomson AB (2010). Beta-glucan extracts inhibit the *in vitro* intestinal uptake of long-chain fatty acids and cholesteroland down-regulate genes involved in lipogenesis and lipid transport in rats. J. Nutr. Biochem. 21 (8): 695–701.

Dudgeon-Bollinger AL, Fastnaught CE, Berglund PT (1997). Extruded snack products from waxy hull-less barley. Cereal Foods World. 42: 762–66.

Edney MJ, Marchylo BA, MacGregor AW (1991). Structure of total barley beta-glucan. J. Inst. Brew. 97: 39–44.

El Khoury D, Cuda C, Luhovyy BL, Anderson GH (2012). Beta glucan: health benefits in obesity and metabolic syndrome. J. Nutr. Metab. 2012: 851362.

Faghfoori Z, Navai L, Shakerhosseini R, Somi MH, Nikniaz Z, Norouzi MF (2011). Effects of an oral supplementation of germinated barley foodstuff on serum tumour necrosis factor-{alpha}, interleukin-6 and -8 in patients with ulcerative colitis intervention periods. Ann. Clin. Biochem. 48 (3): 233–37.

FDA (2006). FDA. CFR 101.81 Health claims: Soluble fiber from certain foods and risk of coronary heart disease (CHD). Washington, DC.

Gao R, Wang Y, Wu Z, Ming J, Zhao G (2012). Interaction of Barley β-Glucan and Tea Polyphenols on Glucose Metabolism in Streptozotocin-Induced Diabetic Rats. J. Food Sci. 77 (6): H128–34.

German B, Xu R, Walzem R, Kinsella JE, Knuckles B, Nakamura M, Yokoyama W (1996). Effects of dietary fats and barley fiber on total cholesterol and lipoprotein cholesterol distribution in plasma of hamsters. Nutr. Res. 16: 1239–49.

Hanai H, Kanauchi O, Mitsuyama K, Andoh A, Takeuchi K, Takayuki I, Araki Y, Fujiyama Y, Toyonaga A, Sata M, Kojima A, Fukuda M, Bamba T (2003). Treatment of ulcerative colitis patients by long-term administration of germinated barley foodstuff: multi-center open trial. Int. J. Mol. Med. 12 (5): 701–704.

Hoang MH, Houng SJ, Jun HJ, Lee JH, Choi JW, Kim SH, Kim YR, Lee SJ (2011). Barley intake induces bile acid excretion by reduced expression of intestinal ASBT and NPC1L1 in C57BL/6J mice. J. Agric. Food Chem. 59 (12): 6798–805.

Ikegami, S., Tomita, M., Honda, S., Yamaguchi, M., Mizukawa, R., Suzuki, Y., Ishii, K., Ohsawa, S. and Kiyooka, N., *et al.* (1996) Effect of boiled barley-rice-feeding in hyper-cholesterolemic and normo-lipidemic subjects. Plant. Foods Hum. Nutr. 49: 317–328.

Jenkins AL, Jenkins DJA, Zdravkovic U, Wursch P, Vuksan V (2002). Depression of the glycemic index by high levels of β-glucan fiber in two functional foods tested in type 2 diabetes. Eur. J. Clin. Nutr. 56: 622–28.

Jenkins DJ, Srichaikul K, Wong JM, Kendall CW, Bashyam B, Vidgen E, Lamarche B, Rao AV, Jones PJ, Josse RG, Jackson CJ, Ng V, Leong T, Leiter LA (2010). Supplemental barley protein and casein similarly affect serum lipids in hypercholesterolemic women and men. J. Nutr. 140 (9): 1633–37.

Jones PJH, Asp N-G, Silva P (2008). Evidence for health claims on foods: how much is enough? Introduction and general remarks. J. Nutr. 138: 1189S – 91S.

Jose-Cunilleras E, Taylor LE, Hinchcliff KW (2004). Glycemic index of cracked corn, oat groats and rolled barley in horses. J. Anim. Sci. 82 (9): 2623–29.

Judd PA, Truswell AS (1981). The effects of rolled oats on blood lipids and fecal steroid excretion in man. Am. J. Clin. Nutr. 34: 2061–67.

Kahlon TS, Chow FI, Knuckles BE, Chiu MM (1993). Cholesterol-lowering effects in hamsters of β-glucan-enriched barley fraction, dehulled whole barley, rice bran, and oat bran and their combinations. Cereal Chem. 70: 435–40.

Kalra S, Jood S. (2000). Effect of dietary barley β-glucan on cholesterol and lipoprotein fractions in rats. J. Cereal Sci. 31: 141–45.

Kanauchi O, Mitsuyama K, Andoh A, Iwanaga T. (2008). Modulation of intestinal environment by prebiotic germinated barley foodstuff prevents chemo-induced colonic carcinogenesis in rats. Oncol. Rep. 20 (4): 793–801.

Kanauchi O, Mitsuyama K, Homma T, Takahama K, Fujiyama Y, Andoh A, Araki Y, Suga T, Hibi T, Naganuma M, Asakura H, Nakano H, Shimoyama T, Hida N, Haruma K, Koga H, Sata M, Tomiyasu N, Toyonaga A, Fukuda M, Kojima A, Bamba T. (2004). Germinated barley foodstuff prolongs remission in patients with ulcerative colitis. Int. J. Mol. Med. 13 (5): 643–47.

Keenan JM, Goulson M, Shamliyan T, Knutson N, Kolberg L, Curry L (2007). The effects of concentrated barley b-glucan on blood lipids and other CVD risk factors in a population of hypercholesterolemic men and women. Br. J. Nutr. 97: 1162–68.

Kiryluk J, Kawka A, Gasiorowski H, Chalcarz A, Aniola J (2000). Milling of barley to obtain beta-glucan enriched products. Nahrung. 44: 238–41.

Lahouar L, Ghrairi F, El Felah M, Salem HB, Miled AH, Hammami M, Achour L (2011). Effect of dietary fiber of "Rihane" barley grains and azoxymethane on serum and liver lipid variables in Wistar rats. J. Physiol. Biochem. 67 (1): 27–34.

Lairon D (2001). Dietary fiber and dietary lipids. In: McCleary BV, Prosky L, editors. Advanced dietary fiber technology. London: Blackwell Science. pp. 177–85.

Lazaridou A, Biliaderis CG (2007). Molecular aspects of cereal beta-glucan functionality: Physical properties, technological applications and physiological effects. J. Cereal Sci. 46:101–118.

Lia A, Andersson H, Mekki N, Juhel C, Senft M, Lairon D. (1997). Postprandial lipemia in relation to sterol and fat excretion in ileostomy subjects given oat-bran and wheat test meals. Am. J. Clin. Nutr. 66: 357–65.

Lia A, Hallmans G, Sandberg AS, Sundberg B, Aman P, Andersson H. (1995). Oat beta-glucan increases bile acid excretion and a fiber-rich barley fraction increases cholesterol excretion in ileostomy subjects. Am. J. Clin. Nutr. 62: 1245–51.

Liljeberg HG, Granfeldt YE, Björck IM (1996). Products based on a high fiber barley genotype, but not on common barley or oats, lower postprandial glucose and insulin responses in healthy humans. J. Nutr. 126 (2): 458–66.

Lupton JR, Morin JL, Robinson MC (1993). Barley bran flour accelerates gastrointestinal transit time. J. Am. Diet. Assoc. 93 (8): 881–85.

Lupton JR, Robinson MC, Morin JL (1994). Cholesterol-lowering effect of barley bran flour and oil. J. Am. Diet. Assoc. 94: 65–70.

Madhujith T, Shahidi F (2007). Antioxidative and antiproliferative properties of selected barley (Hordeum vulgarae L.) cultivars and their potential for inhibition of low-density lipoprotein (LDL) cholesterol oxidation. J. Agric. Food Chem. 55 (13): 5018–24.

Mahdi GS, Naismith DJ (1991). Role of chromium in barley in modulating the symptoms of diabetes. Ann. Nutr. Metab. 35 (2): 65–70.

Mahdi GS, Naismith DJ, Price RG, Taylor SA, Risteli J, Risteli L (1994). Modulating influence of barley on the altered metabolism of glucose and of basement membranes in the diabetic rat. Ann. Nutr. Metab. 38 (2): 61–67.

Marconi E, Graziano M, Cubadda R (2000). Composition and utilization of barley pearling by-products for making functional pastas rich in dietary fiber and beta-glucans. Cereal Chem. 77: 133–39.

Martinez VM, Newman RK, Newman CW (1992). Barley diets with different fat sources have hypocholesterolemic effects in chicks. J. Nutr. 122 (5): 1070–76.

McIntosh GH, Jorgensen L, Royle P (1993). The potential of an insoluble dietary fiber-rich source from barley to protect from DMH-induced intestinal tumours in rats. Nutr. Cancer. 19 (2): 213–21.

McIntosh GH, Le Leu RK, Royle PJ, Young GP (1996). A comparative study of the influence of differing barley brans on DMH-induced intestinal tumours in male Sprague-Dawley rats. J. Gastroenterol. Hepatol. 11 (2): 113–19.

McIntosh GH, Whyte J, McArthur R, Nestel PJ (1991). Barley and wheat foods: influence on plasma cholesterol concentrations in hypercholesterolemic men. Am. J. Clin. Nutr. 53: 1205–209.

Moriartey S, Temelli F, Vasanthan T (2011). Effect of storage conditions on the solubility and viscosity of β-glucan extracted from bread under *in vitro* conditions. J. Food Sci. 76 (1): C1–7.

Naismith DJ, Mahdi GS, Shakir NN (1991). Therapeutic value of barley in the management of diabetes. Ann. Nutr. Metab. 35 (2): 61–64.

Newman RK, Lewis SE, Newman CW, Boik RJ, Ramage RT (1989a). Hypocholesterolemic effect of barley foods on healthy men. Nutr. Rep. Int. 39: 749–60.

Newman RK, Newman CW, Graham H (1989b). The hypocholesterolemic function of barley β-glucans. Cereal Foods World 34: 883–86.

Nilsson A, Granfeldt Y, Ostman E, Preston T, Björck I. (2006). Effects of GI and content of indigestible carbohydrates of cereal-based evening meals on glucose tolerance at a subsequent standardised breakfast. European Journal of Clinical Nutrition. 60 (9): 1092–99.

Oakenfull DG, Hood RL, Sidhu GS, Saini HS (1991). Martin, D. J. Wrigley, CW. eds. Effects of barley and isolated barley β-glucans on plasma cholesterol in the rat. Proceedings of Cereals International. 1991. 344–49 Brisbane, Australia.

Oda T, Aoe S, Imanishi S, Kanazawa Y, Sanada H, Ayano Y (1994). Effects of dietary oat, barley, and guar gums on serum and liver lipid concentrations in diet-induced hypertriglyceridemic rats. J. Nutr. Sci. Vitaminol. (Tokyo). 40 (2): 213–17.

Pereira MA, O'Reilly E, Augustsson K, Fraser GE, Goldbourt U, Heitmann BL, Hallmans G, Knekt P, Liu S, *et al.* (2004). Dietary fiber and risk of coronary heart disease – a pooled analysis of cohort studies. Arch. Intern. Med. 164: 370–76.

Pins J, Keenan JM, Curry LL, Goulson MJ, Kolberg LW (2005). Extracted barley beta-glucan improves CVD risk factors and other biomarkers in a population of generally healthy hypercholesterolemic men and women. Prev. Control. 1: 131.

Pins JJ, Kaur H (2006). A review of the effects of barley B-glucan on cardiovascular and diabetic risk. Cereal Foods World. 51: 8–11.

Pins JJ, Kaur H, Dodds E, Keenan JM (2007). The effects of cereal fibers and barley foods rich in beta-glucan on cardiovascular disease and diabetes risk. In: Marquart L, Jacobs DR Jr, McIntosh GH, Poutanen K, Reicks M, editors. Whole grains and health. London: Blackwell. pp. 75.- 85.

Poppitt SD, van Drunen JD, McGill AT, Mulvey TB, Leahy FE (2007). Supplementation of a high-carbohydrate breakfast with barley beta-glucan improves postprandial glycaemic response for meals but not beverages. Asia Pac. J. Clin. Nutr. 16 (1): 16.-.24.

Ranhotra GS, Gelroth JA, Leinen SD, Bhatty RS (1998). Dose response to soluble fiber in barley in lowering blood lipids in hamster. Plant. Foods Hum. Nutr. 52 (4): 329–36.

Shimizu C, Kihara M, Aoe S, Araki S, Ito K, Hayashi K, Watari J, Sakata Y, Ikegami S (2008). Effect of high β-glucan barley on serum cholesterol concentrations and visceral fat area in Japanese men—a randomized, double-blinded, placebo-controlled trial. Plant Foods Hum. Nutr. 63: 21–25.

Simon, André (1963). Guide to Good Food and Wines: A Concise Encyclopedia of Gastronomy Complete and Unabridged p. 150 Collins, London.

Smith KN, Queenan KM, Thomas W, Fulcher RG, Slavin JL (2008). Physiological effects of concentrated barley beta-glucan in mildly hypercholesterolemic adults. J. Am. Coll. Nutr. 27 (3): 434–40.

Son BK, Kim JY, Lee SS. (2008). Effect of adlay, buckwheat and barley on lipid metabolism and aorta histopathology in rats fed an obesogenic diet. Ann. Nutr. Metab. 52 (3): 181–87.

Storsley JM (2001). Characterization of non-starch polysaccharides from hull-less barley. M.Sc. Thesis, University of Manitoba.

Talati R, Baker WL, Pabilonia MS, White CM, Coleman CI (2009). The effects of barley-derived soluble fiber on serum lipids. Ann. Fam. Med. 7 (2): 157–63.

Tiwari U, Cummins (2011). E.Meta-analysis of the effect of β-glucan intake on blood cholesterol and glucose levels. Nutrition. Apr 5. [Epub ahead of print].

Tosh S (2007). Factors affecting bioactivity of cereal beta-glucans. In: Salovaara H, Gates F, Tenkanen Meditors. Dietary fiber components and functions. Wageningen: Academic Press. pp. 75–89.

Turunen K, Tsouvelakidou E, Nomikos T, Mountzouris KC, Karamanolis D, Triantafillidis J, Kyriacou A (2011). Impact of beta-glucan on the faecal microbiota of polypectomized patients: A pilot study. Anaerobe. Apr. 16.

USDA (2012). National Nutrient Database for Standard Reference, Release. 25.

Vervuert I, Bothe C, Coenen M (2007). Glycaemic and insulinaemic responses to mechanical or thermal processed barley in horses. J. Anim. Physiol. Anim. Nutr (Berl). 91 (5-6): 263–68.

Vervuert I, Voigt K, Hollands T, Cuddeford D, Coenen M (2008). Effects of processing barley on its digestion by horses. Vet. Rec. 162 (21): 684–88.

Vitaglione P, Lumaga RB, Montagnese C, Messia MC, Marconi E, Scalfi L (2010). Satiating effect of a barley beta-glucan-enriched snack. J. Am. Coll. Nutr. 29 (2): 113–21.

Wang L, Newman RK, Newman CW, Jackson LL, Hofer PJ (1993). Tocotrienol and fatty acid composition of barley oil and their effects on lipid metabolism. Plant. Foods Hum. Nutr. 43 (1): 9–17.

Wilson TA, Nicolosi RJ, Delaney B, Chadwell K, Moolchandani V, Kotyla T, Ponduru S, Zheng GH, Hess R, Knutson N, Curry L, Kolberg L, Goulson M,Ostergren K (2003). Reduced and high molecular weight barley beta-glucans decrease plasma total and non-HDL-cholesterol in hypercholesterolemic Syrian golden hamsters. J. Nutr. 133 (2): 468–75.

Wilson TA, Nicolosi RJ, Delaney B, Chadwell K, Moolchandani V, Kotyla T, Ponduru S, Zheng GH, Hess R, *et al.* (2004). Reduced and high molecular weight barley β-glucans decrease plasma total and non-HDL-cholesterol in hypercholesterolemic Syrian golden hamsters. J. Nutr. 134: 2617–22.

Wood PJ (2002). Relationships between soluble properties of cereal beta-glucans and physiological effects–a review. Trends Food Sci. Technol. 13: 313–20.

Wood PJ, Beer MU, Butler G (2000). Evaluation of role of concentration and molecular weight of oat beta-glucan in determining effect of viscosity on plasma glucose and insulin following an oral glucose load. Br. J. Nutr. 84: 19–23.

Wood PJ, Weisz J, Blackwell BA (1994). Structural studies of (1!3), (1!4)- β-D-glucans by ^{13}C-nuclear magnetic resonance spectroscopy and by rapid analysis of cellulose-like regions using high-performance anion-exchange chromatography of oligosaccharides released by lichenase. Cereal Chem. 71: 301–307.

Wood PJ (2007). Rheology and physiology of soluble fibers: what are the relationships and what use can be made of them? In: Salovaara H, Gates F, Tenkanen M, editors. Dietary fiber components and functions. Wageningen: Academic. pp.113–26.

Wursch P, Pi-Sunyer FX (1997). The role of viscous soluble fiber in the metabolic control of diabetes. A review with special emphasis on cereal rich in beta-glucan. Diabetes Care. 20: 1774–80.

Yang JL, Kim YH, Lee HS, Lee MS, Moon YK (2003). Barley beta-glucan lowers serum cholesterol based on the up-regulation of cholesterol 7alpha-hydroxylase activity and mRNA abundance in cholesterol-fed rats. J. Nutr. Sci. Vitaminol. (Tokyo). 49 (6): 381–87.

Yu YM, Cang WC, Liu CS, Tsai CM (2004). Effect of young barley leaf extract and adlay on plasma lipids and LDL oxidation in hyperlipidemic smokers. Biol Pharm Bull. 27 (6): 802–805.

Zhang, J.-X., Lundin, E., Reuterving, C.-O., Hallmans, G., Stenling, R., Westerlund, E. and Aman, P (1994). Effects of rye bran, oat bran and soya-bran fibre on bile composition, gallstone formation, gall-bladder morphology and serum cholesterol in Syrian golden hamsters (Mesocricetus auratus). Br. J. Nutr. 71: 861–70.

Chapter 14

Flax Seeds

(*Linum usitatissimum*)

Flax (also known as common flax or linseed) is native to the region extending from the eastern Mediterranean to India and was probably first domesticated in the Fertile Crescent. Flax was extensively cultivated in ancient Ethiopia and ancient

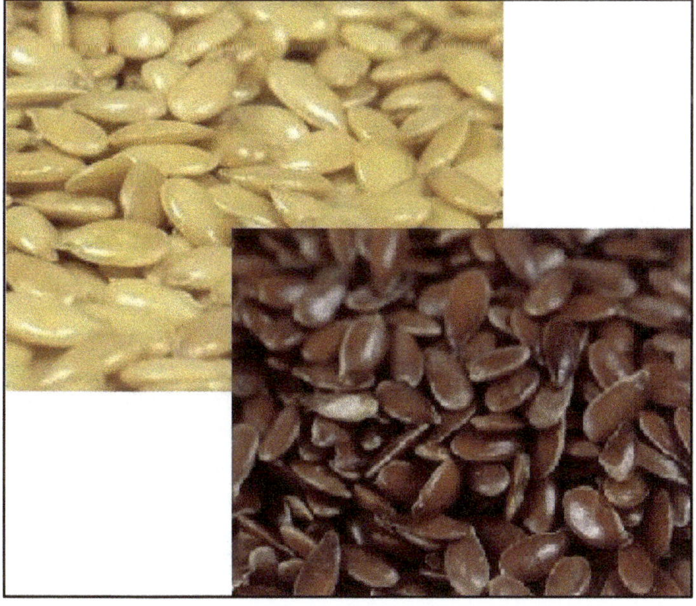

Golden Flax Seeds/Brown Flax Seeds

Egypt. In a prehistoric cave in the Republic of Georgia, dyed Flax fibers have been found in 30,000 BC (Balter, 2009; Kvavadze *et al.*, 2009) implicating that flax is the first domesticated species in human history. New Zealand Flax is not related to Flax but was named after it, as both plants are used to produce fibers. As the source of linen fiber, flax has been cultivated since at least 5000 BC (Oomah, 2001).

Varieties

Flax seeds are basically of two varieties: (1) Brown and (2) Yellow or Golden with similar nutritional characteristics and equal number of short-chain ω-3 fatty acids. The exception is a type of yellow Flax called solin (trade name Linola), which has a completely different oil profile and very low omega-3 Fatty acid content. Both the varieties have been for consumed for thousands of years.

Traditional Uses

The Latin name for flaxseed species is 'Usitatissimum' which means 'most useful', pointing to the several traditional uses of the plant and their importance for human life. Accordingly, besides being used as nutritious food, linseed oil which is extracted from flaxseeds is used as edible oil, nutritional supplement, and also as an ingredient in many wood finishing products. Flax is also grown as an ornamental plant in gardens.

Nutritional Value of Flax Seeds

One hundred grams of ground flax seed supply about 450 kilocalories, 41 grams of fat, 28 grams of fiber, and 20 grams of protein. Flax seed sprouts are edible, with a slightly spicy flavour. Whole flax seeds are chemically stable. Ground flaxseed can go rancid at room temperature in as little as one week (Alpers and Sawyer-Morse, 1996).

Nutritional Value per 100 g

Nutrient	*Amount*	*Nutrient*	*Amount*
Pantothenic acid (mg)	0.985	Vitamin B_6 (mg)	0.473
Vitamin C (mg)	0.6	Thiamine (mg)	1.64
Riboflavin (mg)	0.16	Niacin (mg)	3.08
Calcium (mg)	255	Iron (mg)	5.73
Magnesium (mg)	392	Potassium (mg)	813
Zinc (mg)	4.34	Energy (kcal)	534
Carbohydrates (g)	28.88	Dietary fiber (g)	27.30
Fat (g)	42.16	Fatty acids, total saturated (g)	3.663
Fatty acids, total monounsaturated	7.527	Fatty acids, total polyunsaturated (g)	28.730
Protein (g)	18.29		

USDA (2012).

Flaxseed is one of the richest plant sources of the ω-3 fatty acid alpha-linolenic acid (ALA, C18:3 ù-3) (Gebauer *et al.*, 2006). The oil contains 55 – 60 per cent alpha-linolenic acid (Kaithwas *et al.*, 2011; Hall *et al.*, 2006). Flax seed is the richest food source of phytohormone lignans, one of the major groups of phyto-estrogens (Thompson *et al.*, 1991) with secoisolariciresinol diglucoside (SDG) as the major lignan. Apart from SDG, flaxseed is a potential source of other phenolic compounds (Giada, 2010) natural phenolic glucosides, p-coumaric acid glucoside and ferulic acid glucoside (Strandås *et al.*, 2008).

Therapeutic Benefits of Flax Seeds

Traditionally, flaxseed has been grown for its oil. Flaxseed has been playing a major role in the field of diet and disease due to its potential health benefits associated with high content of α-linolenic acid, the phytoestrogen, lignans and soluble fiber. Health care professionals recommend flaxseeds due to their numerous health benefits in diabetes, CVD, cancer etc.

According to the U.S. Department of Agriculture, flaxseeds contain 27 identifiable cancer preventive compounds, and thus offer many benefits. Lignans have been implicated as having antitumourigenic (Thompson *et al.*, 1996a,b), estrogenic and/ or antiestrogenic (Collins *et al.*, 1997) and antioxidant (Prasad, 1997a,b; Prasad, 2000a; Kitts *et al.*, 1999) properties. The ALA content of flaxseed was found to be the primary component that provided the antiarrhythmic action (Ander *et al.*, 2004) which may explain the lower incidence of sudden death in subjects ingesting ALA (Albert *et al.*, 2005). In experimental animal trials, SDG significantly reduced high-fat diet-induced visceral and liver fat accumulation, hyperlipidemia, hypercholesterolemia, hyperinsulinemia and hyperleptinemia (Fukumitsu *et al.*, 2008). The mechanism proposed for these actions was the regulation of adipogenesis-related gene expression induced by flaxseed lignans.

Antioxidant and Anti-inflammatory

Secoisolariciresinol diglucoside exhibits significant antioxidant effects and inhibits DNA scissions, lipid peroxidation and decreases ROS (Newairy *et al.*, 2009; Lee *et al.*, 2008; Prasad, 2000a,b; 2001; Kitts *et al.*, 1999). Dietary flaxseed, flaxseed oil, or flaxseed lignan decreased inflammation, oxidative lung damage, lipid peroxidation, and hyperinsulinemia in animals (Ogborn *et al.*, 2006; Lee *et al.*, 2009; Velasquez *et al.*, 2003; Fukumitsu *et al.*, 2008). Diet supplemented with flax and pumpkin seeds mixture accelerated the antioxidant enzymes activities observed in diabetic rats and significantly decreased kidney malonaldialdehyde levels. Kidney histological sections showed glomerular hypertrophy and tubular dilatation. Thus, the flax and pumpkin seeds mixture may be helpful to prevent diabetes and its complications (Makni *et al.*, 2010, 2011).

Flaxseed supplementation decreased TBARS ($p = 0.0215$) and HOMA-IR ($p = 0.0382$) but did not change plasma inflammatory biomarkers. The study provided a weak support that decreased insulin resistance might have been secondary to antioxidant activity of flaxseed and suggested further investigation (Rhee and Brunt, 2011). Flax seed is protective against pulmonary ischemia-reperfusion injury in an experimental murine model and that it affects ROS generation and ROS detoxification via pathways not limited to upregulation of antioxidant enzymes such as HO-1 (Lee *et al.*, 2008). Lee-Hilz *et al.* (2006) points to the possibility that the flavonoid component of flax seed may be acting in a pro-oxidant manner to upregulate cytoprotective enzymes such as NQO-1 and GST. They showed that the reduction potential of flavonoids directly correlates with the induction of ARE-mediated gene transcription. The relationship between FS lignans and flax seed flavonoids is complex. Flaxseed oil suppresses oxygen radical production by white blood cells, prolongs bleeding time, and in higher doses suppresses serum levels of inflammatory mediators and does not lower serum lipids (Prasad, 2009 a).

Several investigators reported significant anti-inflammatory effects of flaxseeds (Cohen *et al.*, 2005; Dupasquier *et al.*, 2007; Ogborn *et al.*, 2006; Caughey *et al.*, 1996; Paschos *et al.*, 2005; Kaithwas *et al.*, 2011). Flaxseed oil, flaxseed lignan, or whole flaxseed supplementation significantly decreased serum TNF-α, IL-1 β, IL-6, CRP, glucose, or glycosylated haemoglobin concentrations or increased insulin sensitivity in humans (Caughey *et al.*, 1996; Zhang *et al.*, 2008; Pan *et al.*, 2007; Hallund *et al.*, 2008; Bloedon *et al.*, 2008). The oil also inhibited arachidonic acid-induced inflammation, suggesting its capacity to inhibit both cyclooxygenase and lipoxygenase pathways of arachidonate metabolism.

Singh *et al.* (2012) demonstrated the anti-arthritic and disease modifying activity of flax seed fixed oil and believed that dietary incorporation of flax seed oil may be beneficial in the prevention and management of rheumatoid arthritis and other chronic inflammatory disorders.

Antidiabetic

Flaxseeds or its oil are found to be beneficial in diabetes, as a hypoglycaemic agent and for prevention or management of complications of diabetes. Studies have shown that SDG from flaxseed can prevent the development of type 1 diabetes by approximately 71 per cent (Prasad, 2000 b) and type 2 diabetes by 80 per cent in animal models with induced diabetes (Prasad, 2001). Statistically significant improvements in glycemic control were also observed in type 2 diabetic patients treated for 12 weeks with 360 mg/day of flaxseed-derived lignan supplement (Pan *et al.*, 2007). The Long-chain PUFAs and lignans of flaxseeds can increase cell membrane fluidity, enhance the number of insulin receptors and the affinity of insulin to its receptors, suppress TNF-α, IL-6, macrophage migration inhibitory factor and leptin synthesis, increase the number of glucose transporter type 4 receptors, serve as endogenous ligands of peroxisome proliferator-activated receptors, modify lipolysis and regulate the balance between pro- and antioxidants (Das, 2005).

Haliga *et al.* (2007) reported that dietary flaxseed supplementation may reduce the incidence of diabetic macrovascular complications through improvement of lipid profile as the same induced significant reductions in hepatic cholesterol (-39.5 per cent) and triglycerides levels (-28.8 per cent). Tao *et al.* (2008) found that dietary intake of ALA (highest quintile greater than 2.11 g/day) was positively associated with lower odds of peripheral neuropathy. In an animal model, Velasquez *et al.* (2003) reported that flaxseed meals reduced proteinuria and ameliorated nephropathy in type 2 diabetes mellitus. In type 2 diabetic patients, 5 g/day of flaxseed oil consumption has been associated with a significant reduction of plasmin alpha-2-plasmin inhibitor complex level, plasminogen activator inhibitor-1 activity and thrombin anti-thrombin III complex level thus preventing thrombosis in diabetics after two weeks of intervention (Tohgi, 2004). Pan *et al.* (2009a) suggested from their study that lignan might modulate C-reactive protein levels in type 2 diabetics. These results need to be confirmed by further large clinical trials of longer duration.

Offspring from mothers fed with flaxseeds (F mothers) had higher body mass since lactation until adulthood. At 21 days of age, they presented lower total and subcutaneous fat mass, higher leptinemia, lower total cholesterol, lower triacylglycerol and lower insulinemia ($p<0.05$). At 180 days, offspring from F mothers had lower glycemia, higher insulinemia and lower adiponectin ($p<0.05$) concentrations and they did not show any changes in body composition (Figueiredo *et al.*, 2009).

Hypolipidemic and Cardioprotective

Human studies have shown that flaxseed can modestly reduce serum total and low-density lipoprotein cholesterol concentrations, reduce postprandial glucose absorption, decrease some markers of inflammation, and raise serum levels of the ω-3 fatty acids- ALA and eicosapentaenoic acid (Bloedon and Szapary, 2004).

Flax seeds may lower cholesterol levels, especially in women (Pan *et al.*, 2009b). In general, flaxseed-enriched diets have been reported to induce anywhere from 0 per cent to 18 per cent decreases in LDL and 0 per cent to 11 per cent decreases in TC (Bloedon and Szapary, 2004), most studies reported no changes in HDL levels in response to dietary flax-seed (Cunnane *et al.*, 1995; Clark *et al.*, 2001; Lemay *et al.*, 2002; Arjmandi *et al.*, 1998; Lucas *et al.*, 2002).

Prasad (1999) reported that rabbits receiving secoisolariciresinol diglucoside, had reduced hypercholesterolemic atherosclerosis that could be partly attributed to lowered total- and low-density lipoprotein (LDL)-cholesterol concentrations. Flax lignan complex was effective in slowing down the progression of atherosclerosis by 31 per cent, and this effect was associated with a reduction in oxidative stress (Prasad, 2009b).

However, the hypocholesterolemic effects of whole flaxseed can also be attributed to its α-linolenic acid and fiber components (Cunnane *et al.*, 1995; Bierenbaum *et al.*, 1993; Jenkins *et al.*, 1999). The mechanism involved in hyperlipidemic effect of flaxseeds was explained as reduction in serum total cholesterol and LDL cholesterol and that the antiatherogenic activity of flaxseed is independent of its α-linolenic acid content (Prasad *et al.*, 1998). Soluble fiber mucilage present in flaxseed may also contribute to the observed hypo-cholesterolemic properties (Brown *et al.*, 1999; Chen and Anderson, 1986).

Moreover, other constituents present in flaxseed may also play an essential role in lipid metabolism. For instance, the hypocholesterolemic effects of α-linolenic acid have been reported in both animals (Garg *et al.*, 1989) and humans (Chan *et al.*, 1991). Cornish *et al.* (2009) found no differences between groups fed flax seed lignan and the placebo for change in bone measures, body composition, lipoproteins, or cytokines.

Males taking the flaxseed lignan complex reduced metabolic syndrome score relative to men taking placebo, but a similar trend was not seen in females.

Flaxseed consumption was reported to be beneficial as a hypolipidemic agent in post menopausal women too. Lucas *et al.* (2002) have shown that supplementation of flaxseed to the diets of postmenopausal women can lower concentrations of serum total cholesterol and non-HDL cholesterol. Flaxseed given in the form of bread and muffins reduced total cholesterol in postmenopausal women (Arjmandi *et al.*, 1998). It has been suggested that the consumption of up to 50 g flaxseed in its raw form is also safe (Cunnane *et al.*, 1993). Moreover, the lignan SDG is converted by bacteria in the colon of humans and other animals to enterodiol and enterolactone, referred to as mammalian lignans. These exhibit weak estrogenic activity as they can bind to estrogen receptors on cell membranes (Nesbitt *et al.*, 1999).

In a crossover study in which hyperlipidemic men and postmenopausal women were fed 50 g of partially defatted flaxseed daily for 3 weeks, Jenkins *et al.* (1999) observed overall reductions of 5.5 and 9.7 per cent in serum total- and LDL-cholesterol concentrations, respectively and concluded that flaxseed gum is likely the major active ingredient responsible for the lipid-lowering action of flaxseed. They also confirmed that supplementing the diet with partially defatted flaxseed results in reductions in serum LDL-cholesterol concentrations similar to those observed with full-fat flaxseed by *Cunnane et al. (1993; 1995) and Bierenbaum et al. (1993).* Dietary flaxseed significantly improves lipid profile in hyperlipidemic patients and may favourably modify cardiovascular risk factors (Manda°escu *et al.*, 2005).

Recently, Patade *et al.* (2008) found that mild to moderate hypercholesterolemic Native American postmenopausal women who consumed flaxseed (30 g/day) for three months exhibited a reduction of TC by 7 per cent and LDL cholesterol by 10 per cent without changes in HDL cholesterol or TG concentrations. Zhang *et al.* (2008) also found significant reductions in TC (22 per cent) and LDL cholesterol levels (24 per cent) in hypercholesterolemic subjects after an eight-week dietary supplementation with 600 mg/day of secoisolariciresinol diglucoside (SDG), a lignan derived from flaxseed. These results suggest that specific subgroups of patients could obtain more beneficial hypolipidemic effects from flaxseed or its components.

Flaxseed has gained much importance in recent times as ethnomedicine due to its wide pharmacological actions. Although its therapeutic potential, as antioxidant, primarily as hydroxyl radical scavenger, anticancer, antidiabetic antiviral, bactericidal, anti-inflammatory, and antiatherosclerotic agent is known (Zanwar *et al.*, 2010; Rajesha *et al.*, 2006; Chen *et al.*, 2002; Prasad, 1997a; 2000a; b; Collins *et al.*, 2003; Kinniry *et al.*, 2006), very few studies evaluating its cardioprotective potential are presently available (Penumathsa *et al.*, 2007; 2008). Based on the clinical trials, epidemiological investigations and experimental studies, Rodriguez-Leyva *et al.* (2010) reviewed the available work on flax seeds and CVD to identify the known cardiovascular effects of flaxseed and to importantly emphasize the need for further research in this area.

Clinical trials (Chan *et al.*, 1991) have provided further evidence that consumption of α-linolenic acid-rich oils such as flaxseed oil may offer greater protection against cardiovascular disease than linoleic acid-rich oils through their effects on platelet functions. Flaxseed is an alternative to marine products as it is one of the richest sources of the plant-based and ω-3 fatty acids, alpha-linolenic acid (ALA). Based on the results of clinical trials, epidemiological investigations and experimental studies, ingestion of ALA has been suggested to have a positive impact on CVD. Because of its high ALA content, the use of flax seed has been advocated to combat CVD (Rodriguez-Leyva *et al.*, 2010). The results are persuasive because most of these studies gathered data from large sample populations and/or over relatively long collection periods. Allman *et al.* (1995) have shown some changes in platelet aggregation as a function of flaxseed ingestion.

In the Lyon Diet Heart Study (de Lorgeril *et al.*, 1999), ALA was associated with a decreased risk of recurrent fatal and nonfatal myocardial infarction, and a 73 per cent reduction in risk of primary end points (cardiac mortality and morbidity) between the experimental and control groups. In a double-blinded, placebo-controlled study (Singh *et al.*, 1997) conducted in India, 120 patients with suspected acute myocardial infarction were followed and supplemented with 2.9 g/day of ALA (enriched oil). After one year of follow-up, both cardiac death and nonfatal myocardial infarction were significantly lower in this group of patients compared with those on placebo. ALA may involve a potent anti-inflammatory action.

Atherosclerosis was significantly prevented by flaxseed supplementation in the hypercholesterolemic rabbit (Dupasquier *et al.*, 2006) and in the cholesterol-fed, low-density lipoprotein (LDL) receptor-deficient mice (Dupasquier *et al.*, 2007). Flaxseed (0.4 g/day) effectively inhibited the expression of inflammatory markers such as interleukin (IL)-6, mac-3, vascular cell adhesion molecule (VCAM)-1 and the proliferative marker proliferating cell nuclear antigen in aortic atherosclerotic tissue from LDL receptor-deficient mice (Dupasquier *et al.*, 2007). The circulating TG levels were reported to increase in response to a flaxseed diet in older subjects (Cunnane *et al.*, 1995, Djoussé *et al.*, 2005; Singer *et al.*, 1986)) while decreased or did not show any effect in younger subjects (Rallidis *et al.*, 2004; Paschos *et al.*, 2007). The age of the subjects in these studies could have been responsible as younger subjects responded with a decrease in blood TG concentrations after flaxseed (6 g ALA/day) ingestion, whereas older subjects did not (Patenaude *et al.*, 2009). Dupasquier *et al.* (2006) found that a flaxseed-supplemented, ALA-rich diet (12.5 g of flaxseed/day) preserved vascular relaxation from the deleterious effects induced by an atherogenic, high-cholesterol diet suggesting that ALA may directly induce beneficial vascular effects.

Bassett *et al.* (2011) observed that by inclusion of milled flaxseed in an atherogenic diet, brought about a significant reduction in atherosclerosis compared with the groups that consumed cholesterol and/or TFA. ALA was the only component within flaxseed that could inhibit the atherogenic action of cholesterol and/or TFA on its own. Alder *et al.* (2004) demonstrated that dietary flaxseed exerts antiarrhythmic effects during ischemia-reperfusion in rabbit hearts, possibly through shortening of the action potential. Again, Albert *et al.* (2008) provided evidence for an inverse association between ALA intake and the risk of sudden cardiac death among women, supporting the hypothesis that the n-3 fatty acids may have antiarrhythmic properties.

Paschos *et al.* (2007) have reported that 12 weeks of dietary flaxseed supplementation (8 g/day of ALA) resulted in a significant decrease in systolic and diastolic blood pressure in dyslipidemic patients. Conversely, Stuglin and Prasad (2005) found no changes in blood pressure in a shorter four-week intervention using 32.7 g/day of total flaxseed. However, their study examined healthy men and may indicate that pathological conditions are required to detect significant changes in HBP. Thus, studies on high blood pressure (HBP) using flaxseed as a source of ALA are inconclusive.

Spence *et al.* (2003) reported that the rise in blood pressure during mental stress, a strong predictor of atherosclerosis progression, is ameliorated by flaxseed. They also found a decrease in plasma cortisol values in the high-risk post-menopausal women treated with flaxseed. Prasad (2005) observed that lignan complex isolated from flaxseed reduced the extent of hypercholesterolemic atherosclerosis and this effect was associated with marked decreases in oxidative stress, serum total cholesterol, LDL-C and risk ratio, and elevation of serum HDL-C. Secoisolariciresinol diglucoside (SDG) isolated from flaxseed is a lipid-lowering and antioxidant agent. It suppresses the development of hypercholesterolemic atherosclerosis in rabbits. A longer duration of treatment reduces the progression of atherosclerosis to a greater extent, and tends to regress the atherosclerosis (Prasad, 2009 b). Adiponectin, an adipose-specific secretory protein, exhibits antidiabetic and anti-atherogenic properties. The ALA-rich flaxseed oil ingestion in rats exhibited beneficial effects through an increase of the adiponectin level (Sekine *et al.*, 2008). At 250 days old Flax seed supplementation presented significant reduction in body fat mass ($p<0.000$) and higher levels of hemoglobin ($p=0.019$) and albumin ($p=0.030$) than the rats from control group. The long term consumption of flaxseed altered hematologic and immunological indicators in adult Wistar rats (Cardozo *et al.*, 2011).

Nestel *et al.* (1997) reported that in obese human subjects, 20 g/day of ALA from flaxseed oil significantly increased arterial compliance and decreased LDL oxidation when it was compared with an oleic acid and saturated fat intervention. ALA was thought to be the component in flaxseed oil that was responsible for this effect. In overweight adolescents, a significant association among plasma fatty acid composition, metabolic syndrome and low-grade inflammation has been identified (Klein-Platat *et al.*, 2005). ALA levels in plasma cholesterol esters were also inversely related to C-reactive protein (CRP). From these findings, it was suggested that a high intake of long-chain PUFAs, especially ω-3 PUFAs, may protect obese subjects against metabolic syndrome and low-grade inflammation in early adolescence. Consistent with this hypothesis, Faintuch *et al.* (2007) found that morbidly obese patients decreased their white blood cell count, CRP levels, serum amyloid A and fibronectin after two weeks of 5 g/day ALA supplementation from flaxseed.

The omega-3 ALA found in the flaxseed oil fraction also contributes to the antiatherogenic effects of flaxseed via anti-inflammatory and antiproliferative mechanisms. Dietary flaxseed may also protect against ischemic heart disease by improving vascular relaxation responses and by inhibiting the incidence of ventricular fibrillation (Bassett *et al.*, 2009). Kinniry *et al.* (2006) found dietary FS to decrease lung inflammation and lipid peroxidation, suggesting a protective role against pro-oxidant-induced tissue damage *in vivo*. Two independent studies of healthy subjects have shown that inflammatory markers, such as tumour necrosis factor alpha (TNF-α), IL-1-beta, thromboxane B_5 and prostaglandin E_5, were significantly reduced after administration of an ALA-rich diet (13.7 g/day of ALA from flaxseed) (Caughey *et al.*, 1996), as were VCAM-1 and E-selectin after delivery of 2 g/day of ALA (Thies *et al.*, 2001). ALA intake (8 g/day) from a flaxseed source decreases serum concentrations of serum amyloid A, IL-6 (Rallidis *et al.*, 2003), soluble VCAM-1, soluble intercellular adhesion molecule-1, soluble E-selectin (Zhao *et al.*, 2004) as well as the production of TNF-α, IL-1-beta and prostaglandin E_2 by peripheral blood mononuclear cells (Caughey *et al.*, 1996) over a period of four to 12 weeks with doses of ALA greater than 9 g/day.

The study by Barakat and Mahmoud (2011) suggests that both flax/pumpkin and purslane/pumpkin seed mixtures had anti-atherogenic hypolipidemic and immunmodulator effects which were probably mediated by unsaturated fatty acids (including alpha linolenic acid) present in seed mixture.

Interestingly, Flaxseed intake during lactation did not produce histological alterations in prostatic alveolus or in sexual hormones, but programmed to a reduction in lipid profile in adult life with decreased cardiovascular risk (Cardozo *et al.*, 2010 a). Similarly, the cardiotoxic effect of isoprenalin was less in flax lignan concentrate pretreated animals, which was confirmed in histopathological alterations. Haemodynamic, biochemical alteration and histopathological results suggest a cardioprotective protective effect of FLC in isoprenalin induced cardiotoxicity (Zanwar *et al.*, 2011).

Anticarcinogenic

Initial studies suggested that flax seeds taken in the diet may benefit individuals with certain types of breast (Chen *et al.*, 2006; Thompson *et al.*, 2005) and prostate cancers. Lignans have been implicated as having antitumourigenic effect. Inhibition of tumour growth in the breast, prostate, skin, and liver has been observed in animal models suggesting that flaxseed may have other endocrine and non-endocrine effects (Thompson *et al.*, 1996a,b). Lehraiki *et al.* (2010) showed that lignans modulate development of breast cancer cells. The most intense effect was observed for anhydrosecoisolariciresinol, which significantly decreased cell growth at 50 and 100 μM.

Flaxseed inhibited the growth of human estrogen-dependent breast cancer and strengthened the tumour inhibitory effect of tamoxifen at both low and high E2 levels (Chen *et al.*, 2004). Flax seed is rich in mammalian lignan precursors and alpha-linolenic acid, which have been suggested as having anticancer effects. Studies have shown that 10 per cent flax seed inhibited the growth of human estrogen-dependent breast cancer in athymic mice, and it enhanced the inhibitory effect of tamoxifen. Chen *et al.* (2007) and Saggar *et al.* (2010) observed flax seed to inhibit breast tumour growth in a dose-dependent manner and to enhance the inhibitory effect of tamoxifen by modulating the estrogen receptor and growth factor signal transduction pathways. Dietary flaxseed not only inhibited the growth of human breast tumours but also enhanced the effectiveness of tamoxifen in athymic mice with low oestradiol levels.

The n-3 fatty acid-rich cotyledon fraction of flax seed lowered cell proliferation but had no effect on apoptosis; the opposite was observed with tamoxifen. Tumour regression in the flax seed/tamoxifen group was greater compared to the tamoxifen group.

After long-term treatment, flax seed did not stimulate tumour growth and combined with tamoxifen, regressed tumour size in part due to down regulation of the expression of estrogen-related gene products and signal transduction pathways (Chen *et al.*, 2011). Secoisolariciresinol diglucoside has a similar effect as flax seed in reducing tumour growth and in mechanisms of action. The lesser effects of flax seed hull indicated a need for a higher dose to be more effective (Chen *et al.*, 2009).

Consumption of flax, a significant source of dietary estrogens, in addition to their habitual diets increased excretion of enterodiol and enterolactone, but not matairesinol, in a dose-dependent manner in a group of postmenopausal women. Urinary excretion of lignan metabolites is a dose-dependent biomarker of flaxseed intake within the context of a habitual diet (Hutchins *et al.*, 2000). Flaxseed supplementation significantly increased urinary estrogen excretion ($p < 0.0005$) and the urinary 2-hydroxyestrogen and 16 alpha-hydroxyestrone ratio ($p < 0.05$) in a linear, dose-response fashion. There were no significant differences in urinary 16 alpha-hydroxyestrone excretion suggesting that flaxseed may have chemoprotective effects in postmenopausal women (Haggans *et al.*, 1999).

Vascular endothelial growth factor is one key factor in promotion of breast cancer angiogenesis. Dabrosin *et al.* (2002) showed that supplementation of 10 per cent flaxseed, the richest source of mammalian lignans, to mice with established human breast tumours reduced tumour growth and metastasis. Moreover, flaxseed decreased extracellular levels of vascular endothelial growth factor, which may be one mechanistic explanation to the decreased tumour growth and metastasis. Flaxseed has also been shown to reduce the early risk markers for and incidence of mammary and colonic carcinogenesis in animal models (Serraino and Thompson, 1991; 1992; Jenab and Thompson, 1996a,b) and to affect menstrual cycle length in premenopausal women (Phipps, 1993).

Dietary flax seed given post-X-ray thoracic radiation therapy mitigates radiation effects by decreasing pulmonary fibrosis, inflammation, cytokine secretion and lung damage while enhancing mouse survival. Dietary supplementation of flax seed may be a useful adjuvant treatment mitigating adverse effects of radiation in individuals exposed to inhaled radioisotopes or incidental radiation (Christofidou-Solomidou *et al.*, 2011).

Antiulcerogenic and Hepatoprotective

Flax seed fixed oil exhibited significant antiulcer activity against different ulcerogens in experimental animal models. The same significantly inhibited acetylcholine and histamine-induced contraction of guinea pig and rat ileums, respectively, suggesting its anticholinergic and antihistaminic activity which could probably have contributed towards antiulcer activity (Kaithwas and Majumdar, 2010a).

Makni *et al.* (2008) reported that the antiatherogenic and hepatoprotective effects were probably mediated by unsaturated fatty acids present in seed mixture. In control group of rats fed with 1 per cent cholesterol diet (control), lipid parameters decreased significantly, plasma and liver fatty acid composition showed an increase of PUFAs (ALA and LA), and MUFAs (oleic and eicosaenoic acid) and a decrease of SFA (palmitic and stearic acid). In plasma and liver of group fed diet enriched with flax and pumpkin seed mixture, malondialdehyde levels decreased and the efficiency of antioxidant defense system was improved as compared to control group. Liver histological sections showed lipid storage in hepatocytes of control group and an improvement was noted in the experimental group.

Memory

Significant increase in brain weight (39 per cent) and relative brain weight (37 per cent) was verified in pups from mothers fed with flaxseed diet. Maternal diet of flaxseed during pregnancy influences the incorporation of ω-3 fatty acid in the composition of brain tissue, assuring a good development of this organ in newborn rats (Almeida *et al.*, 2011). Rats fed 10 per cent flax seed diet plus casein had lower food intake, protein and weight variation than those fed 10 per cent casein diet. Flaxseed promoted adequate growth and better brain development in animals again explained to be due to increased incorporation of omega-3 into these tissues (Leite, 2011).

Bone Health

Due to structural similarities between lignans and estrogen, it can be postulated that lignans present in flaxseed may also play a role in the maintenance of skeletal health. As far as the effect of flaxseed on bone is concerned, there is a paucity of data. The findings of a study by Babu *et al.* (2000) indicated that feeding whole or defatted flaxseed to weanling female rats for 56 days suppressed serum total Alkaline Phosphatase activity, a nonspecific marker of bone formation. But the findings of a three month study by Lucas *et al.* (2002) indicated that flaxseed has no effect on bone metabolism, as evident by its lack of effects on biomarkers of bone turnover.

But, due to its anti inflammatory effect flaxseed was proved to be beneficial in arthritis. Flax seed fixed oil showed a significant dose-dependent protective effect against Complete Freund's Adjuvant (CFA)-induced arthritis as well. Secondary lesions produced by CFA due to a delayed hypersensitivity reaction were also reduced in a significant manner. Anti-inflammatory activity of the fixed oil can be attributed to the presence of alpha linolenic acid (57.38 per cent, an ω-3 fatty acids, 18:3, n-3) having dual inhibitory effect on arachidonate metabolism resulting in suppressed production of pro-inflammatory n-6 eicosanoids (PGE (2), LTB (4)) and diminished vascular permeability. These observations suggest possible therapeutic potential of the fixed oil of Flax seed in inflammatory disorders like rheumatoid arthritis (Kaithwas and Majumdar, 2010b).

Analgesic and Antipyretic

Flaxseed oil raised the pain threshold to a lesser extent than morphine in tail immersion model, but showed excellent peripherally acting, analgesic activity comparable to aspirin, against acetic acid-induced writhing in mouse. In typhoid, paratyphoid A/B vaccine-induced pyrexia, the oil showed antipyretic activity comparable to aspirin. Dual inhibition of arachidonic acid metabolism, antihistaminic and antibradykinin activities of the oil could account for the biological activity and the active principle could be alpha -linolenic acid an omega-3 (18:3, n-3) fatty acid (Kaithwas *et al.*, 2011).

Other Benefits

Leite *et al.* (2012) observed the food intake, litter size, milk fat content, body weight of the offspring at weaning and weight gain in the group receiving a 25 per cent flaxseed plus 14 per cent casein providing 17 per cent protein and control group receiving a casein-based diet with 17 per cent protein, thus proving that 25 per cent flaxseed promotes an adequate offspring growth.

Moreover, a new potential for flaxseed as a food preservative is under exploration. The fungistatic activity of flaxseed flour was investigated by Xu *et al.* (2008) using the test microorganisms of Strains of *P. chrysogenum, A. flavus, F. graminearum*, and a *Penicillium* sp. isolated from molded noodles. Though there were differences in the degree of mold inhibition among flax seed obtained from different sources and cultivars the authors suggested that flaxseed could be used as a multifunctional food ingredient as it possesses fungistatic activity.

Safety Concerns

When exposed to air or high temperatures used in food preparation, the polyunsaturated fatty acids may undergo thermal or autooxidation. But, studies on oxidation products of intact flaxseed lipids have not shown any harmful effects when flaxseed is included up to 28 per cent, in the baked products.

Also, the presence of cyanogenic glucosides and diglucosides in the flax seeds is a concern as they may release cyanide upon hydrolysis. But, cyanide levels produced as a result of autolysis are below the harmful limits to humans. After oil extraction the meal requires detoxification. However, solvent extraction when used in animal rations was found to reduce the harmful effects of cyanide (Wanasundara and Shahidi (1998).

Cardozo *et al.* (2010 b) found maternal consumption of a flaxseed-based diet during lactation to result in lower body weight at weaning and lower hemoglobin levels in adulthood, when compared with the control group. Flaxseed during perinatal and post-weaning periods improves spatial memory to the detriment of growth. These findings indicate that there must be caution in encouraging the maternal intake of flaxseed during pregnancy and lactation (Fernandes *et al.*, 2011).

Flaxseed supplementation to mothers decreases offspring adiposity and increases pituitary leptin signaling at weaning, but it induces hypertrophic adipocytes and higher thyroid leptin receptor in adulthood. The present data suggest that extensive use of flaxseed during lactation is undesirable (Figueiredo *et al.*, 2012). Also, maternal intake of flaxseed in the diet during lactation produces early insulin sensitivity and hyper-leptinemia. These hormonal imprinting factors could program for selective insulin resistance, since the higher insulin serum concentration was not associated with higher adiposity. These findings, associated with lower serum adiponectin concentration in adulthood, could indicate an increased risk for later development of diabetes mellitus (Figueiredo *et al.*, 2009).

Conclusion

It is indeed gratifying to note that flaxseed has been scientifically credited to be antidiabetic, anticarcinogenic, anti-inflammatory and cardioprotective. However, the safety issues have to be kept in mind while recommending flax seed for therapeutic purposes.

References

Albert CM, Oh K, Whang W, Manson JE, Chae CU, Stampfer MJ, Willett WC, Hu FB. (2005). Dietary alpha-linolenic acid intake and risk of sudden cardiac death and coronary heart disease. Circulation. 112 (21): 3232–38.

Allman MA, Pena NM, Pang D (1995). Supplementation with flaxseed oil versus sunflower oil in healthy young men consuming a low fat diet: Effects on platelet composition and function. Eur. J. Clin. Nutr. 49 (3): 169–78.

Almeida Lenzi KC, Teles Boaventura G, Guzmán Silva MA (2011). Influence of ω-3 fatty acids from the flaxseed (Linum usitatissimum) on the brain development of newborn rats. Nutr. Hosp. 26 (5): 991–96.

Alpers L, Sawyer-Morse MK (1996). Eating Quality of Banana Nut Muffins and Oatmeal Cookies Made With Ground Flaxseed. Journal of the American Dietetic Association. 96 (8): 794–96.

Ander BP, Weber AR, Rampersad PP, Gilchrist JS, Pierce GN, Lukas A (2004). Dietary flaxseed protects against ventricular fibrillation induced by ischemia-reperfusion in normal and hypercholesterolemic rabbits. J. Nutr. 134 (12): 3250–56.

Arjmandi BH, Khan DA, Juma S, Drum ML, Venkatesh S, Sohn E, Wei L, Derman R (1998). Whole flaxseed consumption lowers serum LDL-cholesterol and lipoprotein (a) concentrations in postmenopausal women. Nutr. Res. 18: 1203–14.

Babu US, Mitchell GV, Wiesenfeld P, Jenkins MY, Gowda H (2000). Nutritional and hematological impact of dietary flaxseed and defatted flaxseed meal in rats. Int. J. Food Sci. Nutr. 51 (2): 109–17.

Barakat LA, Mahmoud RH (2011). The antiatherogenic, renal protective and immunomodulatory effects of purslane, pumpkin and flax seeds on hypercholesterolemic rats. N. Am. J. Med. Sci. 3 (9): 411–17.

Bassett CM, McCullough RS, Edel AL, Patenaude A, LaVallee RK, Pierce GN (2011). The α-linolenic acid content of flaxseed can prevent the atherogenic effects of dietary trans fat. Am J Physiol Heart Circ Physiol. 301 (6): H 2220–26.

Bassett CM, Rodriguez-Leyva D, Pierce GN (2009). Experimental and clinical research findings on the cardiovascular benefits of consuming flaxseed. Appl. Physiol. Nutr. Metab. 34 (5): 965–74.

Bierenbaum ML, Reichstein R, Watkins TR (1993). Reducing atherogenic risk in hyperlipemic humans with flaxseed supplementation: a preliminary report. J. Am. Coll. Nutr. 12: 501–504.

Bloedon LT, Balikai S, Chittams J, Cunnane S, Berlin J, Rader D, Szapary PO (2008). Flaxseed and cardiovascular risk factors: results from a double blind, randomized, controlled clinical trial. J. Am. Coll. Nutr. 27: 65–74.

Bloedon LT, Szapary PO (2004). Flaxseed and cardiovascular risk. Nutr. Rev. 62 (1): 18–27.

Brown L, Rosner B, Willett WW, Sacks FM (1999). Cholesterol-lowering effects of dietary fiber: a meta-analysis. Am. J. Clin. Nutr. 69 (1): 30–42.

Cardozo LF, Alves Chagas M, Leal Soares L, Andrade Troina A, Teles Bonaventura G. (2010 a). Exposure to flaxseed during lactation does not alter prostate area or epithelium height but changes lipid profile in rats. Nutr. Hosp. 25 (2): 250–255.

Cardozo LF, Soares LL, Cardozo Brant LH, Chagas MA, Pereira AV, Coca Velarde LG, Teles Boaventura G (2011). Hematologic and immunological indicators are altered by chronic intake of flaxseed in Wistar rats. Nutr. Hosp. 26 (5): 1091–96.

Cardozo LF, Soares LL, Chagas MA, Boaventura GT (2010 b). Maternal consumption of flaxseed during lactation affects weight and hemoglobin level of offspring in rats. J. Pediatr. (Rio J). 86 (2): 126–30.

Caughey GE, Mantzioris E, Gibson RA, Cleland LG, James MJ (1996). The effect on human tumour necrosis factor alpha and interleukin 1 beta production of diets enriched in n-3 fatty acids from vegetable oil or fish oil. Am. J. Clin. Nutr. 63 (1): 116–22.

Chan JK, Bruce VM, McDonald BE (1991). Dietary α-linolenic acid is as effective as oleic acid and linoleic acid in lowering blood cholesterol in normolipidemic men. Am. J. Clin. Nutr. 53 (5): 1230–40.

Chen J, Hui E, Ip T, Thompson LU (2004). Dietary flaxseed enhances the inhibitory effect of tamoxifen on the growth of estrogen-dependent human breast cancer (mcf-7) in nude mice. Clin Cancer Res. 10 (22): 7703–11.

Chen J, Power KA, Mann J, Cheng A, Thompson LU (2007). Flaxseed alone or in combination with tamoxifen inhibits MCF-7 breast tumour growth in ovariectomized athymic mice with high circulating levels of estrogen. Exp. Biol. Med. (Maywood). 232 (8): 1071–80.

Chen J, Saggar JK, Corey P, Thompson LU (2011). Flaxseed cotyledon fraction reduces tumour growth and sensitises tamoxifen treatment of human breast cancer xenograft (MCF-7) in athymic mice. Br. J. Nutr. 105 (3): 339–47.

Chen J, Saggar JK, Corey P, Thompson LU (2009). Flaxseed and pure secoisolariciresinol diglucoside, but not flaxseed hull, reduce human breast tumour growth (MCF-7) in athymic mice. J. Nutr. 139 (11): 2061–66.

Chen WJL, Anderson JW (1986). Hypocholesterolemic effects of soluble fibers. In: Kritchevsky D, Yahouny GV, eds. Dietary fiber: basic and clinical aspects. New York. Plenum Press. 275–89.

Chen JP, Stavro M, Thompson LU (2002). Dietary flaxseed inhibits human breast cancer growth and metastasis and down regulates expression of insulin-like growth factor and epidermal growth factor receptor. Nutr. Cancer. 43: 187–92.

Chen J, Wang L, Thompson LU (2006). Flaxseed and its components reduce metastasis after surgical excision of solid human breast tumour in nude mice. Cancer Lett. 234 (2): 168–75.

Christofidou-Solomidou M, Tyagi S, Tan KS, Hagan S, Pietrofesa R, Dukes F, Arguiri E, Heitjan DF, Solomides CC, Cengel KA (2011). Dietary flaxseed administered post thoracic radiation treatment improves survival and mitigates radiation-induced pneumonopathy in mice. BMC Cancer. 11: 269.

Clark WF, Kortas C, Heidenheim AP, Garland J, Spanner E, Parbtani A (2001). Flaxseed in lupus nephritis: A two-year nonplacebo-controlled crossover study. J. Am. Coll. Nutr. 20 (2Suppl): 143–48.

Cohen S, Moore A, Ward W (2005). Flaxseed oil and inflammation-associated bone abnormalities in interleukin-10 knockout mice. J. Nutr. Biochem. 16: 368–74.

Collins TF, Sprando RL, Black TN, Olejnik N, Wiesenfeld PW, Babu US (2003). Effects of flaxseed and defatted flaxseed meal on reproduction and development in rats. Food Chem. Toxicol. 41: 819 – 34.

Cornish SM, Chilibeck PD, Paus-Jennsen L, Biem HJ, Khozani T, Senanayake V, Vatanparast H, Little JP, Whiting SJ, Pahwa P (2009). A randomized controlled trial of the effects of flaxseed lignan complex on metabolic syndrome composite score and bone mineral in older adults. Appl. Physiol. Nutr. Metab. 34 (2): 89–98.

Cunnane SC, Ganguli S, Menard C, Liede AC, Hamadeh MJ, Chen ZY, Wolever TM, Jenkins DJ (1993). High a linolenic acid flaxseed (Linum usitatissimum): some nutritional properties in humans. Br. J. Nutr. 69 (2): 443–53.

Cunnane SC, Hamadeh MJ, Leide AC, Thompson LU, Wolever TMS, Jenkins DJA (1995). Nutritional attributes of traditional FS in healthy young adults. Am. J. Clin. Nutr. 61 (1): 62–68.

Dabrosin C, Chen J, Wang L, Thompson LU (2002). Flaxseed inhibits metastasis and decreases extracellular vascular endothelial growth factor in human breast cancer xenografts. Cancer Lett. 185 (1): 31–37.

Das UN (2005). A defect in the activity of Δ6 and Δ5 desaturases may be a factor predisposing to the development of insulin resistance syndrome. Prostaglandins Leukot. Essent. Fatty Acids. 72 (5): 343–50.

de Lorgeril M, Salen P, Martin JL, Monjaud I, Delaye J, Mamelle N (1999). Mediterranean diet, traditional risk factors, and the rate of cardiovascular complications after myocardial infarction: Final report of the Lyon Diet Heart Study. Circulation. 99 (6): 779–85.

Djoussé L, Hunt SC, Arnett DK, Province MA, Eckfeldt JH, Ellison RC (2003). Dietary linolenic acid is inversely associated with plasma triacylglycerol: The NHLBI Family Heart Study. Am. J. Clin. Nutr. 78 (6): 1098–102.

Djoussé L, Rautaharju PM, Hopkins PN, Whitsel EA, Arnett DK, Eckfeldt JH, Province MA, Ellison RC (2005). Dietary linolenic acid and adjusted QT and JT intervals in the NHLBI Family Heart Study. J. Am. Coll. Cardiol. 45 (10): 1716–22.

Dupasquier CM, Weber AM, Ander BP, *et al.* (2006). Effects of dietary flaxseed on vascular contractile function and atherosclerosis during prolonged hypercholesterolemia in rabbits. Am. J. Physiol. Heart Circ. Physiol. 291: H2 987–96.

Dupasquier CM, Dibrov E, Kostenuk AL, *et al.* (2007). Dietary flaxseed inhibits atherosclerosis in the LDL receptor deficient mouse in part through anti-proliferative and anti-inflammatory actions. Am. J. Physiol. Heart Circ. Physiol. 293: H 2394–402.

Faintuch J, Horie LM, Barbeiro HV, Barbeiro DF, Soriano FG, Ishida RK, Cecconello I (2007). Systemic inflammation in morbidly obese subjects: Response to oral supplementation with alpha-linolenic acid. Obes. Surg. 17 (3): 341–47.

FAO (2007). Food and Agricultural Organization of the United Nations: Economic and Social Department: The Statistical Division.

Fernandes FS, de Souza AS, do Carmo MG, Boaventura GT (2011). Maternal intake of flaxseed-based diet (Linum usitatissimum) on hippocampus fatty acid profile: implications for growth, locomotor activity and spatial memory. Nutrition. 27 (10): 1040–47.

Figueiredo MS, da Fonseca Passos MC, Trevenzoli IH, Troina AA, Carlos AS, Alves Nascimento-Saba CC, Fraga MC, Manhães AC, de Oliveira E, Lisboa PC, de Moura EG (2012). Adipocyte morphology and leptin signaling in rat offspring from mothers supplemented with flaxseed during lactation. Nutrition. 28 (3): 307–15.

Figueiredo MS, de Moura EG, Lisboa PC, Troina AA, Trevenzoli IH, Oliveira E, Boaventura GT, da Fonseca Passos MC (2009). Flaxseed supplementation of rats during lactation changes the adiposity and glucose homeostasis of their offspring. Life Sci. 85 (9-10): 365–71.

Ford JD, Huang KS, Wang HB, Davin LB, Lewis NG (2001). Biosynthetic pathway to the cancer chemopreventive secoisolariciresinol diglucoside-hydroxymethyl glutaryl ester-linked lignan oligomers in flax (Linum usitatissimum) seed. J. Nat. Prod. 64 (11): 1388–97.

Fukumitsu S, Aida K, Ueno N, Ozawa S, Takahashi Y, Kobori M (2008). Flaxseed lignan attenuates high-fat diet-induced fat accumulation and induces adiponectin expression in mice. Br. J. Nutr. 100 (3): 669–76.

Garg ML, Wierzbicki AA, Thomson ABR, Clandinin MT (1989). Dietary saturated fat level alters the competition between α-linolenic and linoleic acid. Lipids. 24 (4): 334–39.

Gebauer SK, Psota TL, Harris WS, Kris-Etherton PM (2006). n-3 fatty acid dietary recommendations and food sources to achieve essentiality and cardiovascular benefits. Am. J. Clin. Nutr. 83 (6 Suppl): 1526S–35S.

Giada Mde L (2010). Food applications for flaxseed and its components: products and processing. Recent Pat. Food Nutr. Agric. 2 (3): 181–86.

Haggans CJ, Hutchins AM, Olson BA, Thomas W, Martini MC, Slavin JL (1999). Effect of flaxseed consumption on urinary estrogen metabolites in postmenopausal women. Nutr Cancer. 33 (2): 188–95.

Haliga R, Mocanu V, Oboroceanu T, Stitt PA, Luca VC (2007). The effects of dietary flaxseed supplementation on lipid metabolism in streptozotocin-induced diabetic hamsters. Rev. Med. Chir. Soc. Med. Nat. Iasi. 111 (2): 472–76.

Hall C, Tulbek MC, Xu TY (2006). Advances in food and nutrition research, in Flaxseed. Elsevier Inc. pp. 2–3.

Hallund J, Tetens I, Bügel S, Tholstrup T, Bruun J (2008). The effect of a lignan complex isolated from flaxseed on inflammation markers in healthy postmenopausal women. Nutr. Metab. Cardiovasc. Dis. 18: 497–502.

Hutchins AM, Martini MC, Olson BA, Thomas W, Slavin JL (2000). Flaxseed influences urinary lignan excretion in a dose-dependent manner in postmenopausal women. Cancer Epidemiol Biomarkers Prev. 9 (10): 1113–18.

Jenab M., Thompson L. U (1996). The influence of flaxseed and lignans on colon carcinogenesis and β-glucuronidase activity. Carcinogenesis (Lond.), 17: 1343 – 48.

Jenkins DJ, Kendall CW, Vidgen E, Agarwal S, Rao AV, Rosenberg RS, Diamandis EP, Novokmet R, Mehling CC, Perera T, Griffin LC, Cunnane SC (1999). Health aspects of partially defatted flaxseed, including effects on serum lipids, oxidative measures, and ex vivo androgen and progestin activity: a controlled crossover trial. Am. J. Clin. Nutr. 69 (3): 395 – 402.

Kaithwas G, Majumdar DK (2010 a). Therapeutic effect of Linum usitatissimum (flaxseed/linseed) fixed oil on acute and chronic arthritic models in albino rats. Inflammopharmacology. 18 (3): 127–36.

Kaithwas G, Majumdar DK (2010 b). Evaluation of antiulcer and antisecretory potential of Linum usitatissimum fixed oil and possible mechanism of action. Inflammopharmacology. 18 (3): 137–45.

Kaithwas G, Mukherjee A, Chaurasia AK, Majumdar DK (2011). Anti-inflammatory, analgesic and antipyretic activities of Linum usitatissimum L. (flaxseed/linseed) fixed oil. Indian J Exp Biol. 49 (12): 932–38.

Kinniry P, Amrani Y, Vachani A, Solomides CC, Arguiri E, Workman A, Carter J, Christofidou-Solomidou M (2006). Dietary flaxseed supplementation ameliorates inflammation and oxidative tissue damage in experimental models of acute lung injury in mice. J. Nutr. 136 (6): 1545–51.

Kitts DD, Yuan YV, Wijewickreme AN, Thompson LU (1999). Antioxidant activity of the flaxseed lignan secoisolariciresinol diglycoside and its mammalian lignan metabolites enterodiol and enterolactone. Mol. Cell. Biochem. 202 (1-2): 91- 100.

Klein-Platat C, Drai J, Oujaa M, Schlienger JL, Simon C (2005). Plasma fatty acid composition is associated with the metabolic syndrome and low-grade inflammation in overweight adolescents. Am. J. Clin. Nutr. 82 (6): 1178–84.

Kvavadze E, Bar-Yosef O, Belfer-Cohen A, Boaretto E, Jakeli N, Matskevich Z, Meshveliani T. (2009).30,000-Year-Old Wild Flax Fibers. *Science*, 325(5946):1359.

Lee JC, Bhora F, Sun J, Cheng G, Arguiri E, Solomides CC, Chatterjee S, Christofidou-Solomidou M (2008). Dietary flaxseed enhances antioxidant defenses and is protective in a mouse model of lung ischemia-reperfusion injury. Am. J. Physiol. Lung Cell. Mol. Physiol. 294 (2): L 255–65.

Lee J, Krochak R, Blouin A, Kanterakis S, Chatterjee S, Arguiri E, Vachani A, Solomides C, Cengel K, Christofidou-Solomidou M (2009). Dietary flaxseed prevents radiation-induced oxidative lung damage, inflammation and fibrosis in a mouse model of thoracic radiation injury. Cancer Biol. Ther. 8: 47–53.

Lee-Hilz YY, Boerboom AM, Westphal AH, Berkel WJ, Aarts JM, Rietjens IM (2006). Pro-oxidant activity of flavonoids induces EpRE-mediated gene expression. Chem. Res. Toxicol. 19: 1499–505.

Lehraiki A, Attoumbré J, Bienaimé C, Matifat F, Bensaddek L, Nava-Saucedo E, Fliniaux MA, Ouadid-Ahidouch H, Baltora-Rosset S (2010). Extraction of lignans from flaxseed and evaluation of their biological effects on breast cancer MCF-7 and MDA-MB-231 cell lines. J. Med. Food. 13 (4): 834–41.

Leite Ferreira Costa CD, Calvi Lenzi de Almeida K, Guzmán-Silva MA, Azevedo de Meneses J, Teles Boaventura G (2011). Flaxseed and its contribution to body growth and brain of Wistar rats during childhood and adolescence. Nutr. Hosp. 26 (2): 415–20.

Leite CD, Vicente GC, Suzuki A, Pereira AD, Boaventura GT, Dos Santos RM, Velarde LG (2012). Effects of flaxseed on rat milk creamatocrit and its contribution to offspring body growth. J. Pediatr. (Rio J). 88 (1): 74–78.

Lemay A, Dodin S, Kadri N, Jacques H, Forest JC (2002). Flaxseed dietary supplement versus hormone replacement therapy in hypercholesterolemic menopausal women. Obstet. Gynecol. 100 (3): 495–504.

Lucas EA, Wild RD, Hammond LJ, Khalil DA, Juma S, Daggy BP, Stoecker BJ, Arjmandi BH (2002). Flaxseed improves lipid profile without altering biomarkers of bone metabolism in postmenopausal women. J. Clin. Endocrinol. Metab. 87 (4): 1527–32.

Makni M, Fetoui H, Gargouri NK, Garoui el M, Jaber H, Makni J, Boudawara T, Zeghal N (2008). Hypolipidemic and hepatoprotective effects of flax and pumpkin seed mixture rich in omega-3 and omega-6 fatty acids in hypercholesterolemic rats. Food Chem. Toxicol. 46 (12): 3714–20.

Makni M, Fetoui H, Gargouri NK, Garoui el M, Zeghal N (2011). Antidiabetic effect of flax and pumpkin seed mixture powder: effect on hyperlipidemia and antioxidant status in alloxan diabetic rats. J Diabetes Complications. 25 (5): 339–45.

Makni M, Sefi M, Fetoui H, Garoui el M, Gargouri NK, Boudawara T, Zeghal N (2010). Flax and Pumpkin seeds mixture ameliorates diabetic nephropathy in rats. Food Chem. Toxicol. 48 (8-9): 2407–12.

Manda°escu S, Mocanu V, Dãscaliþa AM, Haliga R, Nestian I, Stitt PA, Luca V (2005). Flaxseed supplementation in hyperlipidemic patients. Rev. Med. Chir. Soc. Med. Nat. Iasi. 109 (3): 502–506.

Nesbitt PD, Lam Y, Thompson LU (1999). Human metabolism of mammalian lignan precursors in raw and processed flaxseed. Am. J. Clin. Nutr. 69: 549–55.

Nestel PJ, Pomeroy SE, Sasahara T, Yamashita T, Liang YL, Dart AM, Jennings GL, Abbey M, Cameron JD. (1997). Arterial compliance in obese subjects is improved with dietary plant n-3 fatty acid from flaxseed oil despite increased LDL oxidizability. Arterioscler. Thromb. Vasc. Biol. 17 (6): 1163–70.

Newairy A, Abdou H (2009). Protective role of flax lignans against lead acetate induced oxidative damage and hyperlipidemia in rats. Food Chem. Toxicol. 47: 813–18.

Ogborn M, Nitschmann E, Bankovic-Calic N, Weiler H, Aukema H (2006). Effects of flaxseed derivatives in experimental polycystic kidney disease vary with animal gender. Lipids. 41: 1141–49.

Oomah BD (2001). Flaxseed as a functional food source. J. Sci. Food Agric. 81: 889–94.

Pan A, Demark-Wahnefried W, Ye X, Yu Z, Li H, Qi Q, Sun J, Chen Y, Chen X, Liu Y, Lin X (2009 a). Effects of a flaxseed-derived lignan supplement on C-reactive protein, IL-6 and retinol-binding protein 4 in type 2 diabetic patients. Br. J. Nutr. 101 (8): 1145–49.

Pan A, Sun J, Chen Y, Ye X, Li H, Yu Z, Wang Y, Gu W, Zhang X, Chen X, Demark-Wahnefried W, Liu Y,Lin X (2007). Effects of a flaxseed-derived lignan supplement in type 2 diabetic patients: A randomized, double-blind, cross-over trial. PLoS ONE. 2 (11): e1148.

Pan A, Yu D, Demark-Wahnefried W, Franco OH, Lin X (2009 b). Meta-analysis of the effects of flaxseed interventions on blood lipids. 90 (2): 288–97.

Paschos GK, Magkos F, Panagiotakos DB, Votteas V, Zampelas A (2007). Dietary supplementation with flaxseed oil lowers blood pressure in dyslipidaemic patients. Eur. J. Clin. Nutr. 61 (10): 1201–206.

Paschos G, Yiannakouris N, Rallidis L, Davies I, Griffin B, Panagiotakos D, Skopouli F, Votteas V, Zampelas A (2005). Apolipoprotein E genotype in dyslipidemic patients and response of blood lipids and inflammatory markers to alpha-linolenic acid. Angiology. 56: 49–60.

Patade A, Devareddy L, Lucas EA, Korlagunta K, Daggy BP, Arjmandi BH (2008). Flaxseed reduces total and LDL cholesterol concentrations in Native American postmenopausal women. J. Women's Health (Larchmt). 17 (3): 355–66.

Patenaude A, Rodriguez-Leyva D, Edel AL, Dibrov E, Dupasquier CM, Austria JA, Richard MN, Chahine MN, Malcolmson LJ, Pierce GN (2009). Bioavailability of alpha linolenic acid from flaxseed diets as a function of the age of the subject. Eur. J. Clin. Nutr. 63 (9): 1123–29.

Penumathsa SV, Koneru S, Thirunavukkarasu M, Zhan L, Prasad K. (2007). Secoisolariciresinol diglucoside: relevance to angiogenesis and cardio-protection against ischemia-reperfusion injury. J. Pharmacol. Expt. Therapeutics. 320: 951–59.

Penumathsa SV, Koneru S, Zhan L, John S, Menon VP, Prasad K (2008). Secoisolariciresinol diglucoside induces neovascularization-mediated cardioprotection against ischemia-reperfusion injury in hyper-cholesterolemic myocardium. J. Mol. Cell. Cardiol. 44: 170–79.

Phipps WR, Martini MC, Lampe JW, Slavin JL, Kurzer MS (1993). Effect of flax seed ingestion on the menstrual cycle. J. Clin. Endocrinol. Metab., 77: 1215–19.

Prasad K (1997 a). Hydroxyl radical-scavenging property of secoisolariciresinol diglucoside (SDG) isolated from flax-seed. Mol. Cell. Biochem. 168 (1-2): 117–23.

Prasad K (1997 b). Dietary flax seed in prevention of hyper-cholesterolemic atherosclerosis. Atherosclerosis. 132: 69–76.

Prasad K (1999). Reduction of serum cholesterol and hyper-cholesterolemic atherosclerosis in rabbits by secoisolariciresinol diglucoside isolated from flaxseed. Circulation. 99 (10): 1355–62.

Prasad K (2000 a). Antioxidant activity of secoisolariciresinol diglucoside-derived metabolites, secoisolariciresinol, enterodiol, and enterolactone. Int. J. Angiol. 9 (4): 220–25.

Prasad K (2000 b). Oxidative stress as a mechanism of diabetes in diabetic BB prone rats: Effect of secoisolariciresinol diglucoside (SDG) Mol. Cell. Biochem. 209 (1-2): 89–96.

Prasad K (2001). Secoisolariciresinol diglucoside from flaxseed delays the development of type 2 diabetes in Zucker rat. J. Lab. Clin. Med. 138 (1): 32–39.

Prasad K (2005). Hypo-cholesterolemic and antiatherosclerotic effect of flax lignan complex isolated from flaxseed. Atherosclerosis. 179 (2): 69-75.

Prasad K (2008). Regression of hypercholesterolemic atherosclerosis in rabbits by secoisolariciresinol diglucoside isolated from flaxseed. Atherosclerosis. 197 (1): 34–42.

Prasad K (2009 a). Flaxseed and cardiovascular health. J. Cardiovasc. Pharmacol. 54 (5): 369–77.

Prasad K (2009 b). Flax lignan complex slows down the progression of atherosclerosis in hyperlipidemic rabbits. Cardiovasc. Pharmacol. Ther. 14 (1): 38–48.

Prasad K, Mantha SV, Muir AD, Westcott ND (1998). Reduction of hypercholesterolemic atherosclerosis by CDC-flaxseed with very low α-linolenic acid. Atherosclerosis. 136 (2): 367–75.

Rajesha KN, Murthy C, Kumar KM, Madhusudhan B, Ravishankar GA (2006). Antioxidant potentials of flaxseed by *in vivo* model. J. Agric. Food Chem. 54: 3794–99.

Rallidis LS, Paschos G, Liakos GK, Velissaridou AH, Anastasiadis G, Zampelas A (2003). Dietary alpha-linolenic acid decreases C-reactive protein, serum amyloid A and interleukin-6 in dyslipidaemic patients. Atherosclerosis. 167 (2): 237–42.

Rhee Y, Brunt A (2011). Flaxseed supplementation improved insulin resistance in obese glucose intolerant people: a randomized crossover design. Nutr. J. 10: 44.

Rodriguez-Leyva D, Dupasquier CM, McCullough R, Pierce GN (2010). The cardiovascular effects of flaxseed and its ω-3 fatty acid, alpha-linolenic acid. Can. J. Cardiol. 26 (9): 489–96.

Saggar JK, Chen J, Corey P, Thompson LU (2010). Dietary flaxseed lignan or oil combined with tamoxifen treatment affects MCF-7 tumour growth through estrogen receptor- and growth factor-signaling pathways. Mol. Nutr. Food Res. 54 (3): 415–25.

Sekine S, Sasanuki S, Murano Y, Aoyama T, Takeuchi H (2008). Alpha-linolenic acid-rich flaxseed oil ingestion increases plasma adiponectin level in rats. Int. J. Vitam. Nutr. Res. 78 (4-5): 223–29.

Serraino M, Thompson LU (1991). The effect of flaxseed supplementation on early risk markers for mammary carcinogenesis. Cancer Lett. 60: 135–42.

Serraino M, Thompson LU (1992). The effect of flaxseed supplementation on the initiation and promotional stages of mammary tumourigenesis. Nutr. Cancer. 17: 153–59.

Singer P, Berger I, Wirth M, Godicke W, Jaeger W, Voigt S (1986). Slow desaturation and elongation of linoleic and alpha-linolenic acids as a rationale of eicosapentaenoic acid-rich diet to lower blood pressure and serum lipids in normal, hypertensive and hyperlipemic subjects. Prostaglandins Leukot. Med. 24 (2-3): 173–93.

Singh RB, Niaz MA, Sharma JP, Kumar R, Rastogi V, Moshiri M (1997). Randomized, double-blind, placebo-controlled trial of fish oil and mustard oil in patients with suspected acute myocardial infarction; the Indian experiment of infarct survival – 4. Cardiovasc. Drugs Ther. 11 (3): 485–91.

Singh S, Nair V, Gupta YK (2012).Linseed oil: an investigation of its anti-arthritic activity in experimental models. Phytother. Res. 26 (2): 246–52.

Spence JD, Thornton T, Muir AD, Westcott ND (2003). The effect of flax seed cultivars with differing content of α-linolenic acid and lignans on responses to mental stress. J. Am. Coll. Nutr. 22 (6): 494–501.

Strandås C, Kamal-Eldin A, Andersson R, Åman P (2008). Phenolic glucosides in bread containing flaxseed. Food Chemistry. 110 (4): 997–99,

Stuglin C, Prasad K (2005). Effect of flaxseed consumption on blood pressure, serum lipids, hemopoietic system and liver and kidney enzymes in healthy humans. J. Cardiovasc. Pharmacol. Ther. 10 (1): 23–27.

Tao M, McDowell MA, Saydah SH, Eberhardt MS (2008). Relationship of polyunsaturated fatty acid intake to peripheral neuropathy among adults with diabetes in the National Health and Nutrition Examination Survey (NHANES) 1999–2004. Diabetes Care. 31 (1): 93–95.

Thies F, Miles EA, Nebe-von-Caron G, Powell JR, Hurst TL, Newsholme EA, Calder PC. (2001). Influence of dietary supplementation with long-chain n-3 or n-6 polyunsaturated fatty acids on blood inflammatory cell populations and functions and on plasma soluble adhesion molecules in healthy adults. Lipids. 36 (11): 1183–93.

Thompson LU, Chen JM, Li T, Strasser-Weippl K, Goss PE (2005). Dietary flaxseed alters tumour biological markers in postmenopausal breast cancer. Clin. Cancer Res. 11 (10): 3828–35.

Thompson LU, Rickard SE, Orcheson LJ, Seidl MM. (1996 a). Flaxseed and its lignan and oil components reduce mammary tumour growth at a late stage of carcinogenesis. Carcinogenesis. 17: 1373–76.

Thompson LU, Seidl M, Rickard SE, Orcheson LJ, Fong HHS (1996 b). Anti-tumourigenic effect of mammalian lignan precursor from flaxseed. Nutr. Cancer. 26 (2): 159–65.

Tohgi N (2004). Effect of alpha-linolenic acid-containing linseed oil on coagulation in type 2 diabetes. Diabetes Care. 27 (10): 2563–64.

USDA (2012). National Nutrient Database for Standard Reference, Release 25.

Velasquez MT, Bhathena SJ, Ranich T, Schwartz AM, Kardon DE, Ali AA, Haudenschild CC, Hansen CT (2003). Dietary flaxseed meal reduces proteinuria and ameliorates nephropathy in an animal model of type II diabetes mellitus. Kidney Int. 64 (6): 2100–107.

Wanasundara PK, Shahidi F (1998). Process-induced compositional changes of flaxseed. Adv. Exp. Med. Biol. 434: 307–25.

Xu Y, Hall C 3rd, Wolf-Hall C, Manthey F (2008). Fungistatic activity of flaxseed in potato dextrose agar and a fresh noodle system. Int. J. Food Microbiol. 121 (3): 262–67.

Zanwar AA, Hegde MV, Bodhankar SL (2010). *In vitro* antioxidant activity of ethanolic extract of *Linum usitatissimum*. Pharmacologyonline. 1: 683–96.

Zanwar AA, Hegde MV, Bodhankar SL (2011). Cardioprotective activity of flax lignan concentrate extracted from seeds of Linum usitatissimum in isoprenalin induced myocardial necrosis in rats. Interdiscip. Toxicol. 4 (2): 90–97.

Zhang W, Wang X, Liu Y, Tian H, Flickinger B, Empie MW, Sun SZ (2008). Dietary flaxseed lignan extract lowers plasma cholesterol and glucose concentrations in hyper-cholesterolaemic subjects. Br. J. Nutr. 99 (6): 1301–309.

Zhao G, Etherton TD, Martin KR, West SG, Gillies PJ, Kris-Etherton PM (2004). Dietary alpha-linolenic acid reduces inflammatory and lipid cardiovascular risk factors in hypercholesterolemic men and women. J. Nutr. 134 (11): 2991–97.

Chapter 15

Oats

(*Avena sativa*)

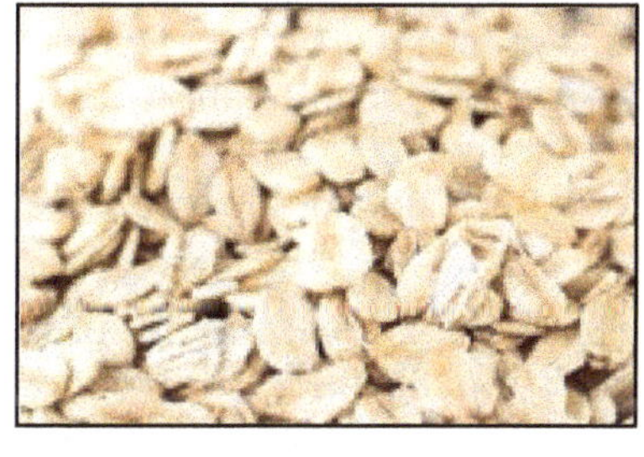

Hippocrates wrote that oats made into porridge or gruel is refreshing and helps hydration. During wars, the Scottish soldiers used to carry a bag of oatmeal as a source of strength. They also believed that it could build and regenerate bones and ligaments.

The modern day oats draw their ancestry from the wild red oat, a plant originated in Asia. Though oats are originally cultivated in southern Europe around 5000 years ago, later on (for the past two thousand years) their cultivation has been noticed in various regions throughout the world. China is a major producer of oats; the annual harvested area of 3,50,000 HA yields approximately 4,65,000 tons, giving an average yield of 1.33 tons/Ha.

The cultivation of oats in Europe was widespread, and oats constituted an important commercial crop since they were a dietary staple for the people of many countries including Scotland, Great Britain, Germany and the Scandinavian countries. In the early 17th century, Scottish settlers brought oats to North America. Today, the largest commercial producers of oats include the Russian Federation, the United States, Germany, Poland and Finland.

Processing of Oats

Oats gain part of their distinctive flavour from the roasting process that they undergo after being harvested and cleaned. Although oats are then hulled, this process does not strip away their bran and their germ allowing them to retain a concentrated part of their fiber and nutrients. Different types of processing methods are followed to evolve the various types of oat products, which are generally used to make breakfast cereals, baked goods and stuffings. Oat groats are just unflattened kernels, while Steel-cut oats are produced by running the grain through steel blades that thinly slices them giving a dense and chewy texture. Old-fashioned oats are steamed and then rolled ones having a flatter shape. Quick-cooking oats are processed like old-fashioned oats, except they are cut finely before rolling. Instant oatmeal is produced by partially cooking the grains and then rolling them very thin with sugar, salt and other ingredients added. Oat bran is the outer layer of the grain under the hull. Oat flour is used in baking often combined with wheat or other gluten-containing flours in making leavened bread.

The effects of various commercial hydrothermal processes (steaming, autoclaving, and drum drying) on levels of selected oat antioxidants showed that steaming and flaking of dehulled oat groats resulted in moderate losses of tocotrienols, caffeic acid, and the avenanthramide Bp (N-(4'-hydroxy)-(E)-cinnamoyl-5-hydroxy-anthranilic acid), while ferulic acid and vanillin increased. The tocopherols and the avenanthramides Bc (N-(3',4'-dihydroxy-(E)-cinnamoyl-5-hydroxy-anthranilic acid) and Bf (N-(4'-hydroxy-3'-methoxy)-(E)-cinnamoyl-5-hydroxy-anthranilic acid) were not affected by steaming. Autoclaving of grains (including the hulls) caused increased levels of all tocopherols and tocotrienols analyzed except beta-tocotrienol, which was not affected. Drum drying of steamed rolled oats resulted in an almost complete loss of tocopherols and tocotrienols, as well as a large decrease in total cinnamic acids and avenanthramides (Bryngelsson *et al.*, 2002). Beta-glucan which is the major fermentable component in both cooked and uncooked rolled oats was not affected by cooking (Lund and Johnson, 1991).

In extruded products, more severe extrusion conditions caused depoly-merization,. The integrity of the cell walls was lost and beta-glucan dispersed throughout the cereal. Differences in the hardness and density of the extruded cereals were also evident as the molecular weight was reduced (Tosh *et al.*, 2010). Sourdough Wheat F/Whole Meal Flour bread, enriched with oat fiber, had higher specific volume, better cell crumb structure and more appreciated acidulous smell, taste and aroma than that with no enrichment with oat fiber. According to Angelov *et al.* (2006) the beta-glucan content in the drink (0.31-0.36 per cent) (whole-grain oat substrate fermented with lactic acid bacteria) remained unchanged both throughout fermentation and storage of the drink. The shelf life of the oat drink stored under refrigeration was estimated to be 21 days.

Nutritive and Phytochemical Composition of Oats

Oats are excellent source of energy, protein, and fat; and hence suitable for very young children and many infants. Oat bran in particular, is good source of B complex vitamins, protein, fat, minerals besides heart healthy soluble fiber beta-glucan (Butt *et al.*, 2008). The specific type of fiber found in oats promotes a healthy digestive system by helping prevent constipation. The dominating fiber fraction in all oat products was hemi-cellulose. Because of the fiber, oats have a low glycemic index and may help reduce the risk of developing type 2 diabetes. Studies also showed that high-fiber foods help control appetite, which is an advantage for those trying to lose weight. They are one of the best sources of Inositol, which is very important for maintaining blood cholesterol level.

Oats have a higher concentration of well-balanced protein (100 gm of oats have around 17 gm of protein) than other cereals–100 gm of oats contain twice as much protein as 100 gm of wheat or cornflakes. Oat protein is nearly equivalent in quality to soy protein, meat, milk, and egg protein as shown by the World Health Organization (Lasztity, 1999) due to a globulin or legume-like protein, avenalin, as the major (80 per cent) storage protein present in oats. Globulins are characterized by solubility in dilute saline. The more typical cereal proteins are gluten and zein, which are prolamins. Avenin, the minor protein of oat is also a prolamine. The protein content of the hull-less oat kernel (groat) ranges from 12–24 per cent, the highest among cereals.

Before even oats were consumed as a food, they were used for medicinal purposes, a use for which they are still honored. The consumption of oats has increased in recent years due to a perceived association with a range of health benefits. Oats are known to be a healthy food for the heart mainly due to their high beta-glucan content. In addition, they contain more than 20 unique polyphenols, avenanthramides, which have shown strong antioxidant activity *in vitro* and *in vivo*.

The polyphenols of oats have also recently been shown to exhibit anti-inflammatory, antiproliferative, and anti-itching activity, which may provide additional protection against coronary heart disease, colon cancer, and skin irritation (Meydani, 2009). Avenanthramides are phenolic compounds present in oats at approximately 300 parts per million (ppm) and have been reported to exhibit antioxidant activity in various cell-types (Sur *et al.*, 2008). Beta-Glucans also exhibit anticoagulant properties. Recently, they have been demonstrated to be anticytotoxic, antimutagenic and antitumourogenic, making them promising candidate as pharmacological promoters of health.

Nutritional Value of Oats – Macro-nutrients (per 100 g)

Nutrient	*Amount*	*Nutrient*	*Amount*
Energy (kcal)	389	Protein (g)	17
Carbohydrate (g)	66	Cystine (g)	0.408
Dietary fiber total (g)	11	Phenylalanine (g)	0.985
–Beta glucan (g)	5	Tyrosine (g)	0.573
–Insoluble (g)	6	Valine (g)	0.937
Total fat (g)	6	Arginine (g)	1.192
–Saturated (g)	1.22	Histidine (g)	0.405
Monounsaturated (g)	2.18	Alanine (g)	0.881
Polyunsaturated (g)	2.54	Aspartic acid (g)	1.448

USDA (2012).

Nutritional Value of Oats – Micro-nutrients (per 100 g)

Nutrient	*Amount*	*Nutrient*	*Amount*
Thiamin (B1) (mg)	0.763	Calcium (mg)	54
Riboflavin (B2) (mg)	0.139	Iron (mg)	4.7
Niacin (mg)	0.961	Magnesium (mg)	177
Pantothenic acid (mg)	1.349	Phosphorus (mg)	523
VitaminB-6 (mg)	0.119	Potassium (mg)	429
Total folate (mcg)	56.0	Sodium (mg)	2.0

USDA (2012).

Oats are generally considered to be very soothing for the nerves. It also contains very high levels of calcium, potassium and magnesium, coupled with Vitamin B-complex. All these vitamins and minerals are very essential for the nervous system.

The B vitamins include thiamin, riboflavin, niacin and folic acid which are used by the body for energy production and maintaining a healthy nervous system. B vitamins also help reduce stress and boost immunity. Due to its folic acid content, oatmeal can reduce the chances of NTDs in fetus.

Among the minerals of oats, phosphorus boosts energy and plays an important role in healthy digestion. Along with calcium it also helps to keep bones and teeth strong and reduces the risk of periodontal disease, and aids in weight maintenance. Selenium works as an antioxidant with vitamin E to help protect the body from free radical damage and thereby against certain cancers; and interestingly some studies suggest that selenium may boost mood. Selenium and Vitamin E present in oats also significantly enhance the human immune response to bacterial infection. This makes oatmeal much preferred during infections. Zinc, present on oats, helps in metabolism, healing wounds and growth of new cells. Oats also contain iron, which helps boost immunity. Magnesium in oats is important not only in energy production, but also in maintaining strong bones and reducing symptoms of premenstrual syndrome.

Therapeutic Value of Oats

Oats are unusual in that the bran is not as physically distinct as in other cereals. This provides a possible benefit in easily providing the high beta-glucan content of the grains in the diet. Oats contain many other phytochemicals as mentioned earlier, including a range of antioxidants that may be associated with several health benefits, although according to Ryan *et al.* (2007) the evidence for such benefits is largely indirect and often confusing and contradictory. Nevertheless, they say that the consumption of oats as part of a balanced diet does seem a reasonable approach. The use of oats is very suitable in cases of depression, insomnia, and physical or nervous fatigue. A mixture of oats, milk and honey reduces stress in the morning and boosts concentration. Complex carbohydrates in oats not only lower the risk of heart disease, but also reduce the risk of stroke and certain cancers and helps lower high blood pressure. Oats also contain tryptophan, a nonessential amino acid that improves mood and thus has also been proven to act as an anti-depressant. Cooked oats relieve fat from the body while unrefined oatmeal can reduce stress.

Oats as Antioxidant Food

Avenanthramides unique to oats may confer health benefits via antioxidant and/or other mechanisms. Oat avenanthramide, generally had the highest antioxidant activity and antigenotoxicity; and comparable to those of ascorbic acid (Lee-Manion *et al.*, 2009; Bratt *et al.*, 2003).

Oats as Anti-inflammatory Food

Avenanthramides, unique polyphenols from oats, decrease the expression of endothelial proinflammatory cytokines at least in part through inhibition of NF-kappaB activation by inhibiting the phosphorylation of IKK and IkappaB, and by suppressing proteasome activity (Guo *et al.*, 2008). Furthermore, cells treated with avenanthramides showed a significant inhibition of tumour necrosis factor-alpha (TNF-alpha) induced NF-kappaB luciferase activity and subsequent reduction of interleukin-8 (IL-8) release. Additionally, topical application of 1-3 ppm avenanthramides mitigated inflammation in murine models of contact hypersensitivity and neurogenic inflammation and reduced pruritogen-induced scratching in a murine itch model. Thus Sur *et al.* (2008) demonstrated that avenanthramides are potent anti-inflammatory agents that appear to mediate the anti-irritant effects of oats.

Oats on Cardiovascular Diseases

Dietary fiber has been suggested to interfere with endogenous cholesterol synthesis in the liver. Marlett *et al.* (1994) demonstrated that oat bran lowers serum cholesterol levels in part by altering bile acid metabolism. In addition, the substantial increase in the proportion of the total bile acid pool that was deoxycholic acid is consistent with the hypothesis that oat bran also decreases cholesterol synthesis. On the other hand, as the cholesterol precursors in serum reflecting endogenous cholesterol synthesis remained almost unchanged, the reduction in the serum cholesterol level by oat bran treatment cannot be ascribed to an inhibition of the endogenous cholesterol synthesis (Uusitupa *et al.*, 1997). The role of oats consumption in the prevention and treatment of both hypertension and hypercholesterolemia was ascertained by He *et al.* (1995). According to Maki *et al.* (2007) consumption of high-fiber oat cereal influenced postprandial triglyceride and free fatty acid levels, which may have implications regarding cardiovascular disease risk. According to Andersson *et al.* (2010) two substrains of mice respond differently to oat bran on plasma cholesterol and this is of practical value and can also help to elucidate mechanisms of the cholesterol-lowering effect of oats. Again Park *et al.* (2009) demonstrated 2,2,6,6-Tetramethyl-1-piperidine oxoammonium ion (TEMPO)-mediated oxidation applied to oat beta-glucans exhibits potential use as an active cholesterol-lowering ingredient.

Consumption of adequate amounts of oats on a consistent basis may decrease the risk of cardiovascular disease by several potential mechanisms: lowering blood lipid levels, improving arterial compliance, reducing low-density lipoprotein oxidation, decreasing plaque formation, scavenging free radicals, and inhibiting platelet aggregation (Hasler *et al.*, 2000). Oat bran supplemented to Western diet lowered plasma cholesterol, reduced levels of some inflammatory markers, and inhibited atherosclerotic lesion development in LDL-receptor-deficient mice. Oats could be considered suitable for a gluten-free diet as they supply high fiber and vitamin B content which are often deficient in such diets (Pulido *et al.*, 2009). Beta-glucan, constituent of soluble fiber of Oats has been proven effective in lowering blood cholesterol thus reducing the risk of cardiovascular disease (CVD). Different physiological effects of beta-glucan are related to its viscosity, attenuation of postprandial plasma glucose and insulin responses, high transport of bile acids towards lower parts of the intestinal tract and high excretion of bile acids thereby lowering of serum cholesterol levels (Butt *et al.*, 2008).

Numerous studies (Amudesan *et al.*, 2003; Berg *et al.*, 2003; Braaten *et al.*, 1994; Brown *et al.*, 1999; Davidson *et al.*, 1991; Karmally *et al.*, 2005; Ripsin *et al.*, 1992; Theuwissen and Mensink, 2007) have shown that oat-containing products reduce LDL cholesterol. Within a practical range of intake, oat bran when added to a fat-modified diet was found to significantly reduce the total cholesterol, low-density lipoprotein cholesterol, and apolipoprotein B. These beneficial effects could be seen independent of co variables such as physical activity or caloric and fat restriction in the diet (Berg *et al.*,2003). Preliminary studies showed that avenanthramides help prevent free radicals from damaging LDL cholesterol.

Dose Recommendations

Daily inclusion of two ounces of oats appeared to facilitate reduction of serum total cholesterol and LDL-C in three hyperlipidemic adults (Van Horn *et al.*, 1991). Increased gut viscosity may prevent dietary cholesterol from reaching the intestinal epithelium. The role of viscosity in determining the cholesterol-lowering effect of soluble fiber has been shown in hamsters (Gallaher *et al.*, 1993) and recently in humans (Reppas *et al.*, 2009) with the use of high-dose (15 g/d) hydroxypropylmethylcellulose. Poulter *et al.* (1994) also found slight reduction in LDL cholesterol on oat based cereal in a crossover study. Beer *et al.* (1995) reported that the cholesterol-lowering capacity of oat gum in healthy young men to be weak. They also suggested that the effect of Oat bran preparations on serum cholesterol levels cannot be estimated only by the beta-glucan content but by measurement of the solubility and viscosity of the beta-glucan. The viscosity of β-glucan solutions is determined by its molecular weight (MW) and solubility (Wood *et al.*, 2000), both of which can be altered by normal methods of processing and storage (Regand *et al.*, 2009). In a later study beta glucan when fed at 1 per cent–10 per cent by weight showed a significant decrease in total and LDL cholesterol levels in mildly hypercholesterolemic subjects (Behall *et al.*, 1997).

The US Food and Drug Administration (Anonymous, 1997) allowed a claim that food products containing oats and that can deliver 3 g β-glucan/d can reduce risk of heart disease. Whereas Queenan and coworkers (2007) demonstrated that 6 grams concentrated oat beta-glucan per day for six weeks produced significant reduction from baseline in total cholesterol (-0.3 +/- 0.1 mmol/L) and LDL cholesterol (-0.3 +/ - 0.1 mmol/L);and the reduction in LDL cholesterol was significantly greater than that of the control group (p = 0.03). However, Biörklund *et al.* (2008) did not find a significant reduction in TC and LDL-C with a daily dose of 4 g of oat beta-glucans incorporated into a healthy ready meal compared with an equal ready meal without beta-glucans.

Six grams of beta-glucan from oats added to the American Heart Association Step II diet and moderate physical activity improved lipid profile and caused a decrease in weight and, thus, reduced the risk of cardiovascular events in overweight male individuals with mild to moderate hypercholesterolemia (Reyna-Villasmil *et al.*, 2007). The European Food Safety Authority recently issued an opinion that a cause and effect relation has been established between the consumption of oat β-glucan and a reduction in blood cholesterol (EFSA, 2009).

The processing required to incorporate oats in foods also influences its lipid lowering ability. An extruded breakfast cereal containing 3 g oat β-glucan/d with a high-MW (2,210,000 g/mol) or medium-MW (530,000 g/mol) lowered LDL cholesterol similarly by H"0.2 mmol/L (5 per cent), but efficacy was reduced by 50 per cent when MW was reduced to 210,000 g/mol. Hence, Wolever *et al.* (2010) suggested that the physicochemical properties of oat β-glucan should be considered when assessing the cholesterol-lowering ability.

Bae *et al.* (2010) found oat beta-glucan hydrolysate, having average molecular weight of 730,000g/mol to be more effective at increasing the excretion of fecal cholesterol and triglyceride than the native beta-glucan, showing its effectiveness in improving the lipid profile.

As Dietary Adjunct/Meal Replacer

Winbald *et al.* (1995) reported that oat bran supplemented diet was effective in lowering serum cholesterol in hyper-cholesterolaemic males who had failed to comply with a conventional lipid lowering diet. Supplementation with oat bran has also been proved to increase plasma HDL-C levels by11.2 per cent in women (n = 18) (p = 0.01), but decrease the total cholesterol/HDL-C ratio by 7.0 per cent (p = 0.002) (Robitaille *et al.*, 2005). The authors concluded that integration of these foods as part of a healthy diet may, therefore, improve the cardiovascular risk profile of women. Since 1 per cent reduction in LDL cholesterol reduces Coronary artery disease (CAD) risk by 1–2 per cent, the 5–6 per cent LDL cholesterol lowering elicited by 3–4 g oat β-glucan *i.e.*3 g of high-MW oat β-glucan/d or 4 g medium MW β-glucan/d or 3 g medium-MW oat β-glucan could reduce the risk of CAD by 5–12 per cent.

Wolever *et al.* (2011) concluded from their study that oat β-glucan reduces LDL-C in both Caucasians and non-Caucasians. Oat consumption was found to be associated with 5 per cent and 7 per cent reductions in total and LDL cholesterol levels, respectively, consistent with earlier conclusions made by the US FDA and United Kingdom Joint Health Claims Initiative (Othman *et al.*, 2011). Interestingly, Charlton *et al.* (2012) recently observed 1-5 g/d of oat Beta glucan was as effective as 3 g/d delivered in different food formats.

In a double-blind, randomized crossover study in adults total cholesterol decreased by 14 per cent on oat bran consumption as compared to 4 per cent in the control group ($P<0.001$). The LDL cholesterol decreased by 16 per cent in the oat bran period compared with 3 per cent in the control period ($P<0.01$), as did total triacylglycerol (21 vs 10 per cent, $P<0.05$) and very-low-density lipoprotein triacylglycerol (33 vs 9 per cent, $P<0.01$). Fecal volume and dry matter were greater on consumption of oat bran diet compared with the control ($P<0.001$), and energy expenditure increased by 37 per cent (1014 vs 638 kJ/day). Addition of oat bran (6 g soluble fiber/day) to a low-fiber diet lowered total and non-HDL cholesterol, as well as hemostatic factors, and may affect energy balance through reduced energy utilization. (Kristensen and Bügel, 2011).

Eussen *et al.* (2011) investigated the effects of oat bran and simultaneous intake of atorvastatin on serum and hepatic lipid levels and found that the oat bran inhibits the intestinal absorption of atorvastatin, and consequently its cholesterol-lowering effects and so they suggest future investigations to focus on food –drug interaction.

The influence of oat bran on the concentration of triglycerides in the blood serum depended on the kind of fats in a diet (Onning *et al.*, 1998; Grajeta, 1999). The diets containing oat bran with lard did not decrease the concentration of these lipids, but the same diets with sunflower oil decreased this concentration significantly (by 22 per cent). Oda *et al.* (1994) observed oat gum to suppress the elevation of serum and liver triglyceride concentrations along with lowering of serum and liver cholesterol concentrations.

Psyllium as well as oat bran are efficacious in lowering plasma LDL cholesterol in both normal and hyper-cholesterolemic individuals as plasma LDL cholesterol concentrations were reduced by an average of 22.6 and 26 per cent in the psyllium and oat bran groups while a non-significant reduction of 8.4 per cent was observed in the hyper-cholesterolemic individuals from the control group. Hypercholesterolemic individuals supplemented with oat bran showed a 28 per cent reduction in plasma triglycerides after 8 weeks (Romero *et al.*, 1998).

Beyond its known effect through lowering blood cholesterol in the prevention of coronary heart disease, avenanthramide-c, which is a unique polyphenol found in oats, arrests SMC proliferation at G1 phase by upregulating the p53-p21cip1 pathway and inhibiting pRB phosphorylation (Nie *et al.*, 2006).

It is also reported (Onning *et al.*, 1999) that oat milk deprived of insoluble fiber has cholesterol-reducing properties as the consumption of oat milk resulted in significantly lower serum total cholesterol (6 per cent, $p = 0.005$) and LDL cholesterol (6 per cent, $p = 0.036$) levels. The decrease in LDL cholesterol was more pronounced if the starting value was higher ($r = -0.55$, $p < 0.001$). The concentration of high-density lipoprotein cholesterol and serum triglycerides did not change significantly after intake of oat milk,

An energy-restricted regimen (a new oat-based soup as the main meal once or twice daily) lead to lower plasma insulin, triglyceride, and low-density lipoprotein cholesterol levels but did not significantly affect the plasma enterostatin concentration in overweight subjects (Rytter *et al.*, 1996).

Keenan *et al.* (2002) found that subjects fed oats experienced a significant reduction in both total cholesterol (9 per cent) and low-density lipoprotein cholesterol

(14 per cent) and also a 7.5 mm Hg reduction in Systolic BP and a 5.5 mm Hg reduction in Diastolic BP. Further, Pins *et al.* (2002) suggested that a diet containing soluble fiber-rich whole oats can significantly reduce the need for antihypertensive medication and improve BP control. Considering the lipid and glucose improvements as well, increased consumption of whole oats may significantly reduce cardiovascular disease risk. According to Saltzman *et al.* (2001) a hypo-caloric diet containing oats consumed over 6 wk resulted in greater improvements in systolic blood pressure and lipid profile than did a hypo-caloric diet without oats.

Oats as Antidiabetic Food

Control of blood glucose and insulin levels is essential in preventing the complications associated with diabetes. Oat beta-glucan slows the rise in blood glucose levels following a meal and delays its decline to pre-meal levels. As the beta-glucan in the soluble fiber of oats is digested, it forms a gel, which causes the viscosity of the contents of the stomach and small intestine to be increased. This in turn slows down digestion and prolongs the absorption of carbohydrates into the bloodstream. Thus dramatic changes in blood sugar levels are avoided. Lund *et al.* (1989) reported that the small intestinal contents from oat-gum-fed or oat-fed rats had a higher wet: dry weight ratio and a higher viscosity than that of the controls. This increased viscosity of the contents of the small intestine may contribute to the low glycaemic index and hypocholesterolaemic effects of oats in man. Oats appear to be amongst the few palatable sources of viscous dietary fibre in the conventional Western diet. Alminger *et al.* (2008) found that the mean serum insulin responses from barley and oat tempe with GI s of 30 and 63 respectively, were significantly lower compared with the glucose load ($P < 0.002$) during the first 60 min. The Insulin Index was also lower for oat tempe compared with barley tempe. Apart from beneficial effects on lipid profile, adding oat bran to the test meals markedly reduced the postmeal insulin rise in human subjects (Dubois *et al.*, 1995). Tapola *et al.* (2005) found the oat bran flour to show a lower 0-120 min area under the glucose response curve (AUC) (47+/-45 mmol min/L) than the glucose load (118+/-40 mmol min/L) ($p<0.002$). Also they found the oat bran flour to decrease the glucose excursion from baseline by 1.6 mmol/l (2.4, 0.8) (mean (95 per cent CI)) and 1.5 mmol/l (2.0, 1.1) at 30 and 45 min after the glucose load, respectively. Thus oat beta glucan had a low glycemic response and acted as an active ingredient decreasing postprandial glycemic response of an oral glucose load in subjects with type 2 diabetes.

Though no gender difference was found by Hallfrisch *et al.* (1995) in the glycemic response to oat extracts. Higher initial glucagon responses were observed in men which decreased after consumption of oat extracts but a similar change was not noticed in women. Tappy *et al.* (1996) has shown that beta-glucan decreased plasma glucose concentrations in both healthy individuals and those with type 2 diabetes, following a single meal. Glucose responses were reduced with 1 per cent and 10 per cent soluble oat extracts in both men and women; however, in women, responses to the 10 per cent extract were lowest.

A 50 per cent reduction in glycemic peak can be achieved with a concentration of 10 per cent beta-glucan in a cereal food (Würsch *et al.*, 1997). A daily consumption of

5 g of oat beta-glucans in a beverage improved the lipid and glucose metabolism, while barley beta-glucans did not (Biörklund *et al.*, 2005), although Granfeldt *et al.* (2008) suggested that a total of 4 g of oats beta glucan to be a critical level for a significant decrease in glucose and insulin responses in healthy people as muesli enriched with 4 g of beta-glucans reduces postprandial glucose and insulin levels to a breakfast based on high glycaemic index products.

The glycemic responses to oat products with increasing amounts of beta-glucan had lower peak values than the reference glucose load. The amount of extractable beta-glucan had a high correlation between the glycemic and insulinemic response. Thus in addition to the total amount of beta-glucan in oat products, the amount of extractable beta-glucan in oat products explains the magnitude of the decrease in glycemic responses to carbohydrate products (Mäkeläinen *et al.*, 2007). The glycemic indices of the prototype beta-glucan cereal (mean+/-s.e.m.; 52+/-5) and beta-glucan bar (43+/-4.1) were significantly lower than the commercial oat bran breakfast cereal (86+/-6) and white bread (100; P<0.05). It was found that the GI of the test foods used in this study decreased by 4.0+/-0.2 units per gram of beta-glucan (Jenkins *et al.*, 2002). Hypoglycaemic effects of oat products might be regulating glucose and fat metabolisms, stimulating hormone secretion, activating the nuclear receptor, and protecting organ function (Shen *et al.*, 2011).

Vervuert *et al.* (2003) indicated that the glucose and insulin responses are not clearly altered by the different types of oat processing. However, the glucose and insulin responses tended to be lower in thermally treated oats when compared with untreated or finely ground oats. Pick *et al.* (2006) had also demonstrated that oat bran concentrate incorporated bread products improved glycemic, insulinemic, and lipidemic responses. Processing oat beta-glucan through enzymatic, rather than by aqueous methods, preserves the viscosity and improves postprandial glycemic control (Panahi *et al.*, 2007). De Angelis *et al.* (2007) demonstrated that the area under the glucose response curve and the value of GI (72 per cent) of Wheat flour bread were significantly (P < 0.05) higher than sourdough Wheat flour or Whole Meal Flour bread enriched with oat fiber (GI = 53.7 per cent). The reduction in GI of the sourdough WF/WMF bread may be due to both fiber content and decreased pH.

The importance of the degree of gelatinization and the product thickness for postprandial glycemic and insulinemic responses was demonstrated by Granfeldt *et al.* (1995; 2000). Rolling of steamed oat grains increased the accessibility of the starch for digestion and absorption compared with boiled intact oat kernels (Granfeldt *et al.*, 1995). All thin (0.5mm) rolled oat flakes elicited high glucose and insulin responses [glycemic index (GI), 88-118; insulinemic index (II), 84-102], not significantly different from white wheat bread (P: > 0.05). In contrast, all varieties of thick (1.0mm) rolled oat flakes gave significantly lower metabolic responses (GI, 70-78; II, 58-77) than the reference bread (P: < 0.05). Thick barley flakes gave high glucose and insulin responses (GI, 94; II, 84), probably because the botanical structure underwent more destruction than the corresponding oat flakes. Minimal processing of oat and barley flakes had a relatively minor effect on GI features compared with the more extensive commercial processing. One exception was thick oat flakes, which in contrast to the corresponding barley flakes, had a low GI. Oat or oat fiber consumption has been shown to reduce postprandial glucose and insulin concentrations (Braaten *et al.*, 1991; 1994), and the reduction in insulin concentration may provide a mechanism by which blood pressure could be reduced (Tuck and Corry, 1991) in response to oat consumption.

Oats in Respiratory Tract Infection

Murphy *et al.* (2008) have shown that consumption of the soluble oat fiber beta-glucan (ObetaG) can offset the increased risk of infection and decreased macrophage antiviral resistance following stressful exercise (Murphy *et al.*, 2007; 2009). However, lung macrophages are reported to be partially responsible for mediating the beneficial effects of ObetaG on susceptibility to respiratory infection following exercise stress (Davis *et al.*, 2004). Early age at introduction of oats was associated with a reduced risk of persistent asthma (hazard ratio (HR); 95 per cent CI) for the first and mid-tertiles compared with the latest tertile which was 0.36 (0.15, 0.85) and 0.37 (0.22, 0.62), respectively, $P < 0.001$) indicating that age at introduction of Oats is inversely and independently associated with development of persistent asthma (Virtanen *et al.*, 2010).

Oats on Immunity

Beta glucan stimulates the immune system, modulating humoral and cellular immunity, and thereby have beneficial effect in fighting infections (bacterial, viral, fungal and parasitic).

Wang *et al.* (2008) extracted the native polysaccharide, a linear (1-3)-, (1-4)-linked beta-glucan (OBG) from the oat bran and synthesized a sulfated derivative OBGS containing 36.5 per cent sulfate. OBGS had potent activity against a primary isolate of human immunodeficiency virus (HIV-1) in peripheral blood mononuclear cells at a concentration (EC (50) =5.98 x 10(-4) μM) approximately 15,000 times below its cytotoxic concentration. OBGS was also active post infection (EC(50)=5.3 x 10(-4) μM) and protected pretreated peripheral mononuclear cells (EC(50)=5.2 x 10(-2) μM) washed free of the compounds prior to infection. Thus, OBGS has potential as a vaginal microbicide and is the first such report for oat bran derived sulfated beta-glucan.

Oats as Anticancer Agent

Oats, like other grains and vegetables, contain hundreds of phytochemicals. Many of them are believed to reduce the risk of cancer. Phytoestrogen compounds, called lignans, in oats have been linked to decreased risk of hormone-related diseases such as breast cancer. Plant lignans are converted by friendly microflora in our intestines into mammalian lignans, including one called enterolactone that is thought to protect against breast and other hormone-dependent cancers as well as heart disease. Most of the research has been focused on breast cancer, but similar effects are expected on other hormone-related cancers such as prostate, endometrium and ovarian cancer. International research has shown that women with a higher intake of dietary fibre have lower circulating estrogen levels, a factor associated with a lower risk of breast cancer. The insoluble fibers in oats are also thought to reduce carcinogens in the gastrointestinal tract by forming bulky stool.

Oats on Celiac Disease

Celiac disease, from Greek "koiliakos", meaning "bowel-related", is a disease often associated with ingestion of wheat, or more specifically a group of proteins labelled prolamines, or more commonly, gluten. The inclusion of oats, known to be a fiber-rich, naturally gluten-free food, would broaden the range of foodstuffs tolerable to celiac patients, though for safety reasons they should be used only by adults until more information is available (Hallert *et al.*, 1999). Oats lack many of the prolamines found in wheat; however, avenin in oats which is a prolamine, is toxic to the intestinal submucosa and can trigger a reaction in some celiacs (CSA, 2006).

In spite of containing avenin, there are several studies suggesting that oats can be a part of a gluten-free diet if it is pure. The first such study was published in 1995 by Janatuinen *et al.*, A follow-up study indicated that it is safe to use oats even for a longer period (Janatuinen *et al.*, 2002). Health Canada and the Canadian Celiac Association (CCA) concluded that the majority of people with celiac disease can tolerate moderate amounts of pure oats (Pulido *et al.*, 2009). Peräaho *et al.* (2004) reported that 73 per cent with celiac disease and 55 per cent with dermatitis herpetiformis consumed oats for the taste, the ease of use, and the low costs; 94 per cent believed that oats diversified the gluten-free diet. Oats could form a potentially useful part of a gluten-free diet, but patients require careful advice and monitoring (Ellis and Ciclitira, 2008).

Størsrud and his colleagues (2003) have also found that including oats can help coeliac patients following a strict gluten-free diet as the same could improve the nutritional value of the diet and were appreciated by the subjects. Consumption of oats does not induce TG2 autoantibody production at mucosal level in children with celiac disease (Koskinen *et al.*, 2009).

According to Holm *et al.* (2006) oats had no detrimental effect in coeliac children in remission, on intestinal histology or serology during the 2-year trial. In most children with coeliac disease, long-term consumption of oats is well tolerated, and it does not result in small bowel mucosal deterioration or immune activation.

Concentrated oat beta-glucan was a fermentable fiber and produced total short chain fatty acids and acetate concentrations similar to inulin and guar gum. Concentrated oat beta-glucan produced the highest concentrations of butyrate at 4, 8, and 12 hours. Thus, a practical dose of beta-glucan can significantly lower serum lipids in a high-risk population and may improve colon health (Queenan *et al.*, 2007).

Fric *et al.* (2011) also opined that oats in a gluten-free diet increase the diet's nutritional value, but their use remains controversial. Contamination with prolamins of other cereals is frequent, and some clinical and experimental studies support the view that a subgroup of celiac patients may be intolerant to pure oats. Hence, emphasis must be laid on selection of oat cultivars with low avenin content, research on such recombinant varieties of oats, development of assay methods to detect avenins in oat products, guidelines for the agricultural processing of oats and the manufacture of oat products, as well as guidelines for following up with celiac patients who consume oats.

Oats on Weight Control

Consumption of a whole-grain ready to eat oat cereal as part of a dietary program for weight loss had favourable effects on fasting lipid levels and waist circumference (Maki *et al.*, 2010). The high amount of soluble fiber in oats forms a gel in the digestive tract. This causes increase in the viscosity of the contents of the stomach and small intestine. The gel delays transit time prolonging the feeling of fullness which helps in weight loss. Also, being low in fat content, oats don't add to body weight as well.

Recent research suggests that children in the age group of 2-18 years old who have a constant intake of oatmeal lowered their risk of obesity. Research confirmed that the children who ate oatmeal were 50 per cent less likely to become overweight, when compared to those children without oat consumption. Some studies suggested that protein has a thermogenic effect that boosts metabolism, which may aid weight loss. According to Beck *et al.* (2009), subjective satiety was increased at a beta-glucan dose of 2.2 g ($p = 0.039$). Subsequent meal intake decreased by greater than 400 kJ with higher beta-glucan dose (>5 g). Improved satiety by Beta-Glucan and release of cholecystokinin are likely to be part of the mechanisms. Peptide Y-Y (PYY) is an anorexigenic hormone implicated in appetite control by beta-glucan. Beck *et al.* (2009) found a significant dose response, with a positive correlation between the amount of beta-glucan consumed and PYY area under the curve ($r(2) = 0.994$, $P = .003$).The optimal dose of beta-glucan appears to lie between 4 and 6 g, with the effects on PYY mediated by viscosity and concentration.

A review of existing data on effects of oats on weight loss suggests that benefits occur early in weight reduction and are at least in part due to negative energy balance and that lipid-lowering effects may partially wane over time despite continued weight loss or maintenance (Mertens and Van Gall 2000, Trials of Hypertension Prevention Collaborative Research Group 1992, Wadden *et al.*, 1999). Further investigation is required to determine whether effects on lipids and blood pressure would persist after weight stabilization.

Sports Performance

Oats have been shown in scientific studies to favourably alter metabolism and enhance performance when ingested 45 minutes to 1 hour before exercise of moderate intensity. Being high in carbohydrates, they are excellent sources useful in boosting performance. Other nutrients present in oats like magnesium, iron and phosphorus; and B complex vitamins help in energy production. Exercise stress was associated with a decrease in macrophage antiviral resistance ($P = 0.007$), which was blocked by ingestion of oats ($P < 0.001$). There were no effects of exercise or oats beta glucan on NK cytotoxicity (Davis *et al.*, 2004).

Other Benefits of Oats

Oats are also exploited for certain cosmetic benefits. Oatmeal bath helps heal dry and flaky skin, eczema and other skin conditions. Skin rashes and insect bites are also healed with mashed oats. Oatmeal scrubs exfoliate your skin and are very beneficial to oily skin.

Safety of Oats

Whether oats should be included in a gluten-free diet has been debated for half a century. In 1995, the largest and most scientifically rigorous study on the safety of oats was published. Investigators concluded that the consumption of oats was safe for adults with celiac disease (Thompson, 2003). Oats can be symptomatically tolerated by most patients with celiac disease; however, the long-term effects of a diet containing oats remain unknown. Patients with celiac disease wishing to consume a diet containing oats should therefore receive regular follow-up, including small bowel biopsy at a specialist clinic for life.

In 2006, Haboubi *et al.*, concluded from his review of the reports that oats can be symptomatically tolerated by most patients with celiac disease; however, the long-term effects of a diet containing oats remain unknown. Patients with celiac disease wishing to consume a diet containing oats should therefore receive regular follow-up, including small bowel biopsy at a specialist clinic for life.

In 1997, the FDA authorized coronary heart disease risk reduction health claim for beta-glucan soluble fiber from oat products. To qualify for this health claim, a food product must contain at least 0.75 grams of beta-glucan soluble fiber from oats per serving. Ideally, patients with celiac disease should be advised to consume only those products tested and found to be free of contamination (Dicky, 2008). Long-term use of oats included in the gluten-free diets of patients with coeliac disease does not stimulate an immunological response locally in the mucosa of the small intestine (Kemppainen *et al.*, 2007).

Conclusion

The extensive scientific evidence available on the therapeutic/health benefits of oats suggest this food to be a readily acceptable meal adjunct.

References

Alminger M, Eklund-Jonsson (2008). Whole-grain cereal products based on a high-fibre barley or oat genotype lower post-prandial glucose and insulin responses in healthy humans. Eur. J. Nutr. 47 (6): 294–300.

Amundesan ÅL, Haugum B, Andersson H (2003). Changes in serum cholesterol and sterol metabolites after intake of products enriched with oat bran concentrate within a controlled diet. Scand. J. Clin. Nutr. 47: 68–74.

Angelov A, Gotcheva V, Kuncheva R, Hristozova T (2006). Development of a new oat-based probiotic drink. Int. J. Food Microbiol. 112 (1): 75–80.

Anonymous (1997). Food labeling: health claims; oats and coronary heart disease. Fed. Regist. 62: 3584–601.

Andersson KE, Svedberg KA, Lindholm MW, Oste R, Hellstrand P (2010). Oats (Avena sativa) reduce atherogenesis in LDL-receptor-deficient mice. Atherosclerosis. 212 (1): 93–99.

Bae IY, Kim SM, Lee S, Lee HG (2010). Effect of enzymatic hydrolysis on cholesterol-lowering activity of oat beta-glucan. N. Biotechnol. 27 (1): 85–88.

Beck EJ, Tosh SM, Batterham MJ, Tapsell LC, Huang XF (2009). Oat beta-glucan increases postprandial cholecystokinin levels, decreases insulin response and extends subjective satiety in overweight subjects. Mol. Nutr. Food Res. 53 (10): 1343–51.

Beer MU, Arrigoni E, Amadò R (1995). Effects of oat gum on blood cholesterol levels in healthy young men. Eur. J. Clin. Nutr. 49 (7): 517–22.

Behall KM, Scholfield DJ, Hallfrisch J (2005). Comparison of hormone and glucose responses of overweight women to barley and oats. J. Am. Coll. Nutr. 24 (3): 182–88.

Berg A, König D, Deibert P, Grathwohl D, Berg A, Baumstark MW, Franz IW (2003). Effect of an oat bran enriched diet on the atherogenic lipid profile in patients with an increased coronary heart disease risk. A controlled randomized lifestyle intervention study. Ann. Nutr. Metab. 47 (6): 306–311.

Biörklund M, Holm J, Onning G (2008). Serum lipids and postprandial glucose and insulin levels in hyperlipidemic subjects after consumption of an oat beta-glucan-containing ready meal. Ann. Nutr. Metab. 52 (2): 83–90.

Biörklund M, van Rees A, Mensink RP, Onning G (2005). Changes in serum lipids and postprandial glucose and insulin concentrations after consumption of beverages with beta-glucans from oats or barley: a randomised dose-controlled trial. Eur. J. Clin. Nutr. 59 (11): 1272–81.

Braaten JT, Wood PJ, Scott FW, Riedel KD, Poste LM, Collins MW (1991). Oat gum lowers glucose and insulin after an oral glucose load. Am. J. Clin. Nutr. 53 (6): 1425–30.

Braaten JT, Wood PJ, Scott FW, Wolynetz MS, Lowe MK, Bradley-White P, Collins MW (1994). Oat β-glucan reduces blood cholesterol concentration in hypercholesterolemic subjects. Eur. J. Clin. Nutr. 48: 465–74.

Bratt K, Sunnerheim K, Bryngelsson S, Fagerlund A, Engman L, Andersson RE, Dimberg LH (2003). Avenanthramides in oats (Avena sativa L.) and structure-antioxidant activity relationships. J. Agric. Food Chem. 51 (3): 594–600.

Brown L, Rosner B, Willett WW, Sacks FM (1999). Cholesterol-lowering effects of dietary fiber: a meta-analysis. Am. J. Clin. Nutr. 69: 30–42.

Bryngelsson S, Dimberg LH, Kamal-Eldin A (2002). Effects of commercial processing on levels of antioxidants in oats (Avena sativa L.). J. Agric. Food Chem. 50 (7): 1890–96.

Butt SM, Tahir-Nadeem M, Khan MK, Shabir R, Butt MS (2008). Oat: unique among the cereals. Eur. J. Nutr. 47 (2): 68–79.

Charlton KE, Tapsell LC, Batterham MJ, O'Shea J, Thorne R, Beck E, Tosh SM (2012). Effect of 6 weeks' consumption of β-glucan-rich oat products on cholesterol levels in mildly hypercholesterolaemic overweight adults. Br. J. Nutr. 107 (7): 1037–47.

CSA (2006). Info on Oats. Celiac Sprue Association/United States of America, Inc. – 09 -26. http://www.csaceliacs.org/InfoonOats.php. Retrieved 2007–09–29.

Davidson MH, Dugan LD, Burns JH, Bova J, Story K, Drennan KB (1991). The hypocholesterolemic effects of β-glucan in oatmeal and oat bran. JAMA. 265: 1833–39.

Davis JM, Murphy EA, Brown AS, Carmichael MD, Ghaffar A, Mayer EP (2004). Effects of oat beta-glucan on innate immunity and infection after exercise stress. Med. Sci. Sports Exerc. 36 (8): 1321–27.

De Angelis M, Rizzello CG, Alfonsi G, Arnault P, Cappelle S, Di Cagno R, Gobbetti M (2007). Use of sourdough lactobacilli and oat fibre to decrease the glycaemic index of white wheat bread. Br. J. Nutr. 98 (6):1196–205.

Dickey W (2008). Making oats safer for patients with coeliac disease. Eur. J. Gastroenterol. Hepatol. 20 (6): 494–95.

Dubois C, Armand M, Senft M, Portugal H, Pauli AM, Bernard PM, Lafont H, Lairon D (1995). Chronic oat bran intake alters postprandial lipemia and lipoproteins in healthy adults. Am. J. Clin. Nutr. 61 (2): 325–33.

Ellis HJ, Ciclitira PJ (2008). Should coeliac sufferers be allowed their oats? Eur. J. Gastroenterol. Hepatol. 20 (6): 492–93.

EFSA (European Food Safety Authority) (2009). Panel on Dietetic Products. Nutrition and allergies (NDA). Scientific opinion on the substantiation of health claims related to beta-glucans and maintenance of normal blood cholesterol concentrations. EFSA J 7: 1254.

Eussen SR, Rompelberg CJ, Andersson KE, Klungel OH, Hellstrand P, Oste R, van Kranen H, Garssen J (2011). Simultaneous intake of oat bran and atorvastatin reduces their efficacy to lower lipid levels and atherosclerosis in LDLr-/- mice. Pharmacol Res. 64 (1): 36–43.

Fric P, Gabrovska D, Nevoral J (2011). Celiac disease, gluten-free diet, and oats. Nutr. Rev. 69 (2): 107–115.

Gallaher DD, Hassel CA, Lee K-J (1993). Relationship between viscosity of hydroxypropyl methylcellulose and plasma cholesterol in hamsters. J. Nutr. 123: 1732–38.

Grajeta H (1999). Effect of amaranth and oat bran on blood serum and liver lipids in rats depending on the kind of dietary fats. Nahrung. 43 (2): 114–17.

Granfeldt Y, Eliasson AC, Björck I (2000). An examination of the possibility of lowering the glycemic index of oat and barley flakes by minimal processing. J. Nutr. 130 (9): 2207–214.

Granfeldt Y, Hagander B, Björck I (1995). Metabolic responses to starch in oat and wheat products. On the importance of food structure, incomplete gelatinization or presence of viscous dietary fibre. Eur. J. Clin. Nutr. 49 (3): 189–99.

Granfeldt Y, Nyberg L, Björck I (2008). Muesli with 4 g oat beta-glucans lowers glucose and insulin responses after a bread meal in healthy subjects. Eur. J. Clin. Nutr. 62 (5): 600–607.

Guo W, Wise ML, Collins FW, Meydani M (2008). Avenanthramides, polyphenols from oats, inhibit IL-1beta-induced NF-kappaB activation in endothelial cells. Free Radic. Biol. Med. 44 (3): 415–29.

Haboubi NY, Taylor S, Jones S (2006). Coeliac disease and oats: a systematic review. Postgrad. Med. J. 82 (972): 672–78.

Hallert C, Olsson M, Störsrud S, Lenner RA, Kilander A, Stenhammar L (1999).[Oats can be included in gluten-free diet]. Lakartidningen. 96 (30-31): 3339–40. [Article in Swedish].

Hallfrisch J, Scholfield DJ, Behall KM (1995). Diets containing soluble oat extracts improve glucose and insulin responses of moderately hypercholesterolemic men and women. Am. J. Clin. Nutr. 61 (2): 379–84.

Hasler CM, Kundrat S, Wool D (2000).Functional foods and cardiovascular disease. Curr. Atheroscler. Rep. 2 (6): 467–75.

He J, Klag MJ, Whelton PK, Mo JP, Chen JY, Qian MC, Mo PS, He GQ (1995). Oats and buckwheat intakes and cardiovascular disease risk factors in an ethnic minority of China. Am. J. Clin. Nutr. 61 (2): 366–72.

Holm K, Mäki M, Vuolteenaho N, Mustalahti K, Ashorn M, Ruuska T, Kaukinen K (2006). Oats in the treatment of childhood coeliac disease: a 2-year controlled trial and a long-term clinical follow-up study. Aliment. Pharmacol. Ther. 23 (10): 1463-1472.

Janatuinen E *et al.* (1995-10-19). A Comparison of Diets with and without Oats in Adults with Celiac Disease. New England Journal of Medicine. http://content.nejm.org/cgi/content/abstract/333/16/1033.

Janatuinen EK, Kemppainen TA, Julkunen RJK, Kosma VM, Mäki M, Heikkinen M, Uusitupa MI (2002). No harm from five year ingestion of oats in celiac disease, Gut. 50. 332–335.

Jenkins AL, Jenkins DJ, Zdravkovic U, Würsch P, Vuksan V (2002). Depression of the glycemic index by high levels of beta-glucan fiber in two functional foods tested in type 2 diabetes. Eur. J. Clin. Nutr. 56 (7): 622–28.

Karmally W, Montez MG, Palmas W Martinez W, Branstetter A, Ramakrishnan R, Holleran SF, Haffner SM, Ginsberg HN (2005). Cholesterol-lowering benefits of oat-containing cereal in Hispanic Americans. J. Am. Diet. Assoc. 105: 967–70.

Keenan JM, Wenz JB, Myers S, Ripsin C, Huang ZQ I1991). Randomized, controlled, crossover trial of oat bran in hyper-cholesterolemic subjects. J. Fam. Pract. 33 (6): 600–608.

Kemppainen T, Janatuinen E, Holm K, Kosma VM, Heikkinen M, Mäki M, Laurila K, Uusitupa M, Julkunen R (2007). No observed local immunological response at cell level after five years of oats in adult coeliac disease. Scand. J. Gastroenterol. 42 (1): 54–59.

Koskinen O, Villanen M, Korponay-Szabo I, Lindfors K, Mäki M, Kaukinen K (2009). Oats do not induce systemic or mucosal autoantibody response in children with coeliac disease. J. Pediatr. Gastroenterol. Nutr. 48 (5): 559–65.

Kristensen M, Bügel S (2011). A diet rich in oat bran improves blood lipids and hemostatic factors, and reduces apparent energy digestibility in young healthy volunteers. Eur. J. Clin. Nutr. 65 (9): 1053–58.

Lasztity, R (1999). The Chemistry of Cereal Proteins. Akademiai. Kiado.(English). ISBN 978-0849327636.

Lee-Manion AM, Price RK, Strain JJ, Dimberg LH, Sunnerheim K, Welch RW (2009). *In vitro* antioxidant activity and antigenotoxic effects of avenanthramides and related compounds. J. Agric. Food Chem. 57 (22): 10619–24.

Lund EK, Gee JM, Brown JC, Wood PJ, Johnson IT (1989). Effect of oat gum on the physical properties of the gastrointestinal contents and on the uptake of D-galactose and cholesterol by rat small intestine *in vitro*. Br. J. Nutr. 62: 91–101.

Lund EK, Johnson IT (1991). Fermentable carbohydrate reaching the colon after ingestion of oats in humans. J. Nutr. 121: 311–17.

Magee, E. (2008). How Food Affects Your Moods. Retrieved August 14, 2009 from WebMD.com.

Mäkeläinen H, Anttila H, Sihvonen J, Hietanen RM, Tahvonen R, Salminen E, Mikola M, Sontag-Strohm T. (2007).The effect of beta-glucan on the glycemic and insulin index. Eur. J. Clin. Nutr.61 (6): 779–85.

Maki KC, Davidson MH, Witchger MS, Dicklin MR, Subbaiah PV (2007). Effects of high-fiber oat and wheat cereals on postprandial glucose and lipid responses in healthy men. Int. J. Vitam. Nutr. Res. 77 (5): 347–56.

Maki KC, Beiseigel JM, Jonnalagadda SS, Gugger CK, Reeves MS, Farmer MV, Kaden VN, Rains TM (2010). Whole-grain ready-to-eat oat cereal, as part of a dietary program for weight loss, reduces low-density lipoprotein cholesterol in adults with overweight and obesity more than a dietary program including low-fiber control foods. J. Am. Diet. Assoc. 110 (2): 205–14.

Marlett JA, Hosig KB, Vollendorf NW, Shinnick FL, Haack VS, Story JA (1994). Mechanism of serum cholesterol reduction by oat bran. Hepatology. 20 (6): 1450–57.

Mertens IL and Van Gall LF (2000). Overweight, obesity, and blood pressure: the effects of modest weight loss. Obes. Res. 8: 270–78.

Meydani M (2009). Potential health benefits of avenanthramides of oats. Nutr Rev. 67 (12): 731–35.

Murphy EA, Davis JM, Brown AS, Carmichael MD, Carson JA, Van Rooijen N, Ghaffar A, Mayer EP (2008). Benefits of oat beta-glucan on respiratory infection following exercise stress: role of lung macrophages. Am. J. Physiol. Regul. Integr. Comp. Physiol. 294 (5): R1593–99.

Murphy EA, Davis JM, Brown AS, Carmichael MD, Ghaffar A, Mayer EP (2007). Oat beta-glucan effects on neutrophil respiratory burst activity following exercise. Med. Sci. Sports Exerc. 39 (4): 639–44.

Murphy EA, Davis JM, Carmichael MD, Mayer EP, Ghaffar A (2009). Benefits of oat beta-glucan and sucrose feedings on infection and macrophage antiviral resistance following exercise stress. Am. J. Physiol. Regul. Integr. Comp. Physiol. 297 (4): R1188–94.

Nie L, Wise M, Peterson D, Meydani M (2006). Mechanism by which avenanthramide-c, a polyphenol of oats, blocks cell cycle progression in vascular smooth muscle cells. Free Radic Biol Med. 41 (5): 702–708.

Oda T, Aoe S, Imanishi S, Kanazawa Y, Sanada H, Ayano Y (1994). Effects of dietary oat, barley, and guar gums on serum and liver lipid concentrations in diet-induced hypertriglyceridemic rats. J. Nutr. Sci. Vitaminol. (Tokyo). 40 (2): 213–17.

Onning G, Akesson B, Oste R, Lundquist I (1998). Effects of consumption of oat milk, soya milk, or cow's milk on plasma lipids and antioxidative capacity in healthy subjects. Ann. Nutr. Metab. 42 (4): 211–20.

Onning G, Wallmark A, Persson M, Akesson B, Elmståhl S, Oste R.(1999).Consumption of oat milk for 5 weeks lowers serum cholesterol and LDL cholesterol in free-living men with moderate hypercholesterolemia. Ann. Nutr. Metab. 43 (5): 301–309.

Othman RA, Moghadasian MH, Jones PJ (2011). Cholesterol-lowering effects of oat β-glucan. Nutr. Rev. 69 (6): 299–309.

Panahi S, Ezatagha A, Temelli F, Vasanthan T, Vuksan V (2007). Beta-glucan from two sources of oat concentrates affect postprandial glycemia in relation to the level of vicosity. J. Am. Coll. Nutr. 26 (6): 639–44.

Park SY, Bae IY, Lee S, Lee HG (2009). Physicochemical and hypocholesterolemic characterization of oxidized oat beta-glucan. J. Agric. Food Chem. 57 (2): 439–43.

Peräaho M, Collin P, Kaukinen K, Kekkonen L, Miettinen S, Mäki M (2004). Oats can diversify a gluten-free diet in celiac disease and dermatitis herpetiformis. Am. Diet. Assoc. 104 (7): 1148–50.

Pick ME, Hawrysh ZJ, Gee MI, Toth E, Garg ML, Hardin RT (1996). Oat bran concentrate bread products improve long-term control of diabetes: a pilot study. J. Am. Diet. Assoc. 96 (12): 1254–61.

Pins JJ, Geleva D, Keenan JM, Frazel C, O'Connor PJ, Cherney LM (2002). Do whole-grain oat cereals reduce the need for antihypertensive medications and improve blood pressure control? J. Fam. Pract. 51 (4): 353–59.

Poulter N, Chang CL, Cuff A, Poulter C, Sever P, Thom S (1994). Lipid profiles after the daily consumption of an oat-based cereal: a controlled crossover trial. Am. J. Clin. Nutr. 59 (1): 66–69.

Pulido OM, Gillespie Z, Zarkadas M, Dubois S, Vavasour E, Rashid M, Switzer C, Godefroy SB (2009). Introduction of oats in the diet of individuals with celiac disease: a systematic review. Adv. Food Nutr. Res. 57: 235–85.

Queenan KM, Stewart ML, Smith KN, Thomas W, Fulcher RG, Slavin JL (2007). Concentrated oat beta-glucan, a fermentable fiber, lowers serum cholesterol in hypercholesterolemic adults in a randomized controlled trial. Nutr. J. 6: 6.

Regand A, Tosh SM, Wolever TMS, Wood PJ (2009). Physicochemical properties of beta-glucan in differently processed oat foods influence glycemic response. J. Agric. Food Chem. 57: 8831–38.

Reppas C, Swidan SZ, Tobey SW, Turowski M, Drressman JB (2009). Hydroxymethylcellulose significantly lowers blood cholesterol in mildly hypercholesterolemic human subjects. Eur. J. Clin. Nutr. 63: 71–77.

Reyna-Villasmil N, Bermúdez-Pirela V, Mengual-Moreno E, Arias N, Cano-Ponce C, Leal-Gonzalez E, Souki A, Inglett GE, Israili ZH, Hernández-Hernández R, Valasco M, Arraiz N (2007). Oat-derived beta-glucan significantly improves HDLC and diminishes LDLC and non-HDL cholesterol in overweight individuals with mild hypercholesterolemia. Am. J. Ther. 14(2): 203–12.

Ripsin CM, Keenan JM, Jacobs DR, *et al.* (1992). Oat products and lipid lowering–a meta analysis. JAMA. 267: 3317–25.

Robitaille J, Fontaine-Bisson B, Couture P, Tchernof A, Vohl MC. (2005). Effect of an oat bran-rich supplement on the metabolic profile of overweight premenopausal women. Ann. Nutr. Metab. 49 (3): 141–48.

Romero AL, Romero JE, Galaviz S, Fernandez ML (1998). Cookies enriched with psyllium or oat bran lower plasma LDL cholesterol in normal and hypercholesterolemic men from Northern Mexico. J. Am. Coll. Nutr. 17 (6): 601–608.

Rottmann LH (2006-09-26). On the Use of Oats in the Gluten-Free Diet. Celiac Sprue Association/United States of America, Inc. (CSA). http://www.csaceliacs.org/library/useofoats.php. Retrieved 2006–10–31.

Ryan D, Kendall M, Robards K (2007). Bioactivity of oats as it relates to cardiovascular disease. Nutr Res Rev. 20 (2): 147–62.

Rytter E, Erlanson-Albertsson C, Lindahl L, Lundquist I, Viberg U, Akesson B, Oste R (1996). Changes in plasma insulin, enterostatin, and lipoprotein levels during an energy-restricted dietary regimen including a new oat-based liquid food. Ann. Nutr. Metab. 40 (4): 212–20.

Saltzman E, Das SK, Lichtenstein AH, Dallal GE, Corrales A, Schaefer EJ, Greenberg AS, Roberts SB (2001). An oat-containing hypocaloric diet reduces systolic blood pressure and improves lipid profile beyond effects of weight loss in men and women. J. Nutr. 131 (5): 1465–70.

Shen RL, Cai FL, Dong JL, Hu XZ (2011). Hypoglycaemic effects and biochemical mechanisms of oat products on streptozotocin-induced diabetic mice. J. Agric. Food. Chem. 59 (16): 8895 – 900.

Størsrud S, Hulthén LR, Lenner RA (2003). Beneficial effects of oats in the gluten-free diet of adults with (special reference to nutrient status, symptoms and subjective experiences. Br. J. Nutr. 90 (1): 101–107.

Sur R, Nigam A, Grote D, Liebel F, Southall MD (2008). Avenanthramides, polyphenols from oats, exhibit anti-inflammatory and anti-itch activity. Arch. Dermatol. Res. 300 (10): 569–74.

Tapola N, Karvonen H, Niskanen L, Mikola M, Sarkkinen E (2005). Glycemic responses of oat bran products in type 2 diabetic patients. Nutr. Metab. Cardiovasc. Dis. 15 (4): 255–61.

Tappy L, Gügolz E, Würsch P (1996). Effects of breakfast cereals containing various amounts of beta-glucan fibers on plasma glucose and insulin responses in NIDDM subjects. Diabetes Care. 19 (8): 831–34.

Theuwissen E and Mensink RP (2007). Simultaneous intake of β-glucan and plant stanol esters affects lipid metabolism in slightly hypercholesterolemia subjects. J. Nutr. 137: 583–88.

Thompson T (2003). Oats and the gluten-free diet. J. Am. Diet. Assoc. 103 (3): 376–79.

Trials of Hypertension Prevention Collaborative Research Group (1992). The effects of nonpharmacologic interventions on blood pressure of persons with high normal levels: results of the Trials of Hypertension Prevention, phase 1. J. Am. Med. Assoc. 267: 1213–20.

Tosh SM, Brummer Y, Miller SS, Regand A, Defelice C, Duss R, Wolever TM, Wood PJ (2010). Processing affects the physicochemical properties of beta-glucan in oat bran cereal. J. Agric. Food Chem. 58 (13): 7723–30.

Tuck ML, Corry DB (1991). Pathophysiology and management of hypertension in diabetes. Annu. Rev. Med. 42: 533–48.

USDA (2012). National Nutrient Database for Standard Reference, Release 25.

Uusitupa MI, Miettinen TA, Sarkkinen ES, Ruuskanen E, Kervinen K, Kesäniemi YA (1997). Lathosterol and other non-cholesterol sterols during treatment of hypercholesterolaemia with beta-glucan-rich oat bran. Eur J Clin Nutr. 51 (9): 607 -611.

Van Horn L, Moag-Stahlberg A, Liu KA, Ballew C, Ruth K, Hughes R, Stamler J (1991). Effects on serum lipids of adding instant oats to usual American diets. Am. J. Public Health. 81 (2): 183–88.

Vervuert I, Coenen M, Bothe C (2003). Effects of oat processing on the glycaemic and insulin responses in horses. J. Anim. Physiol. Anim. Nutr. (Berl). 87 (3-4): 96–104.

Virtanen SM, Kaila M, Pekkanen J, Kenward MG, Uusitalo U, Pietinen P, Kronberg-Kippilä C, Hakulinen T, Simell O, Ilonen J, Veijola R, Knip M (2010). Early introduction of oats associated with decreased risk of persistent asthma and early introduction of fish with decreased risk of allergic rhinitis. Br. J. Nutr. 103 (2): 266–73.

Wadden TA, Anderson DA, Foster GD (1999). Two-year changes in lipids and lipoproteins associated with maintenance of a 5 per cent to 10 per cent reduction in initial weight: some findings and some questions. Obes. Res. 7: 170–78.

Wang SC, Bligh SW, Zhu CL, Shi SS, Wang ZT, Hu ZB, Crowder J, Branford-White C, Vella C (2008). Sulfated beta-glucan derived from oat bran with potent anti-HIV activity. J. Agric. Food Chem. 56 (8): 2624–29.

Winblad I, Joensuu T, Korpela H (1995). Effect of oat bran supplemented diet on hypercholesterolaemia. Scand. J. Prim. Health Care. 13 (2): 118–21.

Würsch P, Pi-Sunyer FX (1997). The role of viscous soluble fiber in the metabolic control of diabetes. A review with special emphasis on cereals rich in beta-glucan. Diabetes Care. 20 (11): 1774–80.

Wolever TM, Gibbs AL, Brand-Miller J, Duncan AM, Hart V, Lamarche B, Tosh SM, Duss R (2011). Bioactive oat β-glucan reduces LDL cholesterol in Caucasians and non-Caucasians. Nutr. J. 10: 130.

Wolever TM, Tosh SM, Gibbs AL, Brand-Miller J, Duncan AM, Hart V, Lamarche B, Thomson BA, Duss R, Wood PJ (2010). Physicochemical properties of oat β-glucan influence its ability to reduce serum LDL cholesterol in humans: a randomized clinical trial. Am. J. Clin. Nutr. 92 (4): 723–32.

Wood PJ, Beer MU, Butler G (2000). Evaluation of role of concentration and molecular weight of oat β-glucan in determining effect of viscosity on plasma glucose and insulin following an oral glucose load. Br. J. Nutr. 84: 19–23.

Chapter 16

Amla

(*Phyllanthus emblica* syn. *Emblica officinalis*/ *Phyllanthus niruri*)

"An Amla a Day Keeps the Doctors Away!"

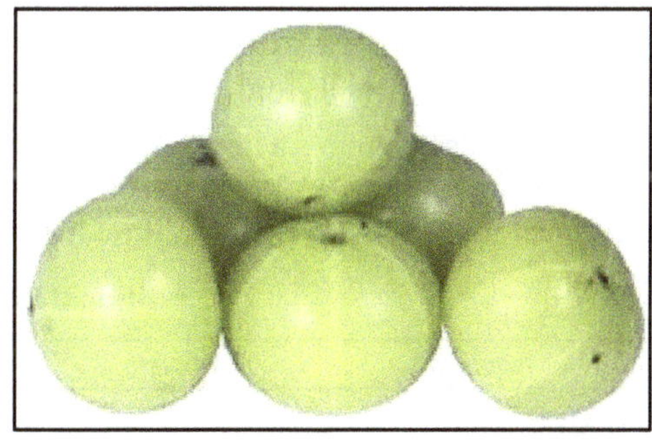

Amla, known as Indian gooseberry is a natural antioxidant and also is a popular home remedy. The amla tree has been worshipped in India from ancient times as the 'Earth Mother', and is said to be nursing humankind. The Indian ayurvedic system of medicine describes amla as a rejuvenating food. Several health benefits such as hypocholesterolemic, antioxidant, anticancer and hepatoprotective effects were attributed to it most of which have been confirmed by the modern medinine.

There are 3 main varieties of amla *viz.*, Banarasi, Francis (Hathijhool) and Chakaiya. These varieties have their own merits and demerits. Banarasi, an early-maturing, is prone to heavy dropping of fruits with poor shelf life. Francis amla suffers from severe incidence of fruit necrosis. Chakaiya fruits are fibrous, smaller in size and also have a tendency to bear heavy crop in alternate years. A matured tree of about 10 years old will yield 50-70 kg of fruit. The yield increases year by year up to 50 years. A well maintained tree will be yielding up to an age of 70 years.

Chemical Constituents of Amla

Amla extract contains plenty of natural bioflavonoids, (which protect and strengthen human cell membranes from oxidative damage) and cytokine-like substances called z-riboside, zeatin, 1-O-galloyl-beta-D-glucose, 3,6-di-O-galloyl-D-glucose, chebulinic acid, quercetin, chebulagic acid, corilagin, 3-ethylgallic acid (3-ethoxy-4,5-dihydroxy-benzoic acid), isostrictiniin and z-nucleotide. The fruit also contains other polyphenols–flavonoids, kaempferol, ellagic acid and gallic acid (Zhang *et al.*, 2003). Habib-ur-Rehman *et al.* (2007) isolated two new flavonoids, (1) kaempferol-3-O-alpha-L-(6''-methyl)-hamnopyranoside and (2) kaempferol-3-O-alpha-L-(6''-ethyl)-hamnopyranoside.). The methanol extract of Amla was found to contain ellagicacid and ascorbic acid as the major compounds by liquid chromatography-mass spectroscopy (LC-MS) analysis (Nampoothiri *et al.*, 2011).

The plant also contains other phenolic compounds, tannins, phyllembelic acid, phyllembelin, rutin, curcuminoids, and emblicol (Krishnaveni and Mirunalini, 2010). Liu *et al.* (2009) found the main components of the essential oil to be beta-caryophyllene, beta-bourbonene, 1-octen-3-ol, thymol, and methyleugenol.

Nutritive Value of Amla

The moisture content of Amla is 91.4 per cent, and it contains 3.4 g fiber, 0.7 g mineral matter, 0.9 g protein, 0.1 g fat, 6.9 g carbohydrate, 0.02 mg Thiamine and 0.08 mg Riboflavin per 100g. Amla extract contains on an average 445 mg/100 g of vitamin C. Some varieties contain 720 mg/100 g of fresh amla pulp or 900 mg/100 ml of amla juice *i.e.* approximately twenty times as much vitamin C as orange juice. Amla has nearly 160 times the concentration of ascorbic acid found in one apple. Although the fruit is reputed to contain high amounts of ascorbic acid (Tarwadi and Agte, 2007), the specific contents are disputed, and the overall antioxidant strength of amla may derive instead from its high density of tannins.

Amla also contains a large amount of most beneficial minerals (34 mg of calcium and 1.2 mg of iron) and amino acids. Being low in sugar and high in fiber, amla becomes an ideal daily fruit for almost everyone.

Nutritional Value per 100 g

Nutrient	*Amount*	*Nutrient*	*Amount*
Energy (kcal)	58	Carbohydrates (g)	13.7
Dietary fiber (g)	3.4	Fat (g)	0.1
Protein (g)	0.5	Calcium (mg)	50
Iron (mg)	1.2	Phosphorus (mg)	20
Sodium (mg)	5.0	Potassium (mg)	225
Thiamine (Vit. B1) (mg)	0.03	Riboflavin (Vit.B2) (mg)	0.01
Vitamin C (mg)	600	Carotene (µg)	9

Gopalan *et al.*, 2010.

Traditional Uses of Amla

Amla fruit is sour and astringent in taste (rasa), with slight sweetness, bitterness and pungency. According to Ayurveda, it is believed to be cooling to the body post digestion. It is also a very important ingredient in the famous Chyavanaprash, and a constituent of Triphala (powder prepared from 3 fruits, one of which is amla). Also, long term use of Indian gooseberry capsules has not shown any adverse effects on human body as it is a natural product and is free of any side effects.

Amla is an important traditional medicine with broad prospects. By cross cultural comparative study, Xia *et al.* (1997) indicated that there are 17 countries in the world using various parts of amla in their medical treatment. The medicinal plant is believed to be good in the treatment of hepatitis, cancer and regulation of stomach function. Amla is also commonly called an adaptogenic herb by various herbalists throughout the world, as it boosts the immune system and is helpful in prevention of immune compromised conditions.

Amla is believed to prevent/cure early aging, skin and eye disorders; and beneficial for hair and respiratory function of human body. Dried fruits have been reported to be useful in haemorrhages, diarrhoea, dysentery, anaemia, jaundice, dyspepsia and cough. Its regular consumption is an antidote for many other ailments/ disorders like acidity, septic fever, biliary colic, vomiting and insomnia. In Chinese traditional therapy, amla fruit is called Yuganzi, which is used to cure throat inflammation. It is acrid, cooling, refrigerant, diuretic and laxative.

Therapeutic Value of Amla

In vivo experimental evidences have shown the potential efficacy of leaves, bark or fruit against clinical conditions such as inflammation, cancer, age-related renal disease, and diabetes (Ganju *et al.*, 2003; Rao *et al.*, 2005). According to Krishnaveni and Mirunalini (2010) various parts of the plant show antidiabetic, hypolipidemic, antibacterial, antioxidant, antiulcerogenic, hepatoprotective, gastroprotective, and chemopreventive properties.

Preclinical studies have shown that amla possesses antipyretic, analgesic, antitussive, antiatherogenic, adaptogenic, cardioprotective, antianaemia, antihypercholesterolemia, wound healing, antidiarrhoeal, antiatherosclerotic, nephroprotective, and neuroprotective properties. In addition, experimental studies have shown that amla and some of its phytochemicals such as gallic acid, ellagic acid, pyrogallol, some norsesquiterpenoids, corilagin, geraniin, elaeocarpusin, and prodelphinidins B1 and B2 also possess anti-neoplastic effects. Amla is also reported to possess radiomodulatory, chemomodulatory, chemopreventive effects, free radical scavenging, antioxidant, anti-inflammatory, antimutagenic and immunemodulatory properties that are efficacious in the treatment and prevention of cancer. Thus, Baliga and D'Souza (2011) summarizing the results of their review on amla emphasized that some aspects suggest future research to establish its activity and utility as a cancer preventive and therapeutic drug in humans.

The various chemical constituents of amla were found to possess different levels of antioxidant potential which is implicated in the therapeutic benefits mentioned above and the available scientific evidences for the therapeutic benefits are shown below.

Amla: The Natural Antioxidant

Cellular damage caused by reactive oxygen species has been implicated in several diseases, and hence natural antioxidants have significant importance in human health. Amla is proved to be useful as potent sources of natural antioxidant (Hazra *et al.*, 2010). The antioxidant activities exhibited by amla extract are superior to those of ascorbic acid itself. For many years, the antioxidant activity of the fruits was attributed to the high content of ascorbic acid; however, this has been questioned while Scartezzini *et al.* (2006) reported that amla contains 0.4 per cent, w/w ascorbic acid.

The Ayurvedic method of processing ("Svaras Bhavana", whereby the therapeutic potential of the plant is enhanced by treating the main herb with its own juice) increases the antioxidant activity and the ascorbic acid (1.28 per cent, w/w) content. They also reported that vitamin C accounts for approximately 45-70 per cent of the antioxidant activity.

Emblicanins are a type of antioxidants found in a. Emblicanin is different from most other antioxidants as it is a prooxidation free cascading antioxidant. Many antioxidants intrinsically have a prooxidant action, especially in the presence of transition metals like iron and copper. Through a series of reactions with oxygen species known as Fenton reaction, iron causes generation of highly toxic hydroxyl radical with subsequent biomolecule damage. It means that the antioxidants which are meant to scavenge free radicals themselves create free radicals. While most antioxidants go directly from an active to an inactive role, Emblicanin utilizes a multilevel cascade of antioxidant compounds resulting in a prolongation of its antioxidant capabilities.

Emblicanin A (one of the key compounds in Emblicanin) aggressively seeks and attacks free radicals. After it neutralizes a free radical, emblicanin A is transformed into emblicanin B, another antioxidant. Emblicanin B in turn also attacks free radicals and is transformed into Emblicanin oligomers. This makes low molecular hydrolyzable tannins emblicanins A and B the best free radical scavenging antioxidant in Amla (Bhutan, 2008). From the estimated ID50 values, by a new procedure developed to separate and quantify the free radical-scavenging activity of individual compounds revealed the increasing order of activity to be emblicanin B > emblicanin A > gallic acid > ellagic acid > ascorbic acid. Probably, the antioxidant activity of amla extract is associated with the presence of hydrolyzable tannins having ascorbic acid-like action (Pozharitskaya, 2007).

But, Majeed *et al.* (2009) found no evidence for the presence of emblicanins A and B in the extract. In addition, according to them the high content of ascorbic acid has also been doubted due to previous non-identification of co-eluting mucic acid gallates.

Emblica officinalis showed greater efficiency in lipid peroxidation and plasmid DNA assay than the other two ingredients in Triphala while Terminalia chebula showed greater radical scavenging activity. Thus Naik *et al.* (2005) reports that the mixture Triphala to be more efficient due to the combined activity of the individual components.

Methanolic as well as ethanolic extracts of amla act as potent α-amylase and α-glucosidase inhibitor. Significant antiglycation activity also confirms the therapeutic potential of these extracts against diabetes. Both the extracts significantly inhibited the oxidation of LDL under *in vitro* conditions. Liquid chromatography-mass spectroscopy (LC-MS) analysis revealed that methanol extract contains ellagic acid and ascorbic acid being the major compound respectively (Nampoothiri *et al.*, 2011).

The extract designated IG-3 was consistently amongst the most effective extracts in the iron (III) reduction and 1,1-diphenyl-2-picrylhydrazyl and superoxide anion radical scavenging assays while the extract designated IG-1 demonstrated the best hydroxyl radical scavenging activity. All extracts appeared to be incapable of chelating iron (II) at realistic concentrations (Poltanov *et al.*, 2009).

Amla contains a high amount of total polyphenol and tannin content. It has a strong antioxidant activity as well as inhibition of TBARS and glycation thus implying that amla is a potential source of natural antioxidants which have free radical scavenging activity and might be used for reducing oxidative stress in diabetes (Kusirisin *et al.*, 2009).

Evaluating its effect on the prooxidant–antioxidant system of liver and the hepatoprotective potential of aqueous extract of the herb *Phyllanthus niruri* on NIM-induced oxidative stress *in vivo* Chatterjee and Sil (2006) revealed that it is probably through its antioxidant property that controls the NIM-induced oxidative stress in the liver.

Antimicrobial Activity

Saeed and Tariq (2007) demonstrated *in vitro* antiviral and antimicrobial properties against *E. coli, K. pneumoniae, K. ozaenae, P. mirabilis, P. aeruginosa, S. typhi, S. paratyphi A, S. paratyphi B and S. marcescens* but did not show any antibacterial activity against Gram negative urinary pathogens. Similarly, Liu *et al.* (2009) found the essential oil of amla to show a broad spectrum of antimicrobial activity against all the tested microorganisms. Gram-positive bacteria were more sensitive to the oils than Gram-negative bacteria. The essential oil obtained by supercritical fluid extraction exhibited a higher antifungal activity compared to the one obtained by hydro distillation.

Rahman *et al.* (2009) observed the chloroform soluble fraction of the methanolic extract to exhibit significant antimicrobial activity against some Gram-positive and Gram-negative pathogenic bacteria and strong cytotoxicity having a LC50 of 10.257 +/- 0.770 mcg/ml (-1). It is thus shown that the chloroform soluble fraction of the ripe fruits of amla containing alkaloids is biologically active.

Coxsackie virus B3 (CVB3) is believed to be a major contributor to viral myocarditis since virus-associated apoptosis plays a role in the pathogenesis of experimental myocarditis. Wang *et al.* (2009) showed that Phyllaemblicin B exerts significant antiviral activities against CVB3 and thus is proved to be a potential therapeutic agent for viral myocarditis.

Pinmai *et al.* (2010) evaluated the *in vitro* and *in vivo* antiplasmodial activity and the cytotoxicity of amla. The presence of flavonoids, hydrolysable tannins, saponin and terpenes in amla was shown to possess antimalarial activity. Aqueous extract of amla exhibited potent antimicrobial activity against *E. cloacae* followed by *E. coli*. The minimum inhibitory concentration of aqueous extract of amla was most active against *K. pneumonia*, whereas that of methanol extract showed maximum activity against *E. coli* (Kumar *et al.*, 2011).

Srikumar *et al.* (2007) reported that both individual and combined aqueous and ethanol extracts of Triphala have antibacterial activity against the bacterial isolates (*P. aeruginosa, K. pneumoniae, S. sonnei, S. flexneri, S. aureus, V. cholerae, S. paratyphi-B, E. coli, E. faecalis, S. typhi*) tested.

Anti-inflammatory Effect

Asmawi *et al.* (1993) reported that the anti-inflammatory action of amla. Leaves and fruits of amla have been used for the anti-inflammatory and antipyretic treatment of rural populations in subtropical and tropical parts of China, India, Indonesia, and the Malay Peninsula. Ihantola-Vormisto *et al.* (1997) reported that the leaves contain as yet unidentified polar compound(s) with potent inhibitory activity on human polymorphonuclear leukocyte and platelet functions and chemically different apolar molecule(s) which inhibit both prostanoid and leukotriene synthesis which confirmed the anti-inflammatory and antipyretic properties of amla.

Arunachalam *et al.* (2011) suggested that the phenolic compounds of *E. officinalis* may serve as potential herbal candidate for amelioration of acute and chronic inflammation due to their modulatory action of free radicals.

Antidiabetic Effect

A significant decrease in blood glucose as well as triglyceride levels and an improvement in the liver function by normalization of the activity of liver specific enzyme alanine transaminase were demonstrated in alloxan-induced diabetic rats fed an aqueous amla fruit extract (Qureshi *et al.*, 2009).

Akhtar *et al.* (2011) reported a significant dose dependant hypoglycaemic hypolipidaemic effect of amla powder in humans. Both normal and diabetic subjects receiving 1, 2 or 3 g of amla powder per day showed significant decrease in fasting and 2-h postprandial blood glucose levels on the 21st day as compared to their baseline values. A significant decrease was also observed in total cholesterol and triglycerides along with significant improvement in HDL-cholesterol and LDL-cholesterol levels in those receiving either 2 or 3 g of amla powder per day.

A mixture of methanolic extracts (75 per cent) of *Terminalia chebula, Terminalia belerica, Emblica officinalis* named as 'Triphala' (equal proportion of above three plant extracts) is being used extensively in Indian system of medicine. Oral administration of the extracts (100 mg/kg body weight) reduced the blood sugar level in normal and in alloxan (120 mg/kg) diabetic rats significantly within 4 h. Continued daily administration of the extract produced a sustained effect (Sabu and Kuttan, 2002).

The oral administration of amla extracts to the diabetic rats slightly improved body weight gain along with significant alleviation of various oxidative stress indices of the serum. The elevated serum levels of 5-hydroxymethylfurfural, (a glycosylated protein and an indicator of oxidative stress) and thiobarbituric acid-reactive substance levels were significantly reduced dose-dependently in the diabetic rats fed amla indicating a reduction in lipid peroxidation. Similarly, the serum level of creatinine, yet another oxidative stress parameter, was also reduced. In addition, significant improvement was also observed in serum albumin and adiponectin levels. These results give the scientific basis for supporting the efficacy of amla in relieving the oxidative stress and improving glucose metabolism in diabetes (Rao *et al.*, 2005).

Methanol extract of amla exhibited maximum scavenging activity against DPPH, superoxide, hydroxyl and nitric oxide radicals. Nampoothiri *et al.* (2011) observed that the methanol extract of amla can act as potent α-amylase and α-glucosidase inhibitor. Significant antiglycation activity also confirmed the therapeutic potential of these extracts against diabetes. The extract also significantly inhibited the oxidation of LDL under *in vitro* conditions.

Uremic patients with diabetes suffer from high levels of oxidative stress due to regular hemodialysis therapy (neutrophil activation induced by hem-incompatibility between the hemodialyser and blood) and complications associated with diabetes. Amla tea ameliorated diabetic nephropathy. In diabetic rats Tiwari *et al.* (2011) found amla to significantly reduce blood glucose, food intake, water intake and urine output as compared to the non diabetic control group. Chen *et al.* (2011b) also reported that oral administration of a 1:1 mixture of (-)-epigallocatechin gallate, (a major component of green tea extract) and amla extract for 3 months significantly improved antioxidant defense as well as diabetic and atherogenic indices in uremic patients with diabetes. Further, they did not observe any significant adverse effect on hepatic function, renal function, or inflammatory responses and hence confirmed the safety and efficacy of this mixture in the treatment of uremic patients with diabetes.

Aldose reductase (AR) has been a drug target because of its involvement in the development of secondary complications of diabetes including cataract. Although numerous synthetic AR inhibitors (ARI) have been tested and shown to inhibit the enzyme, clinically synthetic ARIs have not been very successful. Therefore, Suryanarayana *et al.* (2004; 2007) have assessed the inhibition of AR by constituents of amla both *in vitro* and in-lens organ culture and through the slit lamp microscopic observations and indicated that these supplements delay cataract progression. Tannoids of amla are potent inhibitors of AR. Thus evaluating natural sources such as amla for ARI potential may lead to the development of safer and more effective agents against diabetic retinopathy.

Kumar *et al.* (2009) provided experimental evidence of the preventive and curative effect of amla on nerve function and oxidative stress in animal model of diabetic neuropathy. Since, the fruit is already in clinical use for diabetic patients it may be evaluated for preventive therapy in diabetic patients at risk of developing neuropathy.

Cardioprotective Effect

Flavonoids from amla effectively reduce lipid levels in serum and tissues of hyperlipidemia induced rats by significantly inhibiting hepatic HMG CoA reductase activity. The concerted action of inhibition of synthesis and enhancement of degradation of lipids seems to be the mechanism of hypolipidemic action of amla (Anila and Vijayalakshmi, 2002).

A pilot study on human subjects demonstrated reduction of blood cholesterol levels in both normal and hypercholesterolemic men treated with amla (Jacob *et al.*, 1988). Kim *et al.* (2005) also confirmed that amla is effective in treating hypercholesterolemia and preventing atherosclerosis. Again, Kim *et al.* (2010) reported that fructose-induced metabolic syndrome is attenuated by the poly-phenol-rich fraction of amla.

It also prevents age-related hyperlipidemia through attenuating oxidative stress in the ageing process (Yokozawa *et al.*, 2007b). Bhatia *et al.* (2011) demonstrated the reduction in oxidative stress, prevention of development and progression of hypertension as well as cardiac and renal hypertrophy in DOCA/HS-induced hypertension (via modulation of activated eNOS, endogenous antioxidants, serum NO and electrolyte levels). According to Rajak *et al.* (2004) regular administration of amla causes myocardial adaptation by augmenting endogenous antioxidants and protects rat hearts from oxidative stress associated with ischemic reperfusion injury. Only the ethyl acetate phase showed strong NO scavenging activity *in vitro*, when compared with water and hexane phases. Gallic acid was found to be a major compound in the ethyl acetate extract and Geraniin showed highest NO scavenging activity among the isolated compounds (Kumaran and Karunakaran, 2006). Due to its anti-inflammatory effect, amla showed a trend to reduce the edema in the model of carrageenan- induced paw edema (Dang *et al.*, 2011).

Neuroprotective Effect

Amla is traditionally used for central nervous system disorders. The cognitive impairment seen in epileptics may be a consequence of either the underlying epileptogenic process alone or the use of antiepileptic drugs that cause cognitive impairment as an adverse effect or both. Golecha *et al.* (2010) showed that both 500 and 700 mg/kg intra peritoneal (i.p.) doses of amla extract completely abolished the generalized tonic seizures and also improved the retention latency in passive avoidance task. Further, dose-dependently the extract ameliorated the oxidative stress induced by pentylenetetrazole. Golecha *et al.* (2011) also observed the hydro-alcoholic extract of amla at 700 mg/kg, i.p. dose was most effective in suppressing kainic acid-induced seizures, cognitive decline, and oxidative stress in the brain. The neuroprotective effects, according to these authors, may be due to the antioxidant and anti-inflammatory effects of amla extract. Golechha *et al.* (2012) suggested the fruits of Emblica officinalis to possess memory enhancing, antioxidant and anticholinesterase activity. It may be useful for the treatment of cognitive impairments induced by cholinergic dysfunction. Its potential in the management of dementia and Alzheimer disease needs to be further explored.

Anticarcinogenic Effect

Amla is potential against some cancers (Ngamkitidechakul *et al.,* 2010). Sai Ram *et al.* (2002) observed immunomodulatory effect of amla. Chromium-induced free radical production was inhibited significantly and the antioxidant status was restored back to control level. Amla also inhibited apoptosis and DNA fragmentation induced by chromium. Interestingly, amla relieved the immunosuppressive effects of chromium on lymphocyte proliferation (Sai Ram *et al.,* 2003) and even restored both phagocytosis and Interferon-gamma production considerably. Khan *et al.* (2002) identified pyrogallol to be an active component in the antiproliferative effect of amla extract on human tumour cell lines.

It is interesting to observe that Triphala containing amla was more effective in reducing tumour incidences (Baliga, 2010) compared to its individual constituents. Triphala also significantly increased the antioxidant status of animals which might have contributed to the chemo-prevention. It was inferred that the concomitant use of multiple agents seemed to have a high degree of chemo-prevention potential (Deep *et al.,* 2005). Sandhya *et al.* (2006) also reported that Triphala possesses ability to induce cytotoxicity in tumour cells but spared the normal cells. The differential effect of Triphala on normal and tumour cells seems to be related to its ability to evoke differential response in intracellular Reactive Oxygen Species generation. The differential response of normal and tumour cells to Triphala *in vitro* and the substantial regression of transplanted tumour in mice fed with Triphala points to its potential use as an anticancer drug for clinical treatment. According to Kaur *et al.* (2005) the suppression of the growth of cancer cells in cytotoxic assays may be due to the gallic acid, a major polyphenol observed in Triphala. Chloroform and acetone extracts of Triphala showed inhibition of mutagenicity induced by both direct and S9-dependent mutagens. A significant inhibition of 98.7 per cent was observed with acetone extract against the revertants induced by S9-dependent mutagen, 2-aminofluorene, in co-incubation mode of treatment (Kaur *et al.,* 2002).

Hepatoprotective Effect

Inflammation and oxidative stress contribute to liver injury. As amla is rich in vitamin C, gallic acid, flavonoids, and tannins, it may protect against hepatotoxicity-induced liver injury. Chen and his colleagues (2011a) elucidated the effects of amla (100mg/kg of body weight) supplementation on N-nitrosodiethylamine-induced apoptosis, autophagy, and inflammation in rat livers. Amla decreased N-nitrosodiethylamine-enhanced hepatic apoptosis and autophagy appearances via down-regulation of the Bax/Bcl-2 ratio and Beclin-1 expression. Thus amla supplementation counteracts N-nitrosodiethylamine-induced liver injury via its antioxidant, anti-inflammation, antiapoptosis, and antiautophagic properties.

Amla at an intake level of 10 per cent was shown to modulate hexachlorocyclohexane (HCH) induced impairment in hepatic catalase, glucose-6-phosphate dehydrogenase and superoxide dismutase activities. Prefeeding of amla at 5 and 10 per cent levels appeared to reduce the HCH-induced raise in renal GGT activity. The results showed the elevation of hepatic antioxidant system and reduction of cytotoxic products as a result of prefeeding of amla, which were otherwise affected by the HCH administration (Anilakumar *et al.*, 2007).

Phyllanthus niruri, another variety of amla, just as *Phyllanthus emblica* is a well-known hepatoprotective herbal plant. The protein isolate of *P. niruri* was found to protect liver tissues against carbon tetrachloride-induced oxidative liver damage *in vivo* and somehow stimulating repair mechanism present in the liver (Bhattacharjee and Sil, 2006; 2007).

Gastroprotective Effect

The crude extract of amla which tested positive for alkaloids, tannins, terpenes, flavonoids, sterols and coumarins, caused inhibition of castor oil-induced diarrhea and intestinal fluid accumulation in mice at a dose of 500-700 mg/kg. It showed a combination of Ca^{2+} antagonist and anticholinergic like components in all fractions but with varying potency. The fruit extract possesses anti-diarrheal and spasmolytic activities, mediated possibly through dual blockade of muscarinic receptors and Ca^{2+} channels, thus explaining its medicinal use in diarrhea (Mehmood *et al.*, 2011).

Pretreatment with the butanol extract of the water fraction of amla orally administered for 10 consecutive days at the dose of 100 mg/kg body weight, was found to enhance secretion of gastric mucus and hexosamine ($P<0.001$) in the indomethacin-induced ulceration of rats. The morphological observations also supported a protective effect of the stomach wall from lesion. The antioxidant property appears to be predominantly responsible for this cyto-protective action of the drug (Bandyopadhyay *et al.*, 2000).

Again, oral administration of amla extract at doses 250 mg/kg and 500 mg/kg significantly inhibited the development of gastric lesions in all test models used. It also caused significant decrease of the pyloric-ligation-induced basal gastric secretion, titratable acidity and gastric mucosal injury. Besides, amla extract offered protection against ethanol-induced depletion of stomach wall mucus and reduction in non-protein sulfhydryl concentration. Histopathological analyses were in good agreement with pharmacological and biochemical findings. Thus, Al-Rehaily *et al.* (2002) proved that amla extract possesses antisecretory, antiulcer and cytoprotective properties.

Healing property of amla on gastric ulcer induced by ethanolic extract was dose-specific through the harmonization of the antioxidative property and modulation of anti-inflammatory cytokine level. Amla can therefore be used as a gastroprotective agent in nonsteroidal anti-inflammatory drug-induced gastropathy (Chatterjee *et al.*, 2011).

Another recent animal study reported that treatment with amla reduced severity of acute pancreatitis (induced by L-arginine in rats). It also promoted the spontaneous repair and regeneration process of the pancreas occurring after an acute attack (Sidhu *et al.*, 2011).

Antiaging Effect

According to Chaudhuri (2002) amla helps protect the skin from the damaging effects of free radicals, nonradicals and transition metal-induced oxidative stress. It is thus suitable for use in antiaging, sunscreen and general purpose skin care products. Amla significantly reduced thiobarbituric acidreactive substance levels of serum, renal homogenate, and mitochondria in aged rats, suggesting its preventive effect on oxidative stress during aging. Yokozawa *et al.* (2007 a) found amla extract to reduce the elevated levels of serum creatinine and urea nitrogen in the aged rats. The extract has no pro-oxidation activity induced by iron and/or copper because of its iron and copper chelating ability.

Antiosteoporotic Effect

There is preliminary evidence (*in vitro*) that amla extracts induce apoptosis and modify gene expression in osteoclasts involved in rheumatoid arthritis and osteoporosis (Penolazzi *et al.*, 2008).

Conclusion

It is amazing that amla, one of the richest sources of Vitamin C, has been proved clinically beyond doubt as an excellent remedy for various health issues, although stronger evidence is required for the role of amla in bone health.

References

Akhtar MS, Ramzan A, Ali A, Ahmad M (2011). Effect of Amla fruit (*Emblica officinalis* Gaertn.) on blood glucose and lipid profile of normal subjects and type 2 diabetic patients. Int. J. Food Sci. Nutr. 62 (6): 609–16.

Al-Rehaily AJ, Al-Howiriny TA, Al-Sohaibani MO, Rafatullah S (2002). Gastroprotective effects of 'Amla' *Emblica officinalis* on *in vivo* test models in rats. Phytomedicine. 9 (6): 515–22.

Anila L, Vijayalakshmi NR (2002). Flavonoids from *Emblica officinalis* and *Mangifera indica*-effectiveness for dyslipidemia. J. Ethnopharmacol. 79 (1): 81–87.

Anilakumar KR, Nagaraj NS, Santhanam K (2007). Reduction of exachlorocyclohexane-induced oxidative stress and cytotoxicity in rat liver by *Emblica officinalis* gaertn. Indian J. Exp. Biol. 45 (5): 450–54.

Arunachalam M, Sood S, Singla SK (2011). The anti-inflammatory potential of phenolic compounds from *Emblica officinalis* L. in rat. Inflammopharmacology. 19 (6): 327–34.

Asmawi MZ, Kankaanranta H, Moilanen E, Vapaatalo H (1993). Anti-inflammatory activities of *Emblica officinalis* Gaertn leaf extracts. J. Pharm. Pharmacol. 45 (6): 581–84.

Baliga MS (2010). Triphala, Ayurvedic formulation for treating and preventing cancer: a review. J. Altern. Complement. Med. 16 (12): 1301–308.

Baliga MS, Dsouza JJ (2011). Amla (*Emblica officinalis* Gaertn), a wonder berry in the treatment and prevention of cancer. Eur. J. Cancer Prev. 20 (3): 225–39.

Bandyopadhyay SK, Pakrashi SC, Pakrashi A (2000). The role of antioxidant activity of *Phyllanthus emblica* fruits on prevention from indomethacin induced gastric ulcer. J. Ethnopharmacol. 70 (2): 171–76.

Bhatia J, Tabassum F, Sharma AK, Bharti S, Golechha M, Joshi S, Sayeed Akhatar M, Srivastava AK, Arya DS (2011). *Emblica officinalis* exerts antihypertensive effect in a rat model of DOCA-salt-induced hypertension: role of (p) eNOS, NO and oxidative stress. Cardiovasc. Toxicol. 11 (3): 272–79.

Bhattacharjee R, Sil PC (2006). The protein fraction of *Phyllanthus niruri* plays a protective role against acetaminophen induced hepatic disorder via its antioxidant properties. Phytother. Res. 20 (7): 595–601.

Bhattacharjee R, Sil PC (2007). Protein isolate from the herb, *Phyllanthus niruri* L. (Euphorbiaceae), plays hepatoprotective role against carbon tetrachloride induced liver damage via its antioxidant properties.Food Chem. Toxicol. 45 (5): 817–26.

Bhutan, KK (2008). International Conference on Newer Developments in Drug Discovery from Natural Products and Traditional Medicines–An Overview. P. 16.

Chatterjee A, Chattopadhyay S, Bandyopadhyay SK (2011). Biphasic Effect of *Phyllanthus emblica* L. Extract on NSAID-Induced Ulcer: An Antioxidative Trail Weaved with Immunomodulatory Effect. Evid Based Complement Alternat. Med. 2011: 146808.

Chatterjee M, Sil PC (2006). Hepatoprotective effect of aqueous extract of *Phyllanthus niruri* on nimesulide-induced oxidative stress *in vivo*. Indian J. Biochem. Biophys. 43 (5): 299–305.

Chaudhuri RK (2002). Emblica cascading antioxidant: a novel natural skin care ingredient. Skin Pharmacol. Appl. Skin Physiol. 15 (5): 374–80.

Chen KH, Lin BR, Chien CT, Ho CH (2011a). *Emblica officinalis* Gaertn. attentuates N-nitrosodiethylamine-induced apoptosis, autophagy, and inflammation in rat livers. J. Med. Food. 14 (7-8): 746–55.

Chen TS, Liou SY, Wu HC, Tsai FJ, Tsai CH, Huang CY, Chang YL (2011b). Efficacy of epigallocatechin-3-gallate and Amla (*Emblica officinalis*) extract for the treatment of diabetic-uremic patients. J. Med. Food. 14 (7-8): 718–23.

Dang GK, Parekar RR, Kamat SK, Scindia AM, Rege NN (2011). Anti-inflammatory activity of *Phyllanthus emblica*, *Plumbago zeylanica* and *Cyperus rotundus* in acute models of inflammation. Phytother. Res. 25 (6): 904–908.

Deep G, Dhiman M, Rao AR, Kale RK (2005). Chemopreventive potential of Triphala (a composite Indian drug) on benzo(a)pyrene induced forestomach tumourigenesis in murine tumour model system. J. Exp. Clin. Cancer Res. 24 (4): 555–63.

Ganju L, Karan D, Chanda S, Srivastava KK, Sawhney RC, Selvamurthy W (2003). Immunomodulatory effects of agents of plant origin. Biomed. Pharmacother. 57 (7): 296–300.

Golechha M, Bhatia J, Arya DS (2010). Hydroalcoholic extract of *Emblica officinalis* Gaertn. affords protection against PTZ-induced seizures, oxidative stress and cognitive impairment in rats. Indian J. Exp. Biol. 48 (5): 474–78.

Golechha M, Bhatia J, Ojha S, Arya DS (2011). Hydroalcoholic extract of Emblica officinalis protects against kainic acid-induced status epilepticus in rats: evidence for an antioxidant, anti-inflammatory, and neuroprotective intervention. Pharm. Biol. 49 (11): 1128–36.

Golechha M, Bhatia J, Singh D, Arya DS (2012). Studies on effects of *Emblica officinalis* (Amla) on oxidative stress and cholinergic function in scopolamine induced amnesia in mice, J. Environ. Biol. 33: 95–100.

Gopalan C, Rama Sastri BV, Balasubramanian SC. (Revised and Updated by) Narasinga Rao BS, Deosthale, YG, Pant KC (2000). NIN, ICMR, Hyderabad, India.

Habib-ur-Rehman, Yasin KA, Choudhary MA, Khaliq N, Atta-ur-Rahman, Choudhary MI, Malik S. (2007). Studies on the chemical constituents of *Phyllanthus emblica*. Nat. Prod. Res. 21 (9): 775–81.

Hazra B, Sarkar R, Biswas S, Mandal N (2010). Comparative study of the antioxidant and reactive oxygen species scavenging properties in the extracts of the fruits of *Terminalia chebula, Terminalia belerica* and *Emblica officinalis*. BMC. Complement. Altern. Med. 10: 20.

Ihantola-Vormisto A, Summanen J, Kankaanranta H, Vuorela H, Asmawi ZM, Moilanen E (1997). Anti-inflammatory activity of extracts from leaves of *Phyllanthus emblica*. Planta. Med. 63 (6): 518–24.

Jacob A, Pandey M, Kapoor S, Saroja R (1988). Effect of the Indian gooseberry (Amla) on serum cholesterol levels in men aged 35-55 years. Eur. J. Clin. Nutr. 42 (11): 939–44.

Kaur S, Arora S, Kaur K, Kumar S (2002). The *in vitro* antimutagenic activity of Triphala—an Indian herbal drug. Food Chem. Toxicol. 40 (4): 527–34.

Kaur S, Michael H, Arora S, Härkönen PL, Kumar S (2005). The *in vitro* cytotoxic and apoptotic activity of Triphala—an Indian herbal drug. J. Ethnopharmacol. 97 (1): 15 -20.

Khan MT, Lampronti I, Martello D, Bianchi N, Jabbar S, Choudhuri MS, Datta BK, Gambari R. (2002) Identification of pyrogallol as an antiproliferative compound present in extracts from the medicinal plant *Emblica officinalis*: effects on *in vitro* cell growth of human tumour cell lines. Int. J. Oncol. 21 (1): 187–92.

Kim HJ, Yokozawa T, Kim HY, Tohda C, Rao TP, Juneja LR (2005). Influence of Amla (*Emblica officinalis* Gaertn.) on hypercholesterolemia and lipid peroxidation in cholesterol-fed rats. J. Nutr. Sci. Vitaminol. (Tokyo). 51 (6): 413–18.

Kim HY, Okubo T, Juneja LR, Yokozawa T (2010). The protective role of Amla (*Emblica officinalis* Gaertn.) against fructose-induced metabolic syndrome in a rat model. Br. J. Nutr. 103 (4): 502-12.

Krishnaveni M, Mirunalini S (2010) Therapeutic potential of *Phyllanthus emblica* (Amla): the ayurvedic wonder. J. Basic Clin. Physiol. Pharmacol. 21 (1): 93–105.

Kumar NP, Annamalai AR, Thakur RS (2009). Antinociceptive property of *Emblica officinalis* Gaertn (Amla) in high fat diet-fed/low dose streptozotocin induced diabetic neuropathy in rats. Indian J. Exp. Biol. 47 (9): 737–42.

Kumar A, Tantry BA, Rahiman S, Gupta U (2011). Comparative study of antimicrobial activity and phytochemical analysis of methanolic and aqueous extracts of the fruit of *Emblica officinalis* against pathogenic bacteria. J. Tradit. Chin. Med. 31 (3): 246–50.

Kumaran A, Karunakaran RJ (2006). Nitric oxide radical scavenging active components from *Phyllanthus emblica* L. Plant Foods Hum. Nutr. 61 (1): 1–5.

Kusirisin W, Srichairatanakool S, Lerttrakarnnon P, Lailerd N, Suttajit M, Jaikang C, Chaiyasut C (2009). Antioxidative activity, polyphenolic content and anti-glycation effect of some Thai medicinal plants traditionally used in diabetic patients. Med Chem. 5 (2): 139–47.

Liu X, Zhao M, Luo W, Yang B, Jiang Y (2009). Identification of volatile components in *Phyllanthus emblica* L. and their antimicrobial activity. J. Med. Food. 12 (2): 423–28.

Majeed M, Bhat B, Jadhav AN, Srivastava JS, Nagabhushanam K (2009). Ascorbic acid and tannins from *Emblica officinalis* Gaertn. Fruits—a revisit. J. Agric. Food Chem. 57 (1): 220–25.

Mehmood MH, Siddiqi HS, Gilani AH (2011). The antidiarrheal and spasmolytic activities of *Phyllanthus emblica* are mediated through dual blockade of muscarinic receptors and Ca^{2+} channels. J. Ethnopharmacol. 133 (2): 856–65.

Naik GH, Priyadarsini KI, Bhagirathi RG, Mishra B, Mishra KP, Banavalikar MM, Mohan H (2005). *In vitro* antioxidant studies and free radical reactions of triphala, an ayurvedic formulation and its constituents. Phytother. Res. 19 (7): 582–86.

Nampoothiri SV, Prathapan A, Cherian OL, Raghu KG, Venugopalan VV, Sundaresan A (2011). *In vitro* antioxidant and inhibitory potential of *Terminalia bellerica* and *Emblica officinalis* fruits against LDL oxidation and key enzymes linked to type 2 diabetes. Food Chem. Toxicol. 49 (1): 125–31.

Ngamkitidechakul C, Jaijoy K, Hansakul P, Soonthornchareonnon N, Sireeratawong S (2010). Antitumour effects of *Phyllanthus emblica* L.: induction of cancer cell apoptosis and inhibition of *in vivo* tumour promotion and *in vitro* invasion of human cancer cells. Phytother. Res. 24 (9): 1405–413.

Penolazzi L, Lampronti I, Borgatti M, Khan MT, Zennaro M, Piva R, Gambari R (2008). Induction of apoptosis of human primary osteoclasts treated with extracts from the medicinal plant *Emblica officinalis*. BMC Compl. Altern. Med. 8: 59.

Pinmai K, Hiriote W, Soonthornchareonnon N, Jongsakul K, Sireeratawong S, Tor-Udom S (2010). *In vitro* and *in vivo* antiplasmodial activity and cytotoxicity of water extracts of *Phyllanthus emblica*, *Terminalia chebula*, and *Terminalia bellerica*. J. Med. Assoc. Thai. 93 Suppl. 7: S120–26.

Poltanov EA, Shikov AN, Dorman HJ, Pozharitskaya ON, Makarov VG, Tikhonov VP, Hiltunen R (2009). Chemical and antioxidant evaluation of Indian gooseberry

(*Emblica officinalis* Gaertn., syn. *Phyllanthus emblica* L.) supplements. Phytother. Res. 23 (9): 1309–315.

Pozharitskaya ON, Ivanova SA, Shikov AN, Makarov VG (2007). Separation and evaluation of free radical-scavenging activity of phenol components of Emblica officinalis extract by using an HPTLC-DPPH method. J. Sep. Sci. 30 (9): 1250–54.

Qureshi SA, Asad W, Sultana V (2009). The Effect of *Phyllantus emblica* Linn on Type II Diabetes, Triglycerides and Liver–Specific Enzyme. Pakistan Journal of Nutrition. 8 (2): 125–28.

Rahman S, Akbor MM, Howlader A, Jabbar A (2009). Antimicrobial and cytotoxic activity of the alkaloids of Amlaki (*Emblica officinalis*). Pak. J. Biol. Sci. 12 (16): 1152–55.

Rajak S, Banerjee SK, Sood S, Dinda AK, Gupta YK, Gupta SK, Maulik SK (2004). *Emblica officinalis* causes myocardial adaptation and protects against oxidative stress in ischemic-reperfusion injury in rats. Phytother. Res. 18 (1): 54–60.

Rao TP, Sakaguchi N, Juneja LR, Wada E, Yokozawa T (2005). Amla (*Emblica officinalis* Gaertn.) extracts reduce oxidative stress in streptozotocin-induced diabetic rats. J. Med. Food. 8 (3): 362–68.

Sabu MC, Kuttan R (2002). Antidiabetic activity of medicinal plants and its relationship with their antioxidant property. J. Ethnopharmacol. 81 (2): 155–60.

Saeed S, Tariq P (2007). Antibacterial activities of *Emblica officinalis* and *Coriandrum sativum* against Gram negative urinary pathogens. Pak. J. Pharm. Sci. 20 (1): 32–35.

Sai Ram M, Neetu D, Yogesh B, Anju B, Dipti P, Pauline T, Sharma SK, Sarada SK, Ilavazhagan G, Kumar D, Selvamurthy W (2002). Cytoprotective and immunomodulating properties of Amla (*Emblica officinalis*) on lymphocytes: an *in vitro* study. J. Ethnopharmacol. 81 (1): 5–10.

Sai Ram M, Neetu D, Deepti P, Vandana M, Ilavazhagan G, Kumar D, Selvamurthy W (2003). Cytoprotective activity of Amla (*Emblica officinalis*) against chromium (VI) induced oxidative injury in murine macrophages. Phytother. Res. 17 (4): 430–33.

Sandhya T, Lathika KM, Pandey BN, Mishra KP (2006). Potential of traditional ayurvedic formulation, Triphala, as a novel anticancer drug. Cancer Lett. 231 (2): 206–214.

Scartezzini P, Antognoni F, Raggi MA, Poli F, Sabbioni C (2006). Vitamin C content and antioxidant activity of the fruit and of the Ayurvedic preparation of *Emblica officinalis* Gaertn. J. Ethnopharmacol. 104 (1-2): 113–18.

Sidhu,S, Pandhi P, Malhotra S, Vaiphei Kim, Lal Khanduja K (2011). Beneficial Effects of *Emblica officinalis* in l-Arginine-Induced Acute Pancreatitis in Rats. Journal of Medicinal Food. 14 (1-2): 147–55.

Srikumar R, Parthasarathy NJ, Shankar EM, Manikandan S, Vijayakumar R, Thangaraj R, Vijayananth K, Sheeladevi R, Rao UA (2007). Evaluation of the growth inhibitory activities of Triphala against common bacterial isolates from HIV infected patients. Phytother. Res. 21 (5): 476–80.

Suryanarayana P, Kumar PA, Saraswat M, Petrash JM, Reddy GB (2004). Inhibition of aldose reductase by tannoid principles of *Emblica officinalis*: implications for the prevention of sugar cataract. Mol. Vis. 0: 148–54.

Suryanarayana P, Saraswat M, Petrash JM, Reddy GB (2007). *Emblica officinalis* and its enriched tannoids delay streptozotocin-induced diabetic cataract in rats. Mol. Vis. 13: 1291–97.

Tarwadi K, Agte V (2007). Antioxidant and micronutrient potential of common fruits available in the Indian subcontinent. Int. J. Food Sci. Nutr. 58 (5): 341–49.

Tiwari,V, Kuhad A and Chopra K (2011). *Emblica officinalis* Corrects Functional, Biochemical and Molecular Deficits in Experimental Diabetic Neuropathy by Targeting the Oxido-nitrosative Stress Mediated Inflammatory Cascade" Phytother. Res. Published online in Wiley Online Library (wileyonlinelibrary.com) DOI: 10.1002/ptr.344.

Wang YF, Wang XY, Ren Z, Qian CW, Li YC, Kaio K, Wang QD, Zhang Y, Zheng LY, Jiang JH, Yang CR, Liu Q, Zhang YJ, Wang YF (2009). *Phyllaemblicin B* inhibits *Coxsackie virus* B3 induced apoptosis and myocarditis. Antiviral Res. 84 (2): 150–58.

Xia Q, Xiao P, Wan L, Kong J (1997). [Ethnopharmacology of *Phyllanthus emblica* L]. Zhongguo. Zhong. Yao. Za. Zhi. 22 (9): 515–18, 525, 574. [Article in Chinese].

Yokozawa T, Kim HY, Kim HJ, et al. (2007a). Amla (*Emblica officinalis* Gaertn.) attenuates age-related renal dysfunction by oxidative stress. J. Agric. Food Chem. 55 (19): 7744–52.

Yokozawa T, Kim HY, Kim HJ, Okubo T, Chu DC, Juneja LR (2007b). Amla (*Emblica officinalis* Gaertn.) prevents dyslipidaemia and oxidative stress in the ageing process. Br. J. Nutr. 97 (6): 1187–95.

Zhang LZ, Zhao WH, Guo YJ, Tu GZ, Lin S, Xin LG (2003). [Studies on chemical constituents in fruits of Tibetan medicine *Phyllanthus emblica*]. Zhongguo. Zhong. Yao. Za. Zhi. 28 (10): 940 -43 [Article in Chinese].

Chapter 17

Dates

(*Phoenix dactylifera*)

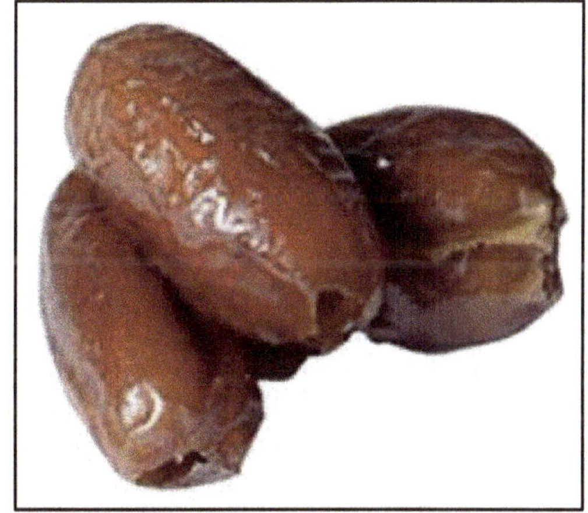

Date palm, a tree native to the Middle East and Africa has been cultivated for thousands of years and its fruits (dates) served as a nutritious meal to the dessert travelers. Its importance is known since biblical times. It is a vital component of the diet in all the Arabian countries. Muslims considered dates as a Holy food and regarded as a symbol associated with Islam. Throughout the month of Ramadan, dates are a common ingredient in the Muslim diet.

The palm tree grows very well in a nearly rainless belt and thus Sahara, as well as the Middle East countries such as Saudi Arabia, Jordan, Iran and Iraq. In three date-producing countries, Morocco, Tunisia and Algeria alone, about 1000 varieties of dates have been reported, many of which seem to be neglected and may have got extinguished. The prized varieties such as Campbell have caught greater attention.

The world production of dates has increased 2.9 times over 40 years while the total world export of dates increased by 1.71 per cent over 40 years (Al-Shahib and Marshall, 2003).

The tree is a dioecious species, with male and female flowers produced on separate trees which are naturally wind pollinated to grow the fruit, but nowadays, artificial pollination is being done for faster cultivation of date fruits. The tree grows thick clusters of date fruits below its fronds by absorbing moisture from springs and under-ground water since there is scarcity of water in the dessert region. The roots of the tree grow deep under the ground to absorb water and other essential nutrients required for the growth of the tree. Unripe date fruit is green in colour, slowly turning yellow-orange as it matures and rich dark brown with a thick, glossy, sticky skin when fully ripe.

Date palms produce between five and ten bunches of dates per tree. A single large bunch may contain more than a thousand dates, and can weigh between 6 to 8 kg. They begin to bear fruit at 3 to 5 years, and reach full production after 10-12 years. Date palms can survive up to 150 years. Interestingly, Ali-Mohamed and Khamis (2004) say that date palm seeds are also used just as coffee seeds for coffee drinks.

Varieties

Popular varieties of date fruit include the Noor and Medjool, Barhi, Barakawi, Golden-princess, Khalas, Halawy, Hilali, Khadrawy and the rare Black sphinx dates. According to Ali-Mohamed and Khamis (2004), the different cultivars of Bahraini date palm (Phoenix dactylifera) seeds are Khalas, Murzban, Khunaizi, Khawajah, Khasaib Asfor, Khaseeb, Garen Gaze, Matteta, Kenta, Rochdi, Mermella, Korkobbi and Eguwa. Some of the varieties cultivated in United Arab Emirates are Khalas, Barhe, Lulu, Shikat alkahlas, Sokkery, Bomaan, Sagay, Shishi, Maghool, Sultana, Fard, Maktoomi, Naptit saif, Jabri, Khodary, Dabbas, Raziz and Shabebe.

Chemical Composition of Dates

Hong *et al.* (2006) documented composition of dates of the cultivar Deglet Noor. Thirteen flavonoid glycosides of luteolin, quercetin, and apigenin, and 6 of their isomeric forms were identified. Both methylated and sulfated forms of luteolin and quercetin are present as mono-, di-, and triglycosylated conjugates whereas apigenin is present as only the diglycoside. Quercetin and luteolin formed primarily O-glycosidic linkages whereas apigenin is present as the C-glycoside. The sugar residues are beta-glycosidically linked. date fruit has various neuro-protective agents such as melatonin (Lipartiti, 1996) and polyphenolic compounds (Mansouri *et al.*, 2005). The polysaccharide consists of a backbone composed of (1→4)-beta-D-mannopyranosyl residues and carries a single (1→6)-alpha-linked D-galactopyranosyl residue (Ishurd *et al.*, 2001).

Nutritive Value of Dates

The importance of the dates in human nutrition comes from its rich composition of carbohydrates, dietary fibers, fatty acids, amino acids, protein, minerals and vitamins. The carbohydrates (44–88 per cent) in dates include mainly glucose and fructose. Habib and Ibrahim (2011) showed a varietal difference in the composition of dates. For example, Khalas variety, considered as premium quality of dates, had significantly higher contents of sugar and selenium and a significantly higher energy value than the other varieties studied (Al-Farsi *et al.*, 2005 b). Compositional analysis by Mrabet *et al.* (2008) showed that the Tunisian date varieties were very rich in reducing sugars (26 to 51 per cent) than Deglet Noor which was rich in sucrose (54 per cent). Date is also a rich source of dietary fiber (6.4–11.5 per cent), with the amount of fiber increasing as the fruit ripens. Dates contain insoluble dietary fiber as a major fraction along with 0.5–3.9 per cent of soluble fiber pectin, both of which have important health benefits. Thus, dates may be considered as an almost ideal food (Al-Shahib and Marshall, 2003). The glycemic index (GI) of different varieties of dates collected from various regions of Oman ranged between 47.6 and 57.7. The regional effects on the GI values of dates were non-significant ($P>0.05$). However, an inverse correlation was observed between the fructose fraction and the GI value of dates (Ali *et al.*, 2009).

Protein content of dates varies from 2.3–5.6 per cent with almost all amino acids, some of which are not present in the most popular fruits such as oranges, apples and bananas. The composition of date flesh is different from that of date seeds. Date seeds contain higher protein and fat as compared to the flesh. The fat content of the fleshy portion of the fruit is 0.2–0.5 per cent, whereas the seed contains 7.7–9.7 per cent of oil which includes both saturated and unsaturated fatty acids. The seeds contain 14 types of fatty acids, but only eight of these fatty acids occur in very low concentration in the flesh. The most abundant fatty acids of the date seed oils were oleic, lauric, myristic, palmitic and stearic acids (Juhaimi *et al.*, 2012). Unsaturated fatty acids are present as palmitoleic, oleic, linoleic and linolenic acids.

Dates are also good sources of micronutrients. Vitamin-A, Thiamine, Riboflavin, Niacin and small amount of Vitamin-C, minerals like Potassium, Boron, Calcium, Cobalt, Copper, Fluorine, Iron, Magnesium, Manganese, Phosphorus, Zinc and Sodium are also found in the flesh of the date fruit. Aluminum, Cadmium, Chloride, Lead and Sulphur are present in the seeds. Dates are also a good source of Selenium and elemental Fluorine (Al-Shahib and Marshall, 2003).

Nutritional Value per 100 g

Nutrient	*Amount*	*Nutrient*	*Amount*
Thiamine (Vit. B1) (mg)	0.050	Riboflavin (Vit.B2) (mg)	0.060
Niacin (Vit. B3) (mg)	1.610	Vitamin B6 (mg)	0.249
Folate (Vit. B9) (µg)	15	Vitamin A (IU)	149
Energy (kcal)	277	Carbohydrates (g)	74.97
Dietary fiber (g)	6.7	Fat (g)	0.15
Protein (g)	1.81	Calcium (mg)	64
Iron (mg)	0.9	Magnesium (mg)	54
Phosphorus (mg)	62	Potassium (mg)	696
Sodium (mg)	1	Zinc (mg)	0.44

USDA, 2012.

Tunisian dates are found to be very rich in vitamin C (24 to 46 mg/100 g) than Deglet Noor variety (1.12 mg/100 g). They were relatively rich in potassium (283 to 733 mg/100 g) but poor in sodium content (0.06 to 0.09 mg/100 g).

Dates are a good source of antioxidants, mainly carotenoids and phenolics. The phenolic content per 100 g is 3942 mg and that of antioxidants is 80400 micromol (Al-Farsi and Lee, 2008). Total concentration of phenolics was higher in the Hallawi by 20–31 per cent as compared to Medjool Dates. The major proportion of the soluble phenolics in both date varieties consisted of phenolic acids, mainly ferulic acid and coumaric acid derivatives, along with chlorogenic and caffeic acid derivatives and a quercetin derivative. Unlike the Medjool Dates, Hallawi Dates contained a significant proportion of catechins as well. Both date varieties possess antioxidant properties *in vitro*, but the ferric ion reducing antioxidant capacity was higher in Hallawi by 24 per cent (Rock *et al.*, 2009). Mrabet *et al.* (2012) recommended that, on the basis of the water- and oil-holding capacities of greater than 17 and 4 mL/g of fiber respectively; and high antiradical capacity (>230 Trolox equiv/kg fiber), some varieties could be included in the formulation of fiber- and antioxidant-rich foods.

Therapeutic Value of Dates

Dates may be considered as an almost ideal food as they provide several potential health benefits. In the folklore, date fruits have been ascribed to have many medicinal properties when consumed either alone or in combination with herbs. It has been used since olden days for treating constipation, intestinal disorders, diarrhea, heart problems, sexual weakness and abdominal cancer. In addition, the date palm fruit possesses many useful properties such as antioxidant and antimutagenic (Vayalil, 2002), antibacterial (Sallal and Ashkenani, 1989), antifungal (Shraideh *et al.*, 1998), antitumoural (Ishurd and Kennedy, 2005) and gastroprotective (Al-Qarawi *et al.*, 2005). Scientific evidences for some of these qualities of dates are discussed below.

Antioxidant

All date varieties serve as a good source of natural antioxidants and could potentially be considered as a functional food or functional food ingredient, although some of their antioxidant constituents are lost during sun-drying (Al-Farsi *et al.*, 2005a). Liolios *et al.* (2009) found the dates to possess strong antioxidant activity due to the presence of phenolic compounds. This antioxidant property of dates has been attributed to its hydroxyl-radical-scavenging activity. It has also been found to significantly inhibit lipid peroxidation and protein oxidation in a dose-dependent manner, thus preventing the formation as well as the accumulation of harmful oxidative substances in the body (Vayalil, 2002). Date sugar exhibited high alpha-glucosidase, alpha-amylase, and ACE inhibitory activities that correlated with high total phenolic content and antioxidant activity.

The antioxidant potential of dates varies with the variety. Chaira *et al.* (2007) found the ethyl acetate extracts from flesh Deglet noor, pit Deglet noor and pit Alig to show an important free radical scavenging activity towards 1-1-diphenyl-2-picrylhydrazyl (DPPH). They also reported that the highest level of flavonoids in the Korkobbi variety is principally responsible for the highest antiradical efficiency of this cultivar. Thus certain nonphenolic factors in dates may also be involved in their significant antioxidant ability (Chaira *et al.*, 2009).

Treatment of dimethoate-induced oxidative stress and nephrotoxicity in rats with date palm fruit extract (Deglet Noor) and also with vitamin C significantly ($p<0.05$) reversed the serum renal markers to their near-normal levels as compared to the nontreated rats. In addition, Deglet Noor extract and vitamin C significantly reduced lipid peroxidation, restored the antioxidant defense enzymes in the kidney, and improved the histopathology changes. Saafi *et al.* (2012) thus proved that date palm fruit may be useful *in vivo* for the prevention of oxidative stress-induced nephrotoxicity.

In addition, pretreatment with date palm fruit extract restored the liver damage induced by dimethoate, as revealed by inhibition of hepatic lipid peroxidation, amelioration of SOD, GPx and CAT activities and improvement of histopathology changes thus proving its usefulness in prevention of hepatotoxicity (Saafi *et al.*, 2011).

Immunomodulator

The immunomodulatory effects of some polyphenols and polysaccharides present in hot water extract of matured date palm fruit (*Phoenix dactylifera* L.) were proved to stimulate the cellular immune system in mice (Karasawa *et al.*, 2011).

Cancer

Dates also possess anti-mutagenic properties. It has been found to inhibit benzo(a)pyrene-induced mutagenecity on *Salmonella* tester strains (TA-98 and TA-100) with a metabolic activation in a dose-dependent manner (Vayalil, 2002). Beta-glucan isolated from Libyan dates were found to exhibit potent antitumour activity; this activity could be correlated to their (1→3)-beta-D-glucan linkages (Ishurd *et al.*, 2002). Such antitumour glucans have also been obtained from a number of other sources, such as yeast, fungi, bacteria, and plants. This is the first study to report antitumour activity for date glucan (Ishurd *et al.*, 2004).

CVD

Dates exhibited antiatherogenic effect by decreasing serum triacylglycerol levels and basal serum oxidative status and increasing the activity of serum HDL-associated antioxidant enzyme paraoxonase-1 without worsening the serum glucose levels and lipid/lipo-protein patterns in healthy subjects (Wasseem *et al.*, 2009). Rock *et al.* (2009) demonstrated that consumption of dates (and mainly the Hallawi variety) by healthy subjects, despite their high sugar content, showed beneficial effects on serum triacylglycerol and oxidative stress and does not worsen serum glucose and lipid/lipoprotein patterns. Thus they opine that dates can be considered as an antiatherogenic food.

The cerebral ischemia in rats induced by occluding bilateral common carotid arteries for 30 minutes caused significant depletion in superoxide dismutase, catalase, glutathione, glutathione peroxidase, glutathione-S-transferase, glutathione reductase and significant increase in lipid peroxidation along with severe neuronal damage in the brain. 15 days pretreatment with methanolic extract of P. dactylifera fruits (100, 300 mg/kg), significantly attenuated all the above alterations except depletion in glutathione peroxidase and glutathione-S-transferase levels induced by cerebral ischemia (Pujari *et al.*, 2011).

Obstetrics

Consumption of dates has traditionally been advised to pregnant and lactating women for its nutritional benefits. Dates consumption during pregnancy has been found to increase the cervical dilatation and spontaneous labor at the time of delivery with a shorter mean latent phase of the first stage of labor and decreased use of oxytocin/prostin to induce labor. Consuming dates during last weeks of pregnancy significantly reduced the need for induction and augmentation of labor and produced a more favourable delivery outcome (Al-Kuran *et al.*, 2011).

Diabetes

The search for substances to protect the nervous system from the degenerative effects of diabetes has high priority in biomedical research. Khalas dates, when eaten alone or in mixed meals with plain yoghurt have low glycaemic indices. Thus, consumption of dates can be expected to be of benefit in glycemic and lipid control of diabetic patients (Miller *et al.*, 2003).

Date fruit extract (DFE) has recently been identified as promising neuroprotective agent in several models of neurodegeneration. DFE counteracted the impairment of the explorative activity of the rats in an open field behavioral test and of the conduction velocity of the sciatic nerve. In addition, pretreatment with DFE significantly reversed each nerve diameter reduction in diabetic rats. The DFE treatment shows efficacy in preventing diabetic complications and for improving pathological parameters of diabetic neuropathy in rats, as compared to the control groups (Zangiabadi *et al.*, 2011). Different altered mechanisms may be involved in the antioxidant and neuro-protective effect of DFE (Asadi-Shekaari *et al.*, 2004; 2008; Vayalil, 2002). Some of the established neuroprotective constitituents of DFE are as follows: melatonin, a potent antioxidant and free radical scavenger (Poeggeler *et al.*, 1993); Vitamin C, an accepted antioxidant agent (Cui *et al.*, 2004); phenolic compounds which are present in cinnamic acids, distinctive flavonoids with strong antioxidant effects (Mansouri *et al.*, 2005); magnesium, an antagonist of NMDA receptors (Lyden and Wahlgren, 2000); Vitamin B_3, a water soluble vitamin with neuroprotective properties (Maynard *et al.*, 2001), manganese, a free radical scavenger; and selenium, an antioxidant factor with synergic effects with vitamin C (Vajragupta *et al.*, 2003).

According to recent studies by Asadi-Shekaari *et al.* (2008) and Panahi *et al.* (2008), DFE significantly inhibited neuronal damage induced by cerebral ischemia most probably due to its antioxidant property.

Ulcer

The aqueous and ethanolic extracts of dates and, to a lesser extent, date pits, were effective in ameliorating the severity of ethanol induced gastric ulceration by decreasing the histamine and gastrin concentrations; and increasing the gastric mucin levels. It is postulated that the basis of the gastro-protective action of date extracts may be multi-factorial, and may include an antioxidant action (Al-Qarawi *et al.*, 2005).

Boghdadi *et al.* (2012) showed a clinical improvement associated with a decline in some inflammation parameters after therapy with dates. Moreover, date palm therapy induced a significant increase in serum and nasal interleukin IL-10 levels.

Antiageing

As date palm kernel is rich in phytohormones, Bauza *et al.* (2002) demonstrated that date palm kernel extract could exhibit a significant antiwrinkle effect in ten healthy women volunteers, between the ages of 46 and 58 years. It can therefore be a useful ingredient in anti aging skin care products.

Safety Issues

Moore *et al.* (2002) identified by sequence analysis *C. cladosporioides* (230 cfu/g) and *S. roseus* in edible dates. Both these organisms have been previously implicated in opportunistic skin infections. So it is emphasized that washing hands following the consumption of dates by hand should be made as a common practice.

Conclusions

Although dates are sugar-packed, many date varieties are low in GI and refute the dogma that dates are similar to candies and regular consumption would develop chronic diseases (Vayalil, 2012). In recent years, an explosion of interest in the numerous health benefits of dates had led to many *in vitro* and animal studies as well as the identification and quantification of various classes of phytochemicals. Based on the available information on the nutritional and phytochemical composition, it is apparent that the dates are highly nutritious and may have several potential health benefits.

References

Ali A, Al-Kindi YS, Al-Said F (2009). Chemical composition and glycemic index of three varieties of Omani dates. Int. J. Food Sci. Nutr. 60 Suppl 4: 51–62.

Al-Farsi M, Alasalvar C, Morris A, Baron M, Shahidi F (2005 a). Comparison of antioxidant activity, anthocyanins, carotenoids, and phenolics of three native fresh and sun-dried date (*Phoenix dactylifera* L.) varieties grown in Oman. J. Agric. Food Chem. 53 (19): 7592–99.

Al-Farsi M, Alasalvar C, Morris A, Baron M, Shahidi F (2005 b). Compositional and sensory characteristics of three native sun-dried date (*Phoenix dactylifera* L.) varieties grown in Oman. J. Agric. Food Chem. 53 (19): 7586–91.

Al-Farsi MA, Lee CY (2008). Nutritional and functional properties of dates: a review. Crit. Rev. Food Sci. Nutr. 48 (10): 877–87.

Ali-Mohamed AY, Khamis AS (2004). Mineral ion content of the seeds of six cultivars of Bahraini date palm (*Phoenix dactylifera*). J. Agric. Food Chem. 52 (21): 6522–25.

Al-Kuran O, Al-Mehaisen L, Bawadi H, Beitawi S, Amarin Z (2011). The effect of late pregnancy consumption of dates fruit on labour and delivery, J. Obstet. Gynaecol. 31 (1): 29–31.

Al-Qarawi AA, Abdel-Rahman H, Ali BH, Mousa HM, El-Mougy SA (2005). The ameliorative effect of dates (*Phoenix dactylifera* L.) on ethanol-induced gastric ulcer in rats. *J. Ethnopharmacol.* 98 (3): 313–17.

Al-Shahib W, Marshall RJ (2003). The fruit of the date palm: its possible use as the best food for the future? Int. J. Food Sci. Nutr. 54 (4): 247–59.

Asadi-Shekaari M, Panahi M, Dabiri SH, Zahed SK, Pour TP (2008). Neuroprotective effects of aqueous date fruit extract on focal cerebral ischemia in rats. *Pakistan J. Med. Sci.* 24 (5): 661–65.

Asadi-Shekari M, Rajab Alian S (2004). Antioxidative effect of aqueous date fruit extract in pc12 cell line. Iranian Journal of Pharmaceutical Research. 3 (1): 72.

Bauza E, Dal Farra C, Berghi A, Oberto G, Peyronel D, Domloge N (2002). Date palm kernel extract exhibits antiaging properties and significantly reduces skin wrinkles. Int. J. Tissue React. 24 (4): 131–36.

Boghdadi G, Marei A, Ali A, Lotfy G, Abdulfattah M, Sorour S (2012). Immunological markers in allergic rhinitis patients treated with date palm immunotherapy. Inflamm Res. 61 (7): 719–24.

Chaira N, Ferchichi A, Mrabet A, Sghairoun M (2007). Chemical composition of the flesh and the pit of date palm fruit and radical scavenging activity of their extracts. Pak. J. Biol. Sci. 10 (13): 2202–207.

Chaira N, Smaali MI, Martinez-Tomé M, Mrabet A, Murcia MA, Ferchichi A (2009). Simple phenolic composition, flavonoid contents and antioxidant capacities in water-methanol extracts of Tunisian common date cultivars (*Phoenix dactylifera* L.). Int. J. Food Sci. Nutr. 60 Suppl 7: 316–29.

Cui K, Luo X, Xu K, Ven Murthy MR (2004). Role of oxidative stress in neuro-degeneration: recent developments in assay methods for oxidative stress and nutraceutical antioxidants. Progress in Neuro-Psychopharmacology and Biological Psychiatry. 28 (5): 771–99.

Habib HM, Ibrahim WH (2011). Nutritional quality of 18 date fruit varieties. Int. J. Food Sci. Nutr. 62 (5): 544–51.

Hong YJ, Tomas-Barberan FA, Kader AA, Mitchell AE (2006). The flavonoid glycosides and procyanidin composition of Deglet Noor dates (*Phoenix dactylifera*). J. Agric. Food Chem. 54 (6): 2405–411.

Ishrud O, Zahid M, Zhou H, Pan Y (2001). A water-soluble galactomannan from the seeds of *Phoenix dactylifera* L. Carbohydr. Res. 335 (4): 297–301.

Ishurd O, Zgheel F, Kermagi A, Flefla M, Elmabruk M (2004). Antitumour activity of beta-D-glucan from Libyan dates. J. Med. Food. 7 (2): 252–55.

Ishurd O, Kennedy JF (2005). The anti-cancer activity of polysaccharide prepared from Libyan dates (*Phoenix dactylifera* L.) Carbohydrate Polymers. 59 (4): 531–35.

Ishurd O, Sun C, Xiao P, Ashour A, Pan Y (2002). A neutral beta-D-glucan from dates of the date palm, *Phoenix dactylifera* L. Carbohydr. Res. 337 (14): 1325–28.

Juhaimi FA, Ghafoor K, Özcan MM (2012). Physical and chemical properties, antioxidant activity, total phenol and mineral profile of seeds of seven different date fruit (*Phoenix dactylifera* L.) varieties. Int. J. Food Sci. Nutr. 63 (1): 84–89.

Karasawa K, Uzuhashi Y, Hirota M, Otani H (2011). A matured fruit extract of date palm tree (*Phoenix dactylifera* L.) stimulates the cellular immune system in mice. J. Agric. Food Chem. 59 (20): 11287–93.

Liolios CC, Sotiroudis GT, Chinou I (2009). Fatty acids, sterols, phenols and antioxidant activity of *Phoenix theophrasti* fruits growing in Crete, Greece. Plant Foods Hum. Nutr. 64 (1): 52–61.

Lipartiti M, Franceschini D, Zanoni R, Gusella M, Giusti P, Cagnoli CM, Kharlamov A, Manev H (1996). Neuro-protective effects of melatonin. Advances in Experimental Medicine and Biology. 398: 315–21.

Lyden P, Wahlgren NG (2000). Mechanisms of action of neuro-protectants in stroke. Journal of Stroke and Cerebrovascular Diseases. 9 (6, part 2): 9–14.

Mansouri A, Embarek G, Kokkalou E, Kefalas P (2005). Phenolic profile and antioxidant activity of the Algerian ripe date palm fruit (*Phoenix dactylifera*). Food Chemistry. 89 (3): 411–20.

Miller CJ, Dunn EV, Hashim IB (2003). The glycaemic index of dates and date/yoghurt mixed meals. Are dates 'the candy that grows on trees'? Eur. J. Clin. Nutr. 57 (3): 427–30.

Moore JE, Xu J, Millar BC, Elshibly S (2002). Edible dates (*Phoenix dactylifera*), a potential source of *Cladosporium cladosporioides* and *Sporobolomyces roseus*: implications for public health. Mycopathologia. 154 (1): 25–28.

Mrabet A, Ferchichi A, Chaira N, Mohamed BS, Baaziz Z, Penny TM (2008). Physico-chemical characteristics and total quality of date palm varieties grown in the southern of Tunisia. Pak. J. Biol. Sci. 11 (7): 1003–1008.

Mrabet A, Rodríguez-Arcos R, Guillén-Bejarano R, Chaira N, Ferchichi A, Jiménez-Araujo A (2012). Dietary Fiber from Tunisian Common Date Cultivars (*Phoenix dactylifera* L.): Chemical Composition, Functional Properties, and Antioxidant Capacity. J. Agric. Food Chem. 60 (14): 3658–64.

Panahi M, Asadi-Shekaari M, Kalantari Pour TP, Safavi A (2008). Aqueous extract of date fruit protects CA1 neurons againt oxidative injury: an ultastructural study. Current Topics in Nutraceutical Research. 6 (3): 125–30.

Poeggeler B, Reiter RJ, Tan DX, Chen LD, Manchester LC (1993). Melatonin, hydroxyl radical-mediated oxidative damage, and aging: a hypothesis. Journal of Pineal Research. 14 (4): 151–68.

Pujari RR, Vyawahare NS, Kagathara VG (2011). Evaluation of antioxidant and neuroprotective effect of date palm (*Phoenix dactylifera* L.) against bilateral common carotid artery occlusion in rats. Indian J. Exp. Biol. 49 (8): 627–33.

Rock W, Rosenblat M, Borochov-Neori H, Volkova N, Judeinstein S, Elias M, Aviram M (2009). Effects of date (*Phoenix dactylifera* L., Medjool or Hallawi Variety) consumption by healthy subjects on serum glucose and lipid levels and on serum oxidative status: a pilot study. J. Agric. Food Chem. 57 (17): 8010–17.

Saafi EB, Arem A, Louedi M, Saoudi M, Elfeki A, Zakhama A, Najjar MF, Hammami M, Achour L (2012). Antioxidant-rich date palm fruit extract inhibits oxidative stress and nephrotoxicity induced by dimethoate in rat. J. Physiol. Biochem. 68 (1): 47–58.

Saafi EB, Louedi M, Elfeki A, Zakhama A, Najjar MF, Hammami M, Achour L (2011). Protective effect of date palm fruit extract (*Phoenix dactylifera* L.) on dimethoate induced-oxidative stress in rat liver. Exp. Toxicol. Pathol. 63 (5): 433–41.

Sallal AK, Ashkenani A (1989). Effect of date extract on growth and spore germination of Bacillus subtilis. *Microbios.* 59 (240–241): 203–210.

Shraideh ZA, Abu-Elteen KH, Sallal AKJ (1998). Ultrastructural effects of date extract on Candida albicans. Mycopathologia. 142 (3): 119–23.

Vajragupta O, Boonchoong P, Sumanont Y, Watanabe H, Wongkrajang Y, Kammasud N (2003). Manganese-based complexes of radical scavengers as neuroprotective agents. Bioorganic and Medicinal Chemistry. 11 (10): 2329–37.

Vayalil PK (2002). Antioxidant and Antimutagenic Properties of Aqueous Extract of Date Fruit (*Phoenix dactylifera* L. Arecaceae) J. Agric. Food Chem, 50 (3): 610–17.

Vayalil PK (2012). Date fruits (*Phoenix dactylifera* Linn): an emerging medicinal food. Crit. Rev. Food Sci. Nutr. 52 (3): 249–71.

Wasseem Rock, Mira Rosenblat, Hamutal Borochov-Neori, Nina Volkova, Sylvie Judeinstein, Mazen Elias and Michael Aviram (2009). Effects of Date (*Phoenix dactylifera* L., Medjool or Hallawi Variety) Consumption by Healthy Subjects on Serum Glucose and Lipid Levels and on Serum Oxidative Status: A Pilot Study, J. Agric. Food Chem., 57 (17): 8010–17.

Zangiabadi N, Asadi-Shekaari M, Sheibani V, Jafari M, Shabani M, Asadi AR, Tajadini H, Jarahi M (2011). Date fruit extract is a neuroprotective agent in diabetic peripheral neuropathy in streptozotocin-induced diabetic rats: a multimodal analysis. Oxid. Med. Cell. Longev. 2011: 976–948.

Chapter 18

Figs

(*Ficus carica* L., *Ficus racemosa*)

Figs, commonly known as *Anjir*, originate from Carica in Asia Minor and the primary fig producers now are America and the Mediterranean regions (Vinson, 1999). Fig is also widely distributed in South Korea. The ideal condition for intensive cultivation of figs is a semi-arid climate with irrigation. Various species of figs are used in traditional medicine. In addition to the fruit the various parts of the plant such as bark, leaves and latex also carry several health benefits. Udumbara (Ficus glomerata Roxb.) is well known drug for its use since ancient times. Atharvaveda considers this as a divine plant and much used in religious sacrifice. It is also called as Yajñodumbara. It grows abundantly in all parts of India. In Ayurveda, bark, leaves and unripe fruits of fig plant are used externally and internally to cure many diseases like Pravahika (Dysentery), Pradara (Menorrhagia), Raktapitta (Haemoptysis) etc. (Subhaktha *et al.*, 2010).

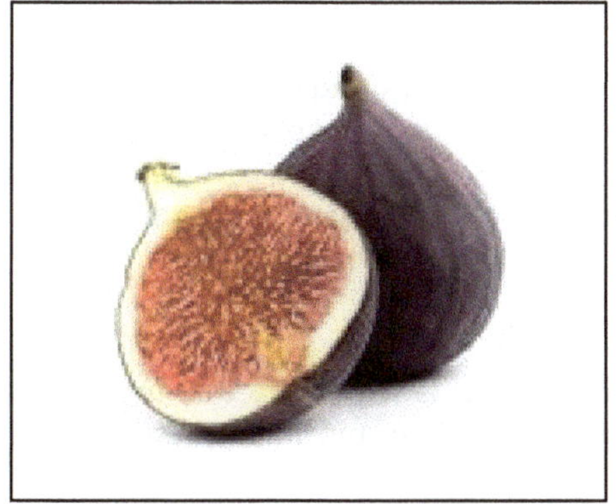

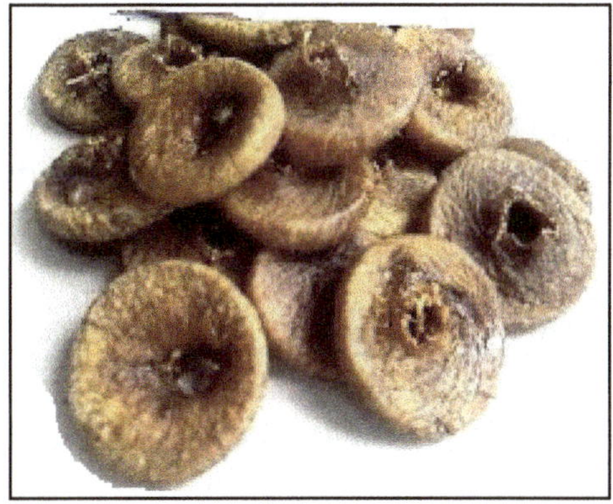

Production

The world production of figs is about one million tons. According to FAO reports (2005) the world's fig production was 1,057,000 tonnes, with Turkey being the top producer (280,000 tonnes), followed by Egypt (170,000 tonnes) and other Mediterranean countries.

Synonyms

Caricae fructus, Feigen, *Ficus benjamina* (weeping fig), *Ficus carica, Ficus glomerata. Ficus racemosa*; Cluster fig, Indian fig, Crattock, Rumbodo, Atteeka, Redwood fig.

Nutritional Value of Figs

Figs contain simple sugars, fiber, fat, amino acids vitamins and minerals (Solomon *et al.*, 2006; Verberic *et al.*, 2006). Among minerals, figs contain substantial levels of potassium, calcium, magnesium, iron, copper, manganese, and sodium (Kim *et al.*, 1981; 1992). Figs are also a good source of flavonoids, polyphenols as well as phytosterols, lanosterol and stigmasterol.

Nutritional Value per 100 g

Nutrient	*Amount*	*Nutrient*	*Amount*
Energy (kcal)	249	Carbohydrates (g)	63.87
Sugars (g)	47.92	Dietary fiber (g)	9.8
Fat (g)	0.93	Protein (g)	3.30
Calcium (mg)	162	Iron (mg)	2.03
Magnesium (mg)	68.0	Phosphorus (mg)	67.0
Potassium (mg)	680	Zinc (mg)	0.55
Thiamine (mg)	0.085	Riboflavin (mg)	0.082
Niacin (mg)	0.619	Pantothenic acid (mg)	0.434
Vitamin B_6 (mg)	0.106	Folate (µg)	9.0
Vitamin C (mg)	1.2		

USDA (2012).

Effect of Processing

There are significant differences in analyzed compounds between fresh and dried figs but properly dried figs can be used as a good source of phenolic compounds (Slatnar *et al.*, 2011). Analysis of individual phenolic compounds revealed a higher content of all phenolic groups in the oven-dried figs. And the total phenolic content and antioxidant activity remained unaffected by the dehydration process.

Traditional Therapeutic Uses

Ficus racemosa commonly known as 'cluster fig' is widely used in Indian folk medicine for the treatment of various diseases/disorders including jaundice, dysentery, diabetes, diarrhea and inflammatory conditions. The leaves of fig plant contain terpenoid, saponin and flavonoid compounds (El-Kholy and Shaban, 1966; Ahmed *et al.*, 1988), which may be related to their alleged antiviral effects on herpes simplex virus (HSV), and hypoglycaemic activity in type-I diabetic patients (Serraclara *et al.*, 1998; Canal *et al.*, 2000).

Figs have been traditionally used for their medicinal benefits for metabolic, cardiovascular, respiratory, and other inflammatory disorders (Duke *et al.*, 2012). The leaves and fruits of *F. carica* are traditionally used as laxative, stimulant and antitussive, (Bellakhdar *et al.*, 1991; Guarrera, 2003). Fig fruit has been a typical component in the health-promoting Mediterranean diet for millennia.

Different parts of Ficus species are commonly used to treat and cure diarrhea. The fruit is mildly laxative, demulcent, digestive, and pectoral. The leaves of this plant have been used as folk medicine for hemorrhoids, neuralgia, warts, diarrhea and carbuncles in Korea and China (Lee, 1996). A decoction prepared from its leaves is used for hemorrhoids, whereas an infusion of its fruits can safely be used as a laxative for children. The leaf decoction is taken as a remedy for diabetes and calcifications in the kidneys and liver (Joseph and Justin, 2011).

Latex is a sticky emulsion that exudes upon damage from specialized canals from several plants. Ficus species possess latex-like material within their vasculatures, affording protection and self-healing from physical attacks. Malic and shikimic acids were present in higher amounts (ca. 26 per cent, each) in the latex. The latex of fig fruit is used in traditional medicine for the treatment of skin infections such as warts and also diseases of possible viral origin (Aref *et al.*, 2011).

F. racemosa is pharmacologically studied for various activities including antidiabetic, antipyretic, anti-inflammatory, antitussive, hepatoprotective, and antimicrobial activities. A wide range of phytochemical constituents have been identified and isolated from various parts of F. racemosa.

Antioxidant

Trolox equivalent antioxidant capacity and ferric reducing power were used as the indicators of antioxidant capacity of figs. Total antioxidant capacities were high in the local figs genotypes compared with the cultivars. Thus it was clear that genotype is the main factor that determines difference in the composition of bioactive compounds in figs and provide information on putative health benefits of locally grown genotypes.The total phenolics content, soluble solids content and titratable acidity greatly vary from 24 to 237 mg of gallic acid equivalent per 100 g fresh weight, 18.60 to 26.30 per cent and 0.16 to 0.47 per cent in local genotypes and the cultivars studied. (Ercisli *et al.*, 2012).

Varietal difference was seen in the antioxidant capacity of figs. Extracts of darker varieties showed higher contents of phytochemicals compared to lighter coloured varieties. Fruit skins contributed most of the above phytochemicals and antioxidant activity compared to the fruit pulp. Antioxidant capacity correlated well with the amounts of polyphenols and anthocyanins (R2 = 0.985 and 0.992, respectively). In the dark-coloured Mission and the red Brown-Turkey varieties, the anthocyanin fraction contributed 36 and 28 per cent of the total antioxidant capacity, respectively. cyanidin-3-O-rutinoside contributed 92 per cent of the total antioxidant capacity of the anthocyanin fraction. Fruits of the Mission variety contained the highest levels of polyphenols, flavonoids, and anthocyanins and exhibited the highest antioxidant capacity (Solomon *et al.*, 2006).

Some recent works have reported that fig antioxidants can protect lipoproteins in plasma from oxidation and produce a significant increase in plasma antioxidant capacity for 4h after consumption (Vinson *et al.*, 2005). Figs are reported to have not only antioxidant effects, but also beneficial effects on cardiovascular, respiratory, and inflammatory diseases (Guarrera, 2005; Jeong and Lachance, 2001). The petroleum ether as well as the methanol extract of *F. racemosa* stem bark improved the antioxidant status considerably as reflected by low TBARS and high GSH values (Ahmed and Urooj, 2010c).

The total extracts of *F. carica* cv. Dottato exhibited a significant dose-dependent anti-radical and inhibition of lipid peroxidation activity, particularly fruits of the first harvest (June) that showed the highest activity with IC 50 of 1.64 mg/mL and 0.004 mg/mL, respectively. Among single fractions, the ethyl acetate fraction from the second harvest (July) showed the highest antiradical activity with an IC 50 value of 0.05 mg/mL while the dichloromethane fraction showed the best inhibition of lipid peroxidation with an IC50 value of 0.02 mg/mL. Dichloromethane fractions showed the highest photodynamic cytotoxicity with an IC 50<5 µg/ml (Marrelli *et al.*, 2012). The stem extract from figs treatment prior to methanol intoxication has significant role in protecting animals from methanol-induced hepatic oxidative damage (Saoudi and Feki, 2012).

Both water extract (WE) and crude hot-water soluble polysaccharide (PS) have notable scavenging activities on DPPH with the EC (50) values of 0.72 and 0.61 mg/ml, respectively. The PS showed higher scavenging activity than WE on superoxide radical (EC 50 of 0.95 mg/ml) and hydroxyl anion radical (scavenging rate 43.4 per cent at concentration of 4 mg/ml). The PS (500 mg/kg) also has a significant increase in the clearance rate of carbon particles and serum hemolysin level of normal mice (Yang *et al.*, 2009).

Hot aqueous extract (FRH) showed significantly higher radical scavenging activity than cold aqueous extract (FRC) and butylated hydroxytoluene (BHT), consequently resulting in a significantly lower IC value than FRC and BHT. Again FRH showed significantly higher activity than FRC though both the extracts exhibited a dose dependent inhibition of porcine kidney and rabbit lung ACE suggesting its potential to be utilized as a therapeutic alternative for hypertension (Ahmed *et al.*, 2010).

The ethanol extract of the fruit *F. racemosa* exhibited significant antioxidant activity in DPPH free radical scavenging assay. 3-O-(E)-Caffeoyl quinate (1) isolated from this plant, also showed significant antioxidant activity (Jahan *et al.*, 2009).

Ethanol extract of the *F. racemosa* Stem Bark (FRE) exhibited significantly higher steady state antioxidant activity than the water extract (FRW). FRE exhibited concentration dependent DPPH, hydroxyl radical and superoxide radical scavenging and inhibition of lipid peroxidation with IC(50) comparable with tested standard compounds. *In vitro* study using micronucleus assay in irradiated Chinese hamster lung fibroblast cells, maximum radioprotection was observed at 20 mcg/ml of FRE. The radioprotection was found to be significant at 1 h prior to 0.5, 1, 2, 3 and 4 Gy gamma-irradiation compared to the respective radiation controls (Veerapur *et al.*, 2009).

The leaves, pulp and peels of two Portuguese white varieties of F. carica exhibited activity against DPPH and nitric oxide radicals in a concentration-dependent way. However, only the leaves presented capacity to scavenge superoxide radical. Leaves were always the most effective part, which seems to be related with phenolics compounds (Oliveira *et al.*, 2009). Racemosic acid showed potent inhibitory activity against COX-1 and 5-LOX *in vitro* with IC50 values of 90 and 18 μM, respectively. Racemosic acid also demonstrated a strong antioxidant activity to scavenge ABTS free radical cations with an IC50 value of 19 μM (Li *et al.*, 2004).

The tests conducted by Orhan *et al.* (2011) revealed that the n-hexane and acetone extracts of the leaves exerted a notable inhibition against both Acetyl Cholinesterase (62.9 +/- 0.9 per cent and 50.8 +/- 2.1 per cent, respectively) and Butyryl Cholinesterase (76.9 +/- 2.2 per cent and 45.6 +/- 1.3 per cent, respectively). However, they had low activity in the antioxidant tests. The chloroform extract was found to be the richest in total flavonoid content (252.5 +/- 1.1 mg/g quercetin equivalent), while the n-butanol extract had the highest total phenol amount (85.9 +/- 3.2 mg/g extract gallic acid equivalent).

The antioxidant potential of latex from figs, checked by distinct *in vitro* chemical assays showed a concentration-dependent activity against DPPH, nitric oxide and superoxide radicals. But the acetylcholinesterase inhibitory capacity was weak (Oliveira *et al.*, 2010a).

Anti-inflammatory

F. racemosa extract (400 mg/kg) exhibited maximum anti-inflammatory effect, that is 30.4, 32.2, 33.9 and 32.0 per cent at the end of 3 h with carrageenin, serotonin, histamine and dextran-induced rat hind paw oedema respectively. In a chronic test the extract (400 mg/kg) showed 41.5 per cent reduction in granuloma weight the effect being comparable to that of phenylbutazone, a prototype of a non-steroidal anti-inflammatory agent (Mandal *et al.*, 2000 a).

The figs leaves are claimed to be effective in various inflammatory conditions like painful or swollen piles, insect sting and bites. Ali *et al.* (2012) validated the traditional claim with pharmacological data. Anti-inflammatory and antioxidant activity of the drug could be due to the presence of steroids and flavanoids, respectively, which are reported to be present in the drug. Furthermore, the anti-inflammatory activity of the drug could be due to its free radical scavenging activity. Further work is also required to isolate and characterize the active constituents responsible for the anti-inflammatory activities.

Antimicrobial

Several reports have shown that the leaf, stem, and woody tissue contain antioxidants and antibiotics (Moon *et al.*, 1997; Ryu *et al.*, 1998).

According to Aref *et al.* (2010) the methanolic extract of *F. carica* latex had no effect against bacteria except for *Proteus mirabilis* but the ethyl acetate extract had inhibition effect on the multiplication of five bacteria species (*E. fecalis, C. freundei, P. aeruginosa, E. coli* and *P. mirabilis*). For the opportunist pathogenic yeasts, ethyl acetate and chlorophormic fractions showed a very strong inhibition (100 per cent); methanolic fraction had a total inhibition against *Candida albicans* (100 per cent) at a concentration of 500 mcg/ml and a negative effect against *C. neoformans. M. canis* was strongly inhibited with methanolic extract (75 per cent) and totally with ethyl acetate extract at a concentration of 750 mg/ml. Hexanoïc extract showed medium results. A strong bactericidal effect the hexane extract of Capri-fig latex was demonstrated by Aref *et al.* (2012). The most sensitive bacteria were *S. saprophyticus* clinical isolate, and *S. aureus* ATCC 25923, with a MIC of 19 µg/ml.

Five extracts (methanolic, hexanic, ethyl acetate, hexane-ethyl acetate (v/v) and chloroformic) of *F. carica* were investigated *in vitro* for their potential antiviral activity against herpes simplex type 1 (HSV-1), echovirus type 11 (ECV-11) and adenovirus (ADV). The hexanic and hexane-ethyl acetate (v/v) extracts inhibited multiplication of viruses by tested techniques at concentrations of 78 µg mL(-1). The hexanic and hexane-ethyl acetate (v/v) extracts inhibited multiplication of viruses by tested techniques at concentrations of 78 µg mL(-1). These two extracts were possible candidates as herbal medicines for herpes virus, echovirus and adenovirus infectious diseases. All extracts had no cytotoxic effect on Vero cells at all tested concentrations (Aref *et al.*, 2011).

Leaf extracts of *F. binjamina* inhibited all viruses *Herpes Simplex Virus*-1 and -2 (HSV-1 and HSV-2) and *Varicella-Zoster* Virus studied, while its fruit extracts inhibited only *Varicella-Zoster* Virus. The greatest antiviral effect was obtained when extracts were added to cells at the time of infection, whereas a partial inhibitory effect was observed when they were added post-infection. There was indirect evidence for strong interactions between the plant extracts and the viruses and weak interactions with the cell surface (Yarmolinsky *et al.*, 2009).

Methanol extracts from the stem bark of figs were active against fungi, gram-positive and gram-negative bacteria thus providing evidence that these might be potential sources of new antimicrobial drug (Kuete *et al.*, 2009). The water extract from the leaves of *Ficus carica* possessed distinct anti-HSV-1 effect. The MTC was 0.5 mg/ml, TDO was 15 mg/ml, and TI was 30.0. It possessed low toxicity and directly killing-virus effect on HSV-1 (Wang *et al.*, 2004).

The milky sap of *F. carica* has a significant toxic effect against early fourth-stage larvae of *Aedes aegypti* L with a lethal concentration [LC (50)] value of 10.2µg/ml and an LC (90) value of 42.3µg/ml. The LC (50) value of the two natural furocoumarins, 5-methoxypsoralen and 8-methoxypsoralen isolated from the milky sap of *F. carica* are 9.4 and 56.3µg/ml, respectively indicating that these compounds play a more important role in the toxicity of the milky sap (Chung *et al.*, 2011).

Mandal *et al.* (2000 b) demonstrated the petroleum ether extract of *F. racemosa* to show a significant antibacterial potential against *Escherichia coli, Basillus pumilis, Bacillus subtilis, Pseudomonas aeruginosa* and *Staphylococcus aureus.*

CVD

Aqueous decoction of fig leaves fed to streptozotocin-induced diabetes led to a decline in the levels of total cholesterol and an decrease in the total cholesterol/HDL cholesterol ratio (with respect to the control group), together with a reduction of the hyperglycaemia (Canal *et al.,* 2000). The acetone extract of *F. racemosa* bark possesses potential cardioprotective activity against doxorubicin-induced cardio-toxicity in rats by scavenging free radicals generated by the administration of the drug (Ahmed and Urooj, 2012).

Velayutham *et al.* (2012) observed that the administration of tannin fraction from *F. racemosa* to significantly reverse the increased blood glucose, total cholesterol, triglycerides, low density lipoprotein. They also found the insulin and high density lipoprotein in the serum were significantly restored. Pérez *et al.* (1999) suggested presence of a single or multiple compounds that influence lipid catabolism in the fig leaf decoction of *F. carica.*

Diabetes

Methanol extract of the stem bark of F. racemosa at the doses of 200 and 400 mg/kg p.o. exhibited significant hypoglycaemic activity in both experimental animal models when compared with the control group and standard antidiabetic agent glibenclamide 10 mg/kg (Rao *et al.,* 2002b). *F. racemosa* bark also exhibited significantly higher glucose-binding capacity than wheat bran (WB) and acarbose (ACB); and consequently showed significantly higher retardation of glucose diffusion compared to WB and ACB. Ahmed and Urooj (2010 d) thus confirmed that F. racemosa bark possesses strong hypoglycaemic effect through inhibition of carbohydrate hydrolyzing enzymes and hence can be utilized as an adjunct in the management of diabetes mellitus. The ethanolic extract of *F. racemosa* bark (300 mg/kg bw) restored the status of blood glucose, lipids and lipoproteins to near normal range in alloxan-induced diabetic rats and these effects were comparable to that of the standard reference drug, glibenclamide (Sophia and Manoharan, 2007).

The decoction of fig leaves (F. carica), supplemented to insulin-dependent diabetics significantly lowered the post-prandial glycemia and the average insulin dose was 12 per cent lower during supplementation (Serraclara *et al.,* 1998). The hypo-glycemic effect in diabetic rats is yet an undefined insulin-like peripheral effect as reported by Perez *et al.* (2000). Pèrez *et al.* (2003) found that both basic and chloroform fraction of *Ficus carica* extract tended to normalize the values of fatty acids and plasma vitamin E values in streptozotocin-induced diabetic rats.

Diarrhea

The ethanolic extracts of F. bengalensis (bark), *F. racemosa* (leaves) and *F. carica* (leaves) significantly inhibited castor oil-induced diarrhea and PGE2-induced enteropooling in rats at 400 and 600 mg/kg. There was a significant dose-dependent decrease in diarrhea produced by all the three models in rats as compared to that of the standard drug group. Ficus species demonstrated significant reductions in fecal output and frequency of droppings in the castor oil-treated rats. The underlying mechanism appears to be spasmolytic and an antienteropooling property. Tannins and flavonoids present in the plant extracts may be responsible for the anti-diarrheal activity (Patil *et al.*, 2012).

Along with excellent antioxidant properties, the stem bark of *F. racemosa* was found to posses antidiabetic property *in vitro and in vivo* in streptozotocin-induced diabetic rats, antihyperglycemic activity *in vivo*, hepatoprotective activity against CCl_4 induced hepatotoxicity and carbohydrate hydrolyzing enzyme inhibitory activity (Ahmed and Urooj, 2008, 2009 a,b,and c, 2010 a, b, c and e).

Cancer

Melanoma and non-melanoma skin cancers are among the most prevalent cancers in the human population. Plant derived natural products have long been and will continue to be an important source for anticancer drug development. In humans, phytosterols and some polyunsaturated fatty acids, such as linoleic acid, are known for their anticarcinogenic properties. The presence of a wide diversity of compounds of distinct classes in *F. carica* latex reveals that it is a potential anticarcinogenic compound (Oliveira *et al.*, 2010a). The close connection between inflammatory/ infectious and cancerous diseases is apparent both from the medieval/ancient to the modern pharmacological knowledge (Lansky *et al.*, 2008). The chemomodulatory effect of *F. racemosa* against ferric nitrilotriaceatate (Fe-NTA) induced renal carcinogenesis and oxidative damage response in rats was reported recently (Khan and Sultana, 2005a).

The presence of racemosic acid, bergenin, tannins, kaempferol, rutin, bergapten, psoralenes, ficusin, coumarin and phenolic glycosides in ethanol extract of *F. racemosa* have shown antioxidant and chemopreventive principles (Baruah *et al.*, 1992; Li *et al.*, 2004). The anticancer active components of fig inhibited 49.3 per cent of the transplanted liver cancer in the mice. The extract obtained by optimized supper critical CO_2 technical method is stable and reasonable, and the extract from fig residues is of the anti-cancer effect (Wang and Ma, 2005).

The *F. carica* extract and the mixture with Armoracia rusticana and Zea mays decreased the level of mutations induced by N-metil-N′-nitro-N-nitrozoguanidin in Vicia faba cells, chlorophyll mutations in *Arabidopsis thaliana* and NaF induced mutability in rat marrow cells. Fig extract and the mixture show the ability to decrease the genotoxicity of environmental mutagens (Agabe-li and Kasimova, 2005).

Khan and Sultana (2005b) showed the chemopreventive effect of *Ficus racemosa* extract (Moraceae) on $KBrO_3$-mediated renal oxidative stress and cell promotion response in rats. Treatment of rats orally with *F. racemosa* extract (200 mg/kg body weight and 400 mg/kg body weight) resulted in a significant decrease in xanthine oxidase, lipid peroxidation and gamma-glutamyl transpeptidase. There was significant recovery of renal glutathione content and antioxidant enzymes. There was also reversal in the enhancement of renal ornithine decarboxylase activity, DNA synthesis and blood urea nitrogen and serum creatinine.

The latex obtained from the fruits *of F. carica* cv. *Dottato* showed the best antiradical activity with an IC50 value of 0.05 mg/ml while the latex obtained from the leaves showed the best antiproliferative on the human tumour cell line (Menichini *et al.*, 2012). A mixture of 6-O-acyl-beta-D-glucosyl-beta-sitosterols, the acyl moeity being primarily palmitoyl and linoleyl with minor amounts of stearyl and oleyl, isolated by Rubnov *et al.* (2001) from fig (Ficuscarica) latex showed *in vitro* inhibitory effects on proliferation of various cancer cell lines. Proteolytic enzymes of fig tree latex could inhibit the proliferation of cancer cell line without any cytotoxic effect on human normal cells. Five mg/ml was the optimum concentration in inhibition of cell line growth. Cancer cell line was more sensitive to *F. carica* latex than normal cells (Hashemi *et al.*, 2011).

Constipation

Constipation is one of the most common functional digestive complaints worldwide. Fig paste (12 g/kg daily, by gavage) for 3 weeks was administered following a 3-week period of constipation induction in dogs. Fig paste significantly increased fecal quantity in constipated dogs, and segmental colonic transit time was also reduced. Thus Oh *et al.* (2011) proved that fig pastes may be useful as a complementary medicine in humans suffering from chronic constipation. Lee *et al.* (2012) also observed similar effect of figs on constipation in rats. Constipation was decreased when fig fruit was fed to rats. Specifically, fecal number, weight, and water content, as well as histological parameters such as thickness and mucin areas in the distal colon were improved. Fig treatment may be a useful therapeutic and preventive strategy for chronic constipation.

Liver Disorders

Hepatoprotective activity of the *F. racemosa* extract of the leaves was seen in rats with induced chronic liver damage by Mandal *et al.* (1999) as the biochemical parameters SGOT, SGPT, serum bilirubin and alkaline phosphatase were all comparable to a standard liver tonic (Neutrosec) in treated rats.

Similarly, methanol extract of *F. racemosa* stem bark exhibited higher hepatoprotective activity than a standard liver tonic (Liv52), while the protective effect of petroleum ether extract was similar to that of Liv52. Histopathological profiles of the liver confirmed the hepato protective effect of *F. racemosa*. Ahmed and Urooz (2010c) observed that F. racemosa possesses potent hepato-protective effects against CCl(4)-induced hepatic damage in rats.

Shade dried leaves of F. carica extracted using petroleum ether (60-80°C) showed significant reversal of biochemical, histological and functional changes induced by rifampicin treatment in rats indicating promising hepatoprotective activity (Gond and Khadabadi, 2008).

Bone Disorders

Park *et al.* (2009) found that the hexane soluble fraction of the common fig *F. carica* (HF6-FC) is a potent inhibitor of osteoclastogenesis in RANKL-stimulated RAW264.7 cells and in bone marrow-derived macrophages (BMMs). HF6-FC exerts its inhibitory effects by suppression of p38 and NF-kappaB but activation of ERK. In addition, HF6-FC significantly decreased the expression of NFATc1 and c-Fos, the master regulator of osteoclast differentiation. Thus they demonstrated that components of HF6-FC may have therapeutic effects on bone-destructive processes such as osteoporosis, rheumatoid arthritis, and periodontal bone resorption. Young *et al.* (2009) also observed that components of HF6-FC may have therapeutic effects on bone-destructive processes such as osteoporosis, rheumatoid arthritis, and periodontal bone resorption.

Memory Enhancer

Alzheimer's disease (AD) is a progressive neurodegenerative disorder resulting in dementia and enhancement of acetylcholine (Ach) levels in brain using acetylcholinesterase inhibitors is one of the most important approaches for the treatment of AD. Cold and hot aqueous extracts of *F. racemosa* stem bark showed dose-dependent inhibition of rat brain acetylcholinesterase with IC_{50} values of 1813 and 1331 mg/mL, respectively (Ahmed and Urooj, 2010 b). Administration of the extract at two levels *viz.*, 250 and 500 mg/kg significantly raised Ach levels in hippocampi of rats compared to control. The percentage enhancement in Ach levels was found to be 22 per cent and 38 per cent, respectively. Further, the extract at both dosage levels elicited significant reduction in transfer latency on elevated plus-maze, which was used as an extero-ceptive behavioral model to evaluate memory in rats. Thus the ACh and memory enhancing activity of *F. racemosa* bark extract can be attributed to the various antioxidant phenolic compounds and the glycoside; racemosic acid (Ahmed *et al.*, 2011). A total of 13 free amino acids some of which are precursors of neurotransmitters were identified in the fig latex (Oliveira *et al.*, 2010b).

In addition to the above, figs/parts of fig plants were found to possess several other health benefits such as anti pyretic, anti diuretic, spasmolytic properties.

The methanol extract of stem bark of *F. racemosa* at doses of 100, 200 and 300 mg/kg body wt. p.o. showed significant dose-dependent reduction in normal body temperature and yeast-provoked elevated temperature. The effect extended up to 5 hrs. after drug administration. The antipyretic effect of the extract was comparable to that of paracetamol (150 mg/kg body wt. p.o.), a standard antipyretic agent (Rao *et al.*, 2002a).

Ratnasooriya *et al.* (2003) provide scientific support for its claimed antidiuretic action. The bark decoction of *F. racemosa* (made as specified in traditional use) in rats using three doses (250, 500 or 1000 mg/kg) significantly impaired the total urine output. The decoction-induced antidiuresis had a rapid onset (within 1 hrs.), peaked at 3 hrs. and lasted through 5 h. However, antidiuretic potential of the decoction was about 50 per cent lower than that of ADH (reference drug).

The methanol extract of F. racemosa demonstrated significant antitussive activity at all tested dose levels when compared with the control as well as codeine phosphate (10 mg), a standard antitussive agent. The extract exhibited maximum inhibition of 56.9 per cent at a dose of 200 mg/kg (p.o.) 90 min after administration (Rao *et al.*, 2003).

Gilani *et al.* (2008) showed the presence of spasmolytic activity in the ripe dried fruit of *F. carica* possibly mediated through the activation of K (+) (ATP) channels along with antiplatelet activity which provides sound pharmacological basis for its medicinal use in the gut motility and inflammatory disorders.

Other Benefits

Parts of fig plant were also found to be useful in food preservation. Aref *et al.* (2011) reported that Saint Pedro *F. carica* L. (Moraceae) crude latex of Kahli amylase was an amylo glucosidase and Bidhi amylase was β-fructose, α (1-4) glucose. Bidhi amylase is a good choice for application in starch, food, detergents and medical industries. The larvicidal activity of crude hexane, ethyl acetate, petroleum ether, acetone, and methanol extracts of the leaf and bark of *F. racemosa* (Moraceae) showed their toxicity against the early fourth-instar larvae of Culex quinquefasciatus (Diptera: Culicidae). The larval mortality was observed after 24-h exposure and the highest larval mortality was found in bark acetone extract (Rahuman *et al.,* 2008). The concentrations required to inhibit the movement of the whole worm and nerve muscle preparation for alcoholic extract of fruits of F. racemosa were 250 and 50 μg/ml, respectively, whereas aqueous extract caused inhibition of the whole worm and nerve muscle preparation at 350 and 150 μg/ml, respectively, suggesting a cuticular barrier. Both alcoholic and aqueous extracts caused death of microfilariae *in vitro.* LC50 and LC90 were 21 and 35 ng/ml, respectively for alcoholic, which were 27 and 42 ng/ml for aqueous extracts (Mishra *et al.,* 2005).

Safety

In spite of all the beneficial effects, the milky sap of the Common fig's green parts acts as an irritant to human skin. Applied externally, fruit latex could cause allergic reaction to sunlight. Therefore it is advisable to contact doctor/in case of any adverse reaction.

References

Agabe-li RA, Kasimova TE (2005). [Antimutagenic activity of *Armoracia rusticana, Zea mays* and *Ficus carica* plant extracts and their mixture]. Tsitol. Genet. 39 (3): 75–79. [Article in Russian].

Ahmed F, Chandra JN, Manjunath S (2011). Acetylcholine and memory-enhancing activity of *Ficus racemosa* bark. Pharmacognosy Res. 3 (4): 246–49.

Ahmed W, Khan AQ, Malik A (1988). Two Triterpenes from the Leaves of *Ficus carica.* Planta. Med. 54: 481.

Ahmed F, Siddesha JM, Urooj A, Vishwanath BS (2010). Radical scavenging and angiotensin converting enzyme inhibitory activities of standardized extracts of *Ficus racemosa* stem bark. Phytother. Res. 24 (12): 1839 – 43.

Ahmed F, Urooj A (2008). Anti-hyperglycemic activity of *Ficus glomerata* stem bark in streptozotocin-induced diabetic rats. Global J. Pharmacol. 2: 41–45.

Ahmed F, Urooj A (2009 a). Antioxidant activity of various extracts of *Ficus racemosa* stem bark. Nat. J. Life Sci. 6: 69–74.

Ahmed F, Urooj A (2009 b). Glucose lowering, hepatoprotective and hypolipidemic activity of stem bark of *Ficus racemosa* in streptozotocin-induced diabetic rats. J. Young Pharm. 1: 160–64.

Ahmed F, Urooj A (2010 d). *In vitro* studies on the hypoglycaemic potential of *Ficus racemosa* stem bark. J. Sci. Food Agric. 90 (3): 397–401.

Ahmed F, Urooj A (2010 a).Traditional uses, medicinal properties, and phyto-pharmacology of *Ficus racemosa*: a review. Pharm. Biol. 48 (6): 672–81.

Ahmed F, Urooj A (2010 b). Anti-cholinesterase activities of cold and hot aqueous extracts of *F. racemosa* stem bark. Pharmacogn. Mag. 6: 142–44.

Ahmed F, Urooj A (2010 c). Hepato-protective effects of *Ficus racemosa* stem bark against carbon tetrachloride-induced hepatic damage in albino rats. Pharm. Biol. 48 (2): 210–16.

Ahmed F, Urooj A (2010 e). Effect of *Ficus racemosa* stem bark on the activities of carbohydrate hydrolyzing enzymes: an *in vitro* study. Pharm. Biol. 48 (5): 518–23.

Ahmed F, Urooj A (2012). Cardioprotective activity of standardized extract of *Ficus racemosa* stem bark against doxorubicin-induced toxicity. Pharm. Biol. 50 (4): 468–73.

Ali B, Mujeeb M, Aeri V, Mir SR, Faiyazuddin M, Shakeel F (2012). Anti-inflammatory and antioxidant activity of *Ficus carica* Linn. leaves. Nat. Prod. Res. 26 (5): 460–65.

Aref HL, Gaaliche B, Fekih A, Mars M, Aouni M, Pierre Chaumon J, Said K (2011). *In vitro* cytotoxic and antiviral activities of *Ficus carica* latex extracts. Nat Prod Res. 25 (3): 310–19.

Aref HL, Mars M, Fekih A, Aouni M, Said K (2012). Chemical composition and antibacterial activity of a hexane extract of Tunisian caprifig latex from the unripe fruit of *Ficus carica*. Pharm. Biol. 50 (4): 407–412.

Aref HL, Mosbah H, Louati H, Said K, Selmi B (2011). Partial characterization of a novel amylase activity isolated from Tunisian *Ficus carica* latex. Pharm. Biol. 49 (11): 1158–66.

Aref HL, Salah KB, Chaumont JP, Fekih A, Aouni M, Said K (2010). *In vitro* antimicrobial activity of four Ficus carica latex fractions against resistant human pathogens (antimicrobial activity of *Ficus carica* latex). Pak. J. Pharm. Sci. 23 (1): 53–58.

Baruah KK, Gohain AK (1992). Chemical composation and nutritive value of Dimaru (*Ficus glomerata* Roxib.) leaves. Ind. J. Nutr. 9: 107–108.

Bellakhdar J, Claisse R, Fleurentin J, Younos C (1991). Repertory of standard herbal drugs in the Moroccan pharmacopoea. Journal of Ethnopharmacology. 35 (2): 123–43.

Canal JR, Torres MD, Romero A, Pérez C (2000). A chloroform extract obtained from a decoction of *Ficus carica* leaves improves the cholesterolaemic status of rats with streptootocin-includede diabetes. Acta. Physiol. Hung. 87: 71–76.

Chung IM, Kim SJ, Yeo MA, Park SW, Moon HI (2011). Immunotoxicity activity of natural furocoumarins from milky sap of *Ficus carica* L. against Aedes aegypti L. Immunopharmacol. Immunotoxicol. 33 (3): 515–18.

Duke JA, Bogenschutz-Godwin MJ, Du Celliar J, Duke PK (2002). Hand Book of Medicinal Herbs. 2nd edition. Boca Raton, Fla, USA: CRC Press.

El-Kholy IS, Shaban MA (1966). Constituents of the leaves of *Ficus carica*, L. II. Isolation of a psi-taraxasteryl ester, rutin, and a new steroid sapogenin. J. Chem. Soc. Perkin. 1. 13: 1140–42.

Ercisli S, Tosun M, Karlidag H, Dzubur A, Hadziabulic S, Aliman Y (2012). Colour and Antioxidant Characteristics of Some Fresh fig (*Ficus carica* L.) Genotypes from Northeastern Turkey. Plant. Foods Hum. Nutr. 2012 May 18.

Gilani AH, Mehmood MH, Janbaz KH, Khan AU, Saeed SA (2008). Ethno pharmacological studies on antispasmodic and antiplatelet activities of Ficus carica. J. Ethnopharmacol. 119 (1): 1- 5.

Gond NY, Khadabadi SS (2008). Hepatoprotective Activity of *Ficus carica* Leaf Extract on Rifampicin-Induced Hepatic Damage in Rats. Indian J. Pharm Sci. 70 (3): 364–66.

Guarrera PM (2003). Food medicine and minor nourishment in the folk traditions of Central Italy (Marche, Abruzzo and Latium) Fitoterapia. 74 (6): 515–544.

Guarrera PM (2005). Traditional phytotherapy in Central Italy (Marche, Abruzzo, and Latium) Fitoterapia. 76 (1): 1–25.

Hashemi SA, Abediankenari S, Ghasemi M, Azadbakht M, Yousefzadeh Y, Dehpour AA (2011). The Effect of fig Tree Latex (*Ficus carica*) on Stomach Cancer Line. Iran. Red. Crescent. Med. J. 13 (4): 272–75.

Jahan IA, Nahar N, Mosihuzzaman M, Rokeya B, Ali L, Azad Khan AK, Makhmur T, Iqbal Choudhary M (2009). Hypoglycaemic and antioxidant activities of *Ficus racemosa* Linn. fruits. Nat Prod Res. 23 (4): 399–408.

Jeong WS, Lachance PA (2001). Phytosterols and fatty acids in fig *(Ficus carica*, var. Mission) fruit and tree components. J. Food Sci. 66 (2): 278–81.

Joseph B, Justin Raj S (2011). Pharmacognostic and phytochemical properties of *Ficus carica* Linn: An overview. International Journal of Pharm.Tech. Research. 3 (1): 8–12.

Khan M, Sultana S (2005a). Chemo-modulatory effect of *Ficus racemosa* extract against chemically induced renal carcinogenesis and oxidative damage response in wistar rats. Life Sci. 77: 1194–210.

Khan N, Sultana S (2005b). Modulatory effect of Ficus racemosa: diminution of potassium bromate-induced renal oxidative injury and cell proliferation response. Basic Clin. Pharmacol. Toxicol. 97 (5): 282–88.

Kim KH (1981). Chemical components of Korean figs and its storage stability. Korean J. Food Sci. Technol. 13 (2): 165–69.

Kim SS, Lee CH, Oh SL, Chung DH (1992). Chemical components in the two cultivars of Korean figs (*Ficus carica* L.) Agric. Chem. Biotechnol. 35 (1): 51–54.

Kuete V, Nana F, Ngameni B, Mbaveng AT, Keumedjio F, Ngadjui BT (2009). Antimicrobial activity of the crude extract, fractions and compounds from stem bark of *Ficus ovata* (Moraceae). J. Ethnopharmacol. 124 (3): 556–61.

Lansky EP, Paavilainen HM, Pawlus AD, Newman RA (2008). Ficus spp. (fig): ethnobotany and potential as anticancer and anti-inflammatory agents. J. Ethnopharmacol. 119 (2): 195–213.

Lee WT (1996). Coloured standard illustrations of Korean plants. Academy Press. Seoul: p. 624.

Lee HY, Kim JH, Jeung HW, Lee CU, Kim DS, Li B, Lee GH, Sung MS, Ha KC, Back HI, Kim SY, Park SH, Oh MR, Kim MG, Jeon JY, Im YJ, Hwang MH, So BO, Shin SJ, Yoo WH, Kim HR, Chae HJ, Chae SW (2012). Effects of *Ficus carica* paste on loperamide-induced constipation in rats. Food Chem. Toxicol. 50 (3-4): 895–902.

Li RW, Leach DN, Myers SP, Lin GD, Leach GJ, Waterman PG (2004). A new anti-inflammatory glucoside from *Ficus racemosa* L. Planta. Med. 70 (5): 421–26.

Mandal SC, Maity TK, Das J, Pal M, Saha BP (1999). Hepato-protective activity of *Ficus racemosa* leaf extract on liver damage caused by carbon tetrachloride in rats. Phytother Res. 13 (5): 430–32.

Mandal SC, Maity TK, Das J, Saba BP, Pal M (2000 a). Anti-inflammatory evaluation of *Ficus racemosa* Linn. leaf extract.J. Ethnopharmacol. 72 (1-2): 87–92.

Mandal SC, Saha BP, Pal M (2000b). Studies on antibacterial activity of *Ficus racemosa* Linn. leaf extract. Phytother. Res. 14 (4): 278–80.

Marrelli M, Menichini F, Statti GA, Bonesi M, Duez P, Menichini F, Conforti F (2012). Changes in the phenolic and lipophilic composition, in the enzyme inhibition and antiproliferative activity of *Ficus carica* L. cultivar Dottato fruits during maturation. Food. Chem. Toxicol. 50 (3-4): 726–33.

Menichini G, Alfano C, Provenzano E, Marrelli M, Statti GA, Somma F, Menichini F, Conforti F (2012). Fig latex (*Ficus carica* L. cultivar Dottato) in combination with UV irradiation decreases the viability of A375 melanoma cells *in vitro*. Anticancer Agents Med. Chem. 2012 Feb 17.

Mishra V, Khan NU, Singhal KC (2005). Potential antifilarial activity of fruit extracts of *Ficus racemosa* Linn. against *Setaria cervi in vitro*. Indian J. Exp. Biol. 43 (4): 346–50.

Moon CK, Kim YG, Kim MY (1997). Studies on the bioactivities of the extractives from *Ficus carica*. J. Inst. Agric. Res. Util. 31: 69–79.

Oh HG, Lee HY, Seo MY, Kang YR, Kim JH, Park JW, Kim OJ, Back HI, Kim SY, Oh MR, Park SH, Kim MG, Jeon JY, Hwang MH, Shin SJ, Chae SW (2011). Effects of *Ficus carica* paste on constipation induced by a high-protein feed and movement restriction in beagles. Lab. Anim. Res. 27 (4): 275–81.

Oliveira AP, Silva LR, Andrade PB, ValentaÞo P, Silva BM, Gonc'alves RF, Pereira JA, Guedes de Pinho P (2010a). Further Insight into the Latex Metabolite Profile of *Ficus carica*. J. Agric. Food Chem. 2010 Oct 5. [Epub ahead of print].

Oliveira AP, Silva LR, Ferreres F, Guedes de Pinho P, Valentão P, Silva BM, Pereira JA, Andrade PB (2010b). Chemical assessment and *in vitro* antioxidant capacity of *Ficus carica* latex.J. Agric. Food Chem. 58 (6): 3393–98.

Orhan IE, Ustün O, Sener B (2011). Estimation of cholinesterase inhibitory and antioxidant effects of the leaf extracts of Anatolian *Ficus carica* var. domestica and their total phenol and flavonoid contents. Nat. Prod. Commun. 6 (3): 375–78.

Park YR, Eun JS, Choi HJ, Nepal M, Kim DK, Seo SY, Li R, Moon WS, Cho NP, Cho SD, Bae TS, Kim BI, Soh Y (2009). Hexane-Soluble Fraction of the Common fig, *Ficus carica*, Inhibits Osteoclast Differentiation in Murine Bone Marrow-Derived Macrophages and RAW 264.7 Cells. Korean J. Physiol. Pharmacol. 13 (6): 417–24.

Patil VV, Bhangale SC, Chaudhari KP, Kakade RT, Thakare VM, Bonde CG, Patil VR (2012). Evaluation of the anti-diarrhoeal activity of the plant extracts of *Ficus species*. Zhong. Xi. Yi. Jie. He. Xue. Bao. 10 (3): 347–52.

Pérez C, Canal JR, Campillo JE, Romero A, Torres MD (1999). Hypo-triglyceridaemic activity of Ficus carica leaves in experimental hypertriglyceridaemic rats. Phytother. Res. 13 (3): 188–91.

Pèrez C, Canal JR, Torres MD (2003). Experimental diabetes treated with *Ficus carica* extract: effect on oxidative stress parameters. Acta. Diabetol. 40 (1): 3–8.

Pérez C, Domínguez E, Canal JR, Campillo JE, Torres MD (2000). Hypo-glycaemic activity of an aqueous extract from *Ficus carica* (fig tree) leaves in streptozotocin diabetic rats. Pharm Biol. 38 (3): 181–86.

Rahuman AA, Venkatesan P, Geetha K, Gopalakrishnan G, Bagavan A, Kamaraj C (2008). Mosquito larvicidal activity of gluanol acetate, a tetracyclic triterpenes derived from *Ficus racemosa* Linn. Parasitol. Res. 103 (2): 333–39.

Rao RB, Anupama K, Swaroop KR, Murugesan T, Pal M, Mandal SC (2002a). Evaluation of anti-pyretic potential of *Ficus racemosa* bark. Phytomedicine. 9 (8): 731–33.

Rao RB, Murugesan T, Sinha S, Saha BP, Pal M, Mandal SC (2002b). Glucose lowering efficacy of *Ficus racemosa* barks extract in normal and alloxan diabetic rats. Phytother. Res. 16 (6): 590–92.

Rao RB, Murugesan T, Pal M, Saha BP, Mandal SC (2003). Antitussive potential of methanol extract of stem bark of *Ficus racemosa* Linn. Phytother. Res. 17 (9): 1117–18.

Ratnasooriya WD, Jayakody JR, Nadarajah T (2003). Antidiuretic activity of aqueous bark extract of Sri Lankan *Ficus racemosa* in rats. Acta. Biol. Hung. 54 (3-4): 357–63.

Rubnov S, Kashman Y, Rabinowitz R, Schlesinger M, Mechoulam R (2001). Suppressors of cancer cell proliferation from fig (*Ficus carica*) resin: isolation and structure elucidation. J. Nat. Prod. 64 (7): 993–99.

Ryu SR, Cho H, Jung JS, Jung ST (1998). The study on the separation, antitumour activity as new substances in fig. J Applied Chem. 2 (2): 961–64.

Saoudi M, El Feki A (2012). Protective Role of *Ficus carica* Stem Extract against Hepatic Oxidative Damage Induced by Methanol in Male Wistar Rats. Evid. Based Complement. Alternat. Med. 2012: 150458.

Serraclara A, Hawkins F, Pérez C, Domínguez E, Campillo JE, Torres MD (1998). Hypoglycaemic action of an oral fig-leaf decoction in type-I diabetic patients. Diabetes Res. Clin. Pract. 39: 19–22.

Slatnar A, Klancar U, Stampar F, Veberic R (2011). Effect of drying of figs (*Ficus carica* L.) on the contents of sugars, organic acids, and phenolic compounds. J. Agric. Food Chem. 59 (21): 11696–702.

Solomon A, Golubowicz S, Yablowicz Z, Grossman S, Bergman M, Gottlieb HE, Altman A, Kerem Z, Flaishman MA (2006). Antioxidant activities and anthocyanin content of fresh fruits of common fig (*Ficus carica* L.). J. Agric. Food Chem. 54 (20): 7717–23.

Sophia D, Manoharan S (2007). Hypolipidemic activities of *Ficus racemosa* Linn. bark in alloxan induced diabetic rats. Afr. J. Tradit. Complement. Altern. Med. 4 (3): 279–88.

Subhaktha PK, Rajasekaran R, Narayana A (2007). Udumbara (*Ficus glomerata* Roxb.): a medico-historical review. Bull. Indian Inst. Hist. Med. Hyderabad. 37 (1): 29–44.

USDA (2012). National Nutrient Database for Standard Reference, Release 25.

Veberic R, Colaric M, Stampar F (2008). Phenolic acids and flavonoids of fig fruit *Ficus carica* in the northern Mediterranean region. Food Chem.106 (1): 153–57.

Veerapur VP, Prabhakar KR, Parihar VK, Kandadi MR, Ramakrishana S, Mishra B, Satish Rao BS, Srinivasan KK, Priyadarsini KI, Unnikrishnan MK (2009). *Ficus racemosa* Stem Bark Extract: A Potent Antioxidant and a Probable Natural Radioprotector. Evid. Based Complement. Alternat. Med. 6 (3): 317–24.

Velayutham R, Sankaradoss N, Ahamed KF (2012). Protective effect of tannins from *Ficus racemosa* in hypercholesterolemia and diabetes induced vascular tissue damage in rats. Asian Pac J Trop Med. 5 (5): 367–73.

Vinson JA (1999). The functional food properties of figs. Cereal Food World. 44 (2): 82–87.

Wang ZB, Ma HL (2005). [Study on anti-cancer components of fig residues with supper critical fluid CO_2 extracting technique]. Zhongguo. Zhong. Yao. Za. Zhi. 30 (18): 1443–47. [Article in Chinese].

Wang G, Wang H, Song Y, Jia C, Wang Z, Xu H (2004). [Studies on anti-HSV effect of *Ficus carica* leaves]. Zhong. Yao. Cai. 27 (10): 754–56. [Article in Chinese].

Yang XM, Yu W, Ou ZP, Ma HL, Liu WM, Ji XL (2009). Antioxidant and immunity activity of water extract and crude polysaccharide from *Ficus carica* L. fruit. Plant. Foods Hum. Nutr. 64 (2): 167–73.

Yarmolinsky L, Zaccai M, Ben-Shabat S, Mills D, Huleihel M (2009). Antiviral activity of ethanol extracts of *Ficus binjamina* and *Lilium candidum in vitro*. N. Biotechnol. 26 (6): 307–13.

Young Ran Park, Jae Soon Eun, Hwa Jung Choi, Manoj Nepal, Dae Keun Kim, Seung-Yong Seo, Rihua Li, Woo Sung Moon, Nam-Pyo Cho, Sung-Dae Cho, Tae Sung Bae, Byung Il Kim, and Yunjo Soh. (2009). Hexane-Soluble Fraction of the Common fig, *Ficus carica*, Inhibits Osteoclast Differentiation in Murine Bone Marrow-Derived Macrophages and RAW 264.7 Cells. Korean J. Physiol. Pharmacol. 13 (6): 417–24.

Chapter 19

Olives

(*Olea europaea*)

The oliv, *Olea europaea*, meaning "Oil from/of Europe" is a species of family Oleaceae, a small tree in the native to the coastal areas of the eastern Mediterranean Basin (the adjoining coastal areas of southeastern Europe, western Asia and northern Africa) as well as northern Iraq, and northern Iran at the south end of the Caspian Sea. The fruit is of major agricultural importance as the source of olive oil.

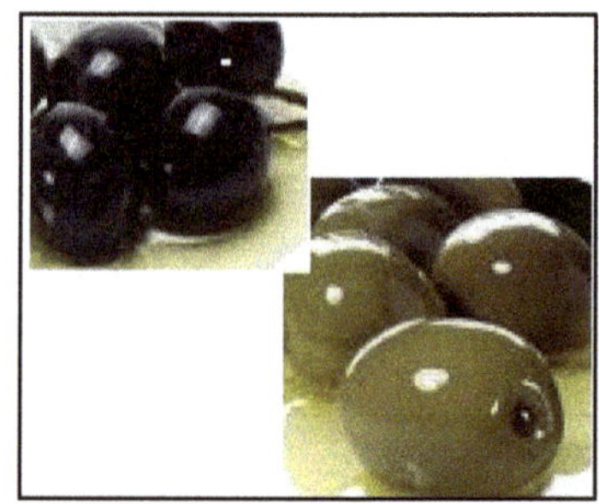

Production

Olives are one of the most extensively cultivated fruit crops in the world and have been cultivated in various parts of the Mediterranean–including Crete and Syria–for at least 5,000 years. According to the Food and Agriculture Organization, 95 per cent of the world's olive is produced in the Mediterranean region. In 2009 there were 9.9 million hectares planted with olive trees, which is more than twice the amount of land devoted to apples, bananas or mangoes. Cultivation area tripled from 2,600,000 to 8,500,000 hectares (6,400,000 to 21,000,000 acres) between 1960 and 2004 and in 2008 reached 10.8 mln Ha.

Olive Varieties

Some of the more popular olive varieties are: manzanilla: Spanish green olive, picholine: French green olive, kalamata: Greek black olive, niçoise: French black olive, ponentine and liguria: Italian black olive and Californian sevillano.

Nutritional Value of Olive

Olives yield 145 Calories, 15–32 g. Fat, 3.84 g. Carbohydrates, 1.03 g. Protein per 100 g (USDA, 2011). Commercial stoned table olives named "alcaparras" from Trás-os-Montes (Portugal) showed 73 per cent water, 14.6 g fat, 77 per cent Oleic acid, 1.1 g protein and 3.4 g ash. 156 Calories and 1.2 g tocopherol on fresh weight basis (Sousa *et al.*, 2011). Olives are a very good source of monounsaturated fat (in the form of oleic acid) and a good source of iron, copper, and dietary fiber. Since olives contain mixed tocopherols, they are also a good source of vitamin E.

The oil content and the other constituents of olive also depend on the stage of maturity. The oil content of olive fruit ranged between 17.5 and 20.25 per cent at the first stage of maturation and from 30.20 and 35 per cent in the last harvest.

Nutritive Value of Olives (Ripe canned) per 100 gms

Nutrient	*Amount*	*Nutrient*	*Amount*
Energy (kcals)	115	Carbohydrate (g)	6.26
Protein (g)	0.84	Fat (g)	10.68
Fatty acids, total saturated (g)	1.415	Calcium (mg)	88
Fatty acids, total monounsaturated (g)	7.888	Fatty acids, total polyunsaturated (g)	0.911
Iron (mg)	3.30	Magnesium(mg)	4
Phosphorus (mg)	3	Potassium (mg)	8
Sodium (mg)	735	Zinc (mg)	0.22
Thiamin (mg)	0.003	Riboflavin (mg)	0.000
Niacin (mg)	0.037	Vitamin A (IU)	403
Vitamin K (μg)	1.4		

USDA (2012).

Chemical/Nutritional Constituents of Olive and Olive Oil

Olives are also a remarkable source of antioxidant and anti-inflammatory phytonutrients. The phytonutrient content of olives depends upon olive variety, stage of maturation, and post-harvest treatment. The different phytochemical constituents in olives are: Simple Phenols–tyrosol, hydroxytyrosol; Terpenes (including secoiridoids and triterpenes)–oleuropein, demethyloleuropein, erythrodiol, uvaol, oleanolic acid, elenoic acid, ligstroside; Flavones–apigenin, luteolin, Hydroxycinnamic acids, caffeic acid, cinnamic acid, ferulic acid, coumaric acid; Anthocyanidins–cyanidins, peonidins; Flavonols–quercetin, kaempferol, Hydroxybenzoic acids, gallic acid, protocatechuic acid, vanillic acid, syringic acid; Hydroxyphenylacetic acids–homovanillic acid, homveratric acid. Olives especially those that have not been subjected to the Spanish brining process contain up to 16 g/ kg of acteosides, hydroxytyrosol, tyrosol and phenyl propionic acids.

Bouaziz *et al.* (2004) observed a correlation between antioxidant activity and total phenolic content of samples which is attributed to the increase of the total phenol level with fruit maturation. The total phenolic content varied from 3.46 to 4.3g per kg^{-1} at the first stage and from 8.7 to 11.5 g per kg^{-1} of fresh fruit weight at the last stage. Total flavonoid content also reached 432.8 g per kg^{-1}. The trolox equivalent at the last stage of maturation of the olive extracts ranged from 2.69 to from 2.15 to 3.03 mmol L^{-1} (Bouaziz *et al.*, 2010).

Muzzalupo *et al.* (2011) showed an inverse correlation between phenols and tocopherol content. In particular, during the ripening phase, tocopherols increased rapidly in olive pericarps while phenolic compounds and chlorophyll levels declined significantly. In the same cultivars at different pericarp ripening stage significant differences were reported in the antioxidant proportions. The significant amounts of these antioxidants confirm the nutritional and medicinal value of olive drupes and its products.

The phytochemical composition of olive oil is different from that of olives. The main active constituents of olive oil include oleic acid, phenolic constituents, and squalene. Olive oil contains variable amounts of triacylglycerols and small quantities of free fatty acids, glycerol, pigments, aroma compounds, sterols, tocopherols, phenols, unidentified resinous components and others (Kiritsakis, 1998).

The main phenolic compounds, hydroxytyrosol and oleuropein, give extra-virgin olive oil its bitter, pungent taste (Omar *et al.*, 2010). Oleuropein is generally the most prominent phenolic compound in olive cultivars and can reach concentrations of up to 140 mg/g on a dry matter basis in young olives (Amiot *et al.*, 1986) and 60–90 mg/g of dry matter in the leaves (Le Tutour, 1992). Oleuropein can be hydrolyzed to hydroxytyrosol, elenolic acid, oleuropein aglycone, and glucose (Corona *et al.*, 2006; Manna *et al.*, 2004).

Olive oil, especially extra virgin, contains smaller amounts of hydroxytyrosol and tyrosol, along with secoiridoids and lignans in abundance. Both olives and olive oil contain substantial amounts of other compounds deemed to be anticancer agents (*e.g.* squalene and terpenoids) as well as the peroxidation-resistant lipid oleic acid (Owen *et al.*, 2004; El and Karakaya, 2009).

Methanolic extracts of olive leaves contain secoiridoids such as oleuropein, ligostroside, dimethyloleuropein, and oleoside (El and Karakaya, 2009); flavonoids, including apigenin, kaempferol, and luteolin; as well as phenolic compounds such as caffeic acid, tyrosol, and hydroxytyrosol (Chiou *et al.*, 2007). Oleuropein, the major phytochemical in olive leaf, is a complex phenol present in large quantities in olive leaves but in lower quantities in olive oil (Soler-Rivas *et al.*, 2000).

Effect of Curing on Composition of Olive

Raw olives are hard and bitter and so they are pickled in brine, or cured in salt or oil. The curing process removes bitter compounds (some of which are healthy polyphenols), softens the fruit, and imbues them with flavour and also with a fair amount of sodium. Water curing, brine curing, oil-curing, dry-curing and lye curing are the most common treatment processes for olives, and each of these treatments can affect the colour and composition of the olives. In the United States, where most olives come from California, they are typically green in colour, picked in an unripe state, lye-cured, and then exposed to air as a way of triggering oxidation and conversion to a black outer colour.

Air drying and drying of olive mill waste (OMW) at 60°C resulted in a substantial decrease in the phenol content and antioxidant capacity and drying at 105° C and freeze-drying produced less degradation. Neither storage at low temperature (4° C) nor the medium of preservation (40 per cent w/w ethanol and 1 per cent w/w acetic acid) for 24 hours could prevent the rapid decrease in phenolic concentrations and antioxidant capacity, when observed for 24 hours in comparison with the OMW samples stored at room temperature (Obied *et al.*, 2008).

Servili *et al.* (2006) found a reduction in the oleuropein, a glucoside secoiridoid responsible for the bitter taste of olive drupes, and increase the hydroxytyrosol concentration of olives upon fermentation with *Lactobacillus pentosus*.

Traditional Therapeutic Uses of Olive

Olive leaves offer an alternative source to study the effects of olive oil polyphenols because the leaf contains the similar polyphenols with only a small amount of oleic acid. Olive tree (*Olea europaea* L.) leaves have been widely used in traditional remedies in European and Mediterranean countries such as Greece, Spain, Italy, France, Turkey, Israel, Morocco, and Tunisia. They have been used in the human diet as an extract, herbal tea, and powder as they contain many potentially bioactive compounds (El and Karakaya 2009). De la Puerta *et al.* (1999) determined the anti-eicosanoid and antioxidant effects of the principal phenolic compounds (oleuropein, tyrosol, hydroxytyrosol and caffeic acid) from the polar fraction of olive oil in leucocytes. The aqueous extract of *O. europaea* leaves displayed wound healing activity and Secoiridoid oleuropein (4.6 per cent) was identified as the major active compound (Koca *et al.*, 2011).

Oleuropein, a chemical constituent of olives, and its major metabolite, hydroxytyrosol, exhibited a range of pharmacological properties beneficial for the cardiovascular system *in vitro*. These actions included inhibition of the proliferation of McCoy cells derived from the synovial fluid in the knee joint (Saenz *et al.*, 1998), enhanced nitric oxide production by mouse macrophages (Visioli *et al.*, 1998a), anti-inflammatory effects (Visioli *et al.*, 1998b, Miles *et al.*, 2005), protected against oxidative myocardial injury induced by ischemia and reperfusion (Manna *et al.*, 2004), decreased blood pressure, inhibited platelet aggregation and eicosanoid production, and scavenged free radicals in addition to inhibition of 5- and 12-lipoxygenases (*Visioli et al., 2002a)*. In addition, oleuropein, was found to posses antiatherogenic (Visioli and Galli, 2001; Carluccio *et al.*, 2003), anticancer (Owen *et al.*, 2000), antimicrobial (Tripoli *et al.*, 2005), and antiviral (Fredrickson, 2000) properties and for these reasons, it is commercially available as food supplement in Mediterranean countries. Koca *et al.* (2011) reported that the leaves and fruits of Olea europaea have been used externally as an emollient for skin ulcers too and for healing of inflammatory wounds.

Antioxidant

Rodríguez *et al.* (2009) presented data to indicate that natural table olives are a rich source of 3,4-dihydroxyphenylglycol and hydroxytyrosol compounds with interesting nutritional and antioxidant properties. A scavenging effect of oleuropein was demonstrated with respect to hypochlorous acid (HOCl) (Visioli *et al.*, 2002b). HOCl is an oxidative substance produced *in vivo* by neutrophil myeloperoxidase at the site of inflammation and can cause damage to proteins including enzymes. Visioli *et al.* (2000) demonstrated that the administration of catecholic phenolic from olive oil (oleuropein) dose-dependently decreases the urinary excretion of 8-iso-PGF2α, indicating lower *in vivo* lipid peroxidation in supplemented volunteers.

Roche *et al.* (2009) found olive phenols (detected in human plasma in olive consumers) and their metabolites to be much more efficient inhibitors of lipid and protein oxidation compared to vitamins C and E. Low postprandial concentrations of olive phenols may help to preserve the integrity of functional proteins and delay the appearance of toxic lipid oxidation products.

It was found that three major constituents–oleuropein (A), luteolin-7-O-glucoside (B) and verbascoside (C) in the extract of the leaves of O. europaea L. possessed potential antioxidant activities. The antioxidant and free radical scavenging properties of olive leaf and its constituents have been described by Lee *et al.* (2009). Olive leaf extract supplemented rats had enhanced vascular relaxant responses to acetylcholine and sodium nitroprusside in the aortic rings derived from the treated rats. Other ex vivo studies have demonstrated the vasodilative effect of oleuropein on isolated rat aorta (Zarzuelo *et al.*, 1991), attributed to L-type Ca^{2+} channel antagonistic effects (Scheffler *et al.*, 2008). *In vivo,* olive leaf extract lowered blood cholesterol (Fki *et al.*, 2005) and lipid (Jemai *et al.*, 2008) concentrations in cholesterol-fed rats and lowered blood pressure in nitro-l-arginine methyl ester-induced hypertensive rats (Khayyal *et al.*, 2002) as well as in normo-tensive rats (Lasserre *et al.*, 1983). The decreased blood lipid concentrations could be due to agonist actions on bile acid-activated TGR5, a metabotropic G-protein–coupled receptor (Sato *et al.*, 2007). Olive leaf extract supplementation also reduced plasma concentrations of uric acid, also one of the major endogenous water-soluble antioxidants (Mene and Punzo, 2008), and malondialdehyde, a marker of lipid peroxidation (Del *et al.*, 2005). The antioxidant activity assay showed that aqueous extract has higher scavenging ability than the n-hexane extract.

Luteolin, another major component of olive leaves, and its derivatives inhibited superoxide anion-mediated impairment of endothelium (Ma *et al.*, 2008), Qian *et al.*, 2009), improved endothelium-dependent relaxation in rat aorta (Qian *et al.*, 2009), inhibited angiotensin-converting enzyme Loizzo *et al., 2007)* and nuclear factor ê light chain enhancer of activated B cell activation, and decreased interleukin-6 and tumour necrosis factor-α release both *in vitro* and *in vivo* (Lopez-Lazaro, 2009).

Olive mill waste (OMW) is rich in biophenols and typically contains 98 per cent of the total phenols in the olive fruit, making value addition to OMW an attractive enterprise (Obied *et al.*, 2005). Olive mill waste water (OMWW) is a major environmental issue in the Mediterranean. Stamatakis *et al.* (2009) confirmed that the PAF inhibitor present in the purified fractions of the biologically active compounds from OMWW resembles the one isolated from olive oil. Thus they offer a new approach on the OMWW handling by offering an alternative use of this waste as starting material for nutritional and/or pharmaceutical purposes in the future. New biophenolic secoiridoids were identified in Australian Frantoio olive mill waste (OMW) extracts. Hydroxytyrosyl acyclodihydroelenolate, the first nonaldehydic acyclic secoiridoid and a second compound as p-coumaroyl-6'-secologanoside (comselogoside) with antioxidant potential have been identified by Obied *et al.* (2007b). The hypocholesterolemic effect of hydroxytyrosol and OMW extract might be due to their abilities to lower serum TC and LDL-C levels as well as slowing the lipid peroxidation process and enhancing antioxidant enzyme activity.

Extracts from both OMW obtained as a by-product from processing of Mission and Frantoio olive fruit and OMW produced from the Mission fruit (containing higher total phenol content) showed broad spectrum antibacterial activity against *S. aureus, B. subtilis, E. coli* and *P. aeruginosa*; whereas individual biophenols (hydroxytyrosol, luteolin, oleuropein) showed more limited activity. Molluscicidal activity was measured against *Isidorella newcombi* and LD (50) values were 424 ppm and 541 ppm for Mission and Frantoio extracts (Obied *et al.*, 2007a).

Review of the human intervention studies showed that olive polyphenols decreased the levels of oxidized-LDL in plasma and positively affected several biomarkers of oxidative damage. The antioxidant effects of olive polyphenols on low-density lipoprotein (LDL) oxidation are observed after a dietary intake of about 10 mg per day. The overall evidence from *in vitro* assays and animal and human studies support the antioxidant effect of olive polyphenols (Raederstorff (2009).

Solid olive residues (SOR) are byproducts of the olive-milling process, but they have an increasing importance in the pharmaceutical industry due to their rich content of biophenols. Such compounds are studied widely for their antioxidant and antimicrobial activities (Mulinacci *et al.*, 2005). The hydroalcoholic extract from solid olive residue (SOR) of c.v. Coratina (polyphenols content 19.7 per cent) and a purified extract (Oleaselecttrade mark) (polyphenols content 35.1 per cent) showed IC (50) 26.96+/-1.53 µg/ml in the DPPH assay, that 10 µg/ml were equivalent to 2.11+/-0.12 µg/ml Trolox (ORAC assay) and IC (50) 1.7+/-0.20 µg/ml in the RBC hemolysis. The Oleaselect extract was 4 to 5 folds more active than the hydroalcoholic extract in all the experimental models, with IC (50) values of 7.36+/-0.38 µg/ml in the DPPH test and of 0.38+/-0.03 µg/ml in RBC; the antioxidant activity in the ORAC assay was slightly greater than that of Trolox (10 µg/ml equivalent to 11.45+/-0.40 µg/ml). Taking into account the total polyphenol content, these results clearly indicate a greater antioxidant activity for the purified extract, due to a cooperative antioxidant interaction among its polyphenol constituents (Aldini *et al.*, 2006).

Anti-inflammatory

Visioli *et al.* (1998 and 2002a) showed that oleuropein increases nitric oxide (NO) production in macrophages challenged with lipopolysaccharide through induction of the inducible form of the enzyme nitric oxide synthase, thus increasing the functional activity of these immunocompetent cells. It is well known that oleuropein elicits anti-inflammatory effects by inhibiting lypoxygenase activity and the production of leukotriene B_4 (De la Puerta *et al.*, 1999). The ethanolic extract did not show a significant anti-inflammatory or analgesic activity, whereas the n-hexane extract displayed 12.7-27.8 per cent inhibition on the carrageenan-induced hind paw edema model at the 400 mg/kg dose, without inducing any apparent acute toxicity as well as gastric damage (Süntar *et al.*, 2010).

Antimicrobial

Among the phenolic and oleosidic compounds in olive brines of the Manzanilla and Gordal varieties, the dialdehydic form of decarboxymethyl elenolic acid linked to hydroxytyrosol showed the strongest antilactic acid bacteria activity, and its presence in brines could explain the growth inhibition of these microorganisms during olive fermentation. An isomer of oleoside 11-methyl ester was also effective against *L. pentosus* and can, therefore, contribute to the antimicrobial activity of olive brines (Medina *et al.*, 2007).

There is a report that olive leaf extracts augment the activity of the HIV-RT inhibitor 3TC (Walker, 1996). The olive leaf extracts were investigated for their antiviral activity against viral hemorrhagic septicemia virus, a salmonid rhabdovirus, and against HIV-1 infection and replication (Micol *et al.*, 2005). Cell-to-cell transmission of HIV was inhibited in a dose-dependent manner with EC_{50}s of 0.2 μg/ml, and HIV replication was inhibited in an *in vitro* experiment (Lee-Huang *et al.*, 2003).

Oleuropein has been shown to have strong antimicrobial activity against both Gram-negative and Gram-positive bacteria (Bisignano *et al.*, 1999; Aziz *et al.*, 1998; Fleming *et al.*, 1973) as well as mycoplasma (Furneri *et al.*, 2002). Phenolic structures similar to oleuropein seem to produce its antibacterial effect by damaging the bacterial membrane and/or disrupting cell peptidoglycans. Caturla *et al.* (2005) used biophysical assays to study the interaction between oleuropein and membrane lipids.

In 2001, Saija and Uccella proposed that the glycoside group modifies the ability to penetrate the cell membrane and get to the target site. Effective interference with the production procedures of certain amino acids necessary for the growth of specific microorganisms has also been suggested. Another mechanism proposed is the direct stimulation of phagocytosis as a response of the immune system to microbes of all types.

Oleuropein and hydrolysis products are able to inhibit the development and production of enterotoxin B by *S. aureus*, the development of *S. enteritidis* and the germination and consequent development of spores of *B. cereus* (Saija and Uccella, 2001; Bisignano *et al.*, 1999; Aziz *et al.*, 1998; Caturla *et al.*, 2005; Furneri *et al.*, 2002; Fleming *et al.*, 1973; Walter *et al.*, 1973; Tassou *et al.*, 1991; Tassou and Nychas 1994; 1995; Tranter *et al.*, 1993). Oleuropein and other phenolic compounds (p-hydroxybenzoic, vanillic and p-coumaric acids) completely inhibit the development of *K. pneumoniae*, *E. coli* and *B. cereus* (Aziz *et al.*, 1998).

Neuroprotective

Mohagheghi *et al.* (2011) reported that oral administration of olive leaf extract reduces infarct volume, brain edema, blood-brain barrier permeability, and improves neurologic deficit scores after transient middle cerebral artery occlusion in rats.

Olive leaf extract inhibits high glucose-induced neural damage and suppresses diabetes-induced thermal hyperalgesia. The mechanisms of these effects may be due, at least in part, to reduced neuronal apoptosis and suggest therapeutic potential of olive leaf extract in attenuation of diabetic neuropathic pain (Kaeidi *et al.*, 2011).

Bazoti *et al.* (2006) have reported that oleuropein decreases or even prevents Aβ aggregation, which is inherent to Alzheimer's disease (AD). The potential effect of oleuropein on brain function in AD is analogous to atherosclerosis because they both are age-dependent diseases in which abnormal accumulation of a normal metabolite (cholesterol and Aβ, respectively) precedes clinical symptoms and leads to Alzheimer's disease (Golde and Eckman, 2001; Hofman *et al.*, 1997).

Cardioprotective

Oleuropein has been shown to be cardioprotective against acute adriamycin cardiotoxicity (Andreadou *et al.*, 2007) and has been shown to exhibit anti-ischemic and hypolipidemic activities (Andreadou *et al.*, 2006). Pharmacological activity of oleuropein includes diverse healing effects due to its vasodilatory (Petkov and Manolov, 1978) antiplatelet aggregation (Petroni *et al.*, 1995) and hypotensive (Ribeiro *et al.*, 1986; Khayyal *et al.*, 2002) properties. Oleuropein reduced infarct size, plasma lipid concentrations, and plasma markers of oxidative stress in cholesterol-fed rabbits (*Andreadou et al., 2006; Al-Azzawie et al., 2006*). A potentially dose dependent inhibition of copper sulphate-induced oxidation of low-density lipoproteins (LDL) was reported by Visioli *et al.* (2002 a; 2006) and Coni *et al.* (2000). The olive leaf extract fed to rats at 500 or 1000 mg/d for 8 weeks exhibited cardioprotective effects. The blood pressure changed significantly within pairs, depending on the dose, with mean systolic differences of d" 6 mmHg (500 mg vs control) and d"13 mmHg (1000 vs 500 mg), and diastolic differences of d" 5 mmHg. Cholesterol levels decreased for all treatments with significant dose-dependent within-pair differences for LDL-cholesterol. Thus, the study confirmed the antihypertensive and cholesterol-lowering action of EFLA943 in humans (Perrinjaquet-Moccetti, 2008). Olive leaf extract reduced the LDL/HDL ratio in doses 50, 75, and 100mg/kg/day in comparison to the control group ($P<0.001$), and offered cerebroprotection from ischemia-reperfusion (Mohagheghi *et al.*, 2011).

Intravenous administration of aqueous and ethanolic extracts of O. africana caused an immediate and dose dependent fall in mean arterial pressure (MAP) and heart rate (HR) in anaesthetised normotensive rats. The aqueous extract was more potent than the ethanolic extract. Orally administered aqueous extract produced lowering of MAP and HR in DOCA-salt hypertensive rats. Propranolol partially blocked the Map lowering effect of *O. africana* (Osim *et al.*, 1999). This effect may be mediated via beta adrenergic receptors. Oral administration of the extract at different dose levels at the same time for a period of 8 weeks showed a dose dependent prophylactic effect against the rise in blood pressure induced by L-NG-Nitroarginine Methyl Ester (L-NAME) best effects being induced by a dose of 100 mg/kg of the extract. In rats previously rendered hypertensive by L-NAME for 6 weeks and then treated with the dose of the extract for a further 6 weeks without discontinuation of L-NAME, normalization of the blood pressure was observed (Khayyal *et al.*, 2002). The antihypertensive effect of the extract may be related to a variety of factors. Hypertensive patients fed *Olea europeae* L. leaf aqueous extract at 400 ng x 4/24 h for 3 months, showed a statistically significant decrease in blood pressure after 15 days treatment with no side effects in a placebo control trial (Cherif *et al.*, 1996).

All the isolates, in a dose 60 mg/kg BW for 6 weeks treatment, prevented the development of severe hypertension and atherosclerosis and also improved the insulin resistance of the experimental animals. Thus, Greek olive leaves, African wild olive leaves and Cape Town cultivar isolates could provide an effective and cheap treatment of the most common type of salt-sensitive hypertension in the African population (Somova *et al.*, 2003).

Antidiabetic

Polyphenols such as oleuropein and hydroxytyrosol from olive leaf extract reverses the chronic inflammation and oxidative stress that induces the cardiovascular, hepatic, and metabolic symptoms in the rat model of diet-induced obesity and diabetes without changing blood pressure (Poudyal *et al.*, 2010). In streptozotocin-induced diabetic rats, olive leaf extract decreased serum concentrations of glucose, lipids, uric acid, creatinine, and liver enzymes (Eidi *et al.*, 2009).

Administration, for 4 weeks, of oleuropein and hydroxytyrosol rich extracts, at 8 and 16 mg/kg body weight of each compound in diabetes induced Wistar rats significantly decreased the serum glucose and cholesterols levels and restored the antioxidant perturbations. The antidiabetic effect of oleuropein and hydroxytyrosol might be due to their antioxidant activities restraining the oxidative stress which is widely associated with diabetes pathologies and complications (Jemai *et al.*, 2009).

Hamden *et al.* (2009) and Fki (2007) demonstrated for the first time that OMW polyphenols and especially purified hydroxytyrosol (HT) are efficient in inhibiting hyper-glycemia and oxidative stress induced by diabetes and suggest that administration of HT may be helpful in the prevention of diabetic complications associated with oxidative stress. Olive leaf extract (100–500 mg/kg) decreased serum concentrations of glucose, lipids, uric acid, creatinine, and liver enzymes in streptozotocin-induced diabetic rats (Eidi *et al.*, 2009).

Anticarcinogenic

Both olives and olive oil contain substantial amounts of anticancer agents (*e.g.* squalene and terpenoids) as well as the peroxidation-resistant lipid, oleic acid (Owen *et al.*, 2004). The protective effects of *Olea europea* L. (olive) leaf and fruit extracts on live cell viability were mediated through the suppression of caspase 3/7 activity. Oleuropein did not decrease the amount of both apoptotic and necrotic cells, whereas extracts significantly protected cells against cytokine-induced death. The molecular mechanism by which olive polyphenols inhibit cytokine-mediated β-cell toxicity appears to be involving the maintenance of redox homeostasis (Cumaoðlu *et al.*, 2011).

Olive leaf extracts showed concentration-dependent anti-proliferative effect as determined by the WST-1 proliferation kit and [(3) H]-thymidine incorporation method. Thus, Fares *et al.* (2011) confirmed that olive leaves extracts exhibit antiproliferative effect on leukemic cells by inducing apoptosis. According to De la Puerta *et al.* (2001), oleuropein has both the ability to scavenge nitric oxide and to cause an increase in the inducible nitric oxide synthase (iNOS) expression in the cell. Goulas *et al.* (2009) demonstrated the antiproliferative activity of oleuropein extracts in cell lines at low micromolar concentrations.

Hamdi and Castellon (2005) showed that oleuropein inhibits growth of LN-18 cells, erythroleukemia and tumour cell lines derived from advanced-grade human tumours, malignant melanoma of the skin-lymph node metastasis and colourectal adenocarcinoma cells in Swiss albino mice with soft tissue sarcoma. Han *et al.* (2009) reported that 200 µg/mL of oleuropein remarkably reduces the viability of MCF-7 cells and decreases the number of MCF-7 cells by inhibiting the rate of cell proliferation and inducing cell apoptosis.

Eythrodiol, uvaol, and oleanolic acid have a significant cytotoxic effect and inhibit proliferation in a dose- and time-dependent manner. At 100 µm, erythrodiol growth inhibition occurred through apoptosis, with the observation of important ROS production and DNA damage, whereas uvaol and oleanolic acid growth inhibition involved cell cycle arrest. The triterpenes protected against oxidative DNA damage at the concentration 10 µM. Uvaol and oleanolic and maslinic acids, tested at 10 and 100 µM, also reduced intracellular ROS level and prevented H(2)O(2)-induced oxidative injury. These results suggest that tested triterpenes may have the potential to provide significant natural defense against human breast cancer (Allouche *et al.*, 2011). Menendez *et al.* (2007) showed that oleuropein aglycone is the most potent phenolic compound in decreasing breast cancer cell viability. Subsequently, Menendez *et al.* (2008a; 2008b; 2009) showed that the secoiridoids deacetoxy oleuropein aglycone, ligstroside aglycone, and oleuropein aglycone, induce strong tumouricidal effects within a micromolar range by selectively triggering high levels of apoptotic cell death in HER2-overexpressing breast carcinomas.

Antiosteoporotic

Oeuropein at 10 to 100µM and hydroxytyrosol at 50 to 100µm inhibited the formation of multinucleated osteoclasts in a dose-dependent manner. Furthermore, both compounds suppressed the bone loss of trabecular bone in femurs of ovariectomized mice (6-week-old BALB/c female mice), while hydroxytyrosol attenuated H_2O_2 levels in MC3T3-E1 cells thus indicating that the olive polyphenols oleuropein and hydroxytyrosol may have critical effects on the formation and maintenance of bone, and can be used as effective remedy in the treatment of osteoporosis symptoms (Hagiwara *et al.*, 2011).

Both oleuropein and olive oil prevented bone loss in ovariectomised rats with inflammation. At necropsy, oleuropein and olive oil consumption had no effect on plasma osteocalcin concentrations (marker of bone formation) or on urinary deoxypyridinoline excretion (marker of bone resorption). In conclusion, oleuropein and olive-oil feeding can prevent inflammation-induced osteopenia in ovariectomised rats (Puel *et al.*, 2004).

Tyrosol and hydroxytyrosol prevented osteopenia by increasing bone formation, probably because of their antioxidant properties. The two doses of olive oil mill waste water had the same protective effect on bone but did not reverse established osteopenia. Puel *et al.* (2006; 2008) reported that a polyphenol, oleuropein at 2.5, 5, 10 or 15 mg/kg body weight per day for 100 days reduced bone loss in ovariectomised rats associated with inflammation, probably by modulating inflammatory parameters.

Other Benefits

Leaves and fruits of *Olea europaea* L.are used for the treatment of various kinds of diseases, *i.e.*, rheumatism and haemorrhoids, and as a vasodilator in vascular disorders for ages in folk medicine. Olive leaf extract (OLE) could potentiate the antinociceptive effect of 5 mg/kg morphine and block low-dose morphine-induced hyperalgesia. Administration of 200 mg/kg OLE (i.p.) caused significant decrease in pain responses in the first and the second phases of formalin test. Thus, the experimental results of Esmaeili-Mahani *et al.* (2010) indicated that olive leaf extract has analgesic property in several models of pain and useful influence on morphine analgesia in rats.

Gupta *et al.* (2010) demonstrated that treatment with olive extract to result in a significant decrease in the immobility time as well as hyperalgesia in a mouse model of immunologically-induced fatigue. There was significant attenuation of oxidative stress as well as serum TNF-α level, strongly indicating the role of oxidative stress and immunological activation in the pathophysiology of chronic fatigue syndrome and highlighting the valuable role of olive extract in combating chronic fatigue syndrome.

Conclusion

The available scientific evidence indicates the nutraceutical importance of oleorupein besides emphasizing the therapeutic benefits of olive leaves and oil.

References

Al-Azzawie HF, Alhamdani MS (2006). Hypoglycaemic and antioxidant effect of oleuropein in alloxan-diabetic rabbits. Life Sci. 78: 1371–77.

Aldini G, Piccoli A, Beretta G, Morazzoni P, Riva A, Marinello C, Maffei Facino R (2006). Antioxidant activity of polyphenols from solid olive residues of c.v. Coratina. Fitoterapia. 77 (2): 121–28.

Allouche Y, Warleta F, Campos M, Sánchez-Quesada C, Uceda M, Beltrán G, Gaforio JJ (2011). Antioxidant, antiproliferative, and pro-apoptotic capacities of pentacyclic triterpenes found in the skin of olives on MCF-7 human breast cancer cells and their effects on DNA damage. J. Agric. Food. Chem. 59 (1): 121–30.

Amiot MJ, Fleuriet A, Macheix JJ (1986). Importance and evolution of phenolic compounds in olive during growth and maturation. J. Agric. Food Chem. 34: 823–26.

Andreadou I, Iliodromitis EK, Mikros E, Constantinou M, Agalias A, Magiatis P, Skaltsounis AL, Kamber E, Tsantili-Kakoulidou A (2006). The olive constituent oleuropein exhibits anti-ischemic, antioxidative, and hypolipidemic effects in anesthetized rabbits. J. Nutr. 136: 2213–19.

Andreadou I, Sigala F, Iliodromitis EK, Papaefthimiou M, Sigalas C, Aligiannis N, Savvari P, Gorgoulis V, Papalabros E, Kremastinos DT (2007). Acute doxorubicin cardiotoxicity is successfully treated with the phytochemical oleuropein through suppression of oxidative and nitrosative stress. J. Mol. Cell. Cardiol. 42: 549–58.

Aziz NH, Farag SF, Mousa LA, Abo-Zaid MA (1998). Comparative antibacterial and antifungal effects of some phenolic compounds. Microbios. 93: 43–54.

Bazoti FN, Bergquist J, Markides K, Tsarbopoulos A (2006). Noncovalent Interaction between Amyloid-β-Peptide (1–40) and Oleuropein Studied by Electrospray Ionization Mass Spectrometry. J. Am. Soc. Mass. Spectrom. 17: 568–75.

Bisignano G, Tomaino A, Lo Cascio R, Crisafi G, Uccella N, Saija A (1999). On the *in vitro* antimicrobial activity of oleuropein and hydroxytyrosol. J. Pharm. Pharmacol. 51: 971–74.

Bouaziz M, Chamkha M, Sayadi S (2004). Comparative study on phenolic content and antioxidant activity during maturation of the olive cultivar Chemlali from Tunisia. J. Agric. Food. Chem. 52 (17): 5476–81.

Bouaziz M, Jemai H, Khabou W, Sayadi S (2010). Oil content, phenolic profiling and antioxidant potential of Tunisian olive drupes. J. Sci. Food. Agric. 90 (10): 1750–58.

Carluccio MA, Siculella L, Ancora MA, Massaro M, Scoditti E, Storelli C, Visioli F, Distante A, De Caterina R (2003). Olive oil and red wine antioxidant polyphenols inhibit endothelial activation: antiatherogenic properties of mediterranean diet phytochemicals. Arterioscler. Thromb. Vasc. Biol. 23: 622–29.

Caturla N, Perez Fons L, Estepa A, Micol V (2005). Differential effects of oleuropein, a biophenol from *Olea europaea,* on anionic and zwiterionic phospholipid model membranes. Chem. Phys. Lipids. 137: 2–17.

Cherif S, Rahal N, Haouala M, Hizaoui B, Dargouth F, Gueddiche M, Kallel Z, Balansard G, Boukef K (1996). [A clinical trial of a titrated Olea extract in the treatment of essential arterial hypertension]. J. Pharm. Belg. 51 (2): 69–71. [Article in French].

Chiou A, Salta FN, Kalogeropoulos N, Mylona A, Ntalla I, Andrikopoulos NK (2007). Retention and distribution of polyphenols after pan-frying of French fries in oils (Cenriched with olive leaf extract. J. Food Sci. 72: S574–84.

Coni E, Benedetto R, Pasquale M, Masella R, Modesti D, Mattei R, Carline EA. (2000). Protective effect of oleuropein, an olive oil biophenol, on low density lipoprotein oxidizability in rabbits. Lipids. 35: 45–54.

Corona G, Tzounis X, Assunta Dessi M, Deiana M, Debnam ES, Visioli F, Spencer JP (2006). The fate of olive oil polyphenols in the gastrointestinal tract: implications of gastric and colonic microflora-dependent biotransformation. Free Radic. Res. 40: 647- 58.

Cumaoðlu A, Ari N, Kartal M, Karasu Ç (2011). Polyphenolic extracts from Olea europea L. protect against cytokine-induced β-cell damage through maintenance of redox homeostasis. Rejuvenation Res. 14 (3): 325–34.

De la Puerta R, Guttierrez VR, Hoult JRS (1999). Inhibition of leukocyte 5-lipoxygenase by phenolics from virgin olive oil. Biochem. Pharmacol. 57: 445–49.

De la Puerta R, Dominguez MEM, Ruiz-Guttierrez V, Flavill JA, Hoult JRS (2001). Effects of olive oil phenolics on scavenging of reactive nitrogen species and upon nitrergic neurotransmission. Life Sci. 69: 1213–22.

Del Rio D, Stewart AJ, Pellegrini N (2005). A review of recent studies on malondialdehyde as toxic molecule and biological marker of oxidative stress. Nutr. Metab. Cardiovasc. Dis. 15: 316–28.

Eidi A, Eidi M, Darzi R (2009). Antidiabetic effect of *Olea europaea* L. in normal and diabetic rats. Phytother. Res. 23: 347–50.

El SN, Karakaya S (2009). Olive tree (*Olea europaea*) leaves: potential beneficial effects on human health. Nutr. Rev. 67 (11): 632–38.

Esmaeili-Mahani S, Rezaeezadeh-Roukerd M, Esmaeilpour K, Abbasnejad M, Rasoulian B, Sheibani V, Kaeidi A, Hajializadeh Z (2010). Olive (*Olea europaea* L.) leaf extract elicits antinociceptive activity, potentiates morphine analgesia and suppresses morphine hyperalgesia in rats. J. Ethnopharmacol. 132 (1): 200–205.

Fares R, Bazzi S, Baydoun SE, Abdel-Massih RM (2011).The antioxidant and anti-proliferative activity of the Lebanese *Olea europaea* extract. Plant. Foods Hum. Nutr. 66 (1): 58–63.

Fki I, Bouaziz M, Sahnoun Z, Sayadi S (2005). Hypocholesterolemic effects of phenolic-rich extracts of Chemlali olive cultivar in rats fed a cholesterol-rich diet. Bioorg. Med. Chem. 13: 5362–70.

Fki I, Sahnoun Z, Sayadi S (2007). Hypocholesterolemic effects of phenolic extracts and purified hydroxytyrosol recovered from olive mill wastewater in rats fed a cholesterol-rich diet. J. Agric. Food Chem. 55 (3): 624–31.

Fleming HP, Walter WM, Jr, Etchells L (1973). Antimicrobial properties of oleuropein and products of its hydrolysis from green olives. Appl. Microbiol. 26: 777–82.

Fredrickson WR, F and S Group, Inc (2002). Method and Composition for Antiviral Therapy with Olive Leaves. U.S. Patent. 2000. 6: 117, 884.

Furneri PM, Marino A, Saija A, Ucella N, Bisignano G. *In vitro* antimycoplasmal activity of oleuropein. Int. J. Antimicrob. Agents. 20: 293–96.

Golde TE, Eckman CB (2001). Cholesterol Modulation as an Emerging Strategy for the Treatment of Alzheimer's Disease. Drug Discov Today. 6: 1049–55.

Goulas V, Exarchou V, Troganis AN, Psomiadou E, Fotsis T, Briasoulis E, Gerothanassis IP (2009). Phytochemicals in olive-leaf extracts and their antiproliferative activity against cancer and endothelial cells. Mol. Nutr. Food Res. 53: 600–608.

Gupta A, Vij G, Chopra K (2010). Possible role of oxidative stress and immunological activation in mouse model of chronic fatigue syndrome and its attenuation by olive extract. J. Neuroimmunol. 226 (1-2): 3–7.

Hagiwara K, Goto T, Araki M, Miyazaki H, Hagiwara H (2011). Olive polyphenol hydroxytyrosol prevents bone loss. Eur. J. Pharmacol. 662 (1-3): 78–84.

Hamden K, Allouche N, Damak M, Elfeki A (2009). Hypoglycaemic and antioxidant effects of phenolic extracts and purified hydroxytyrosol from olive mill waste *in vitro* and in rats. Chem. Biol. Interact. 180 (3): 421–32.

Hamdi HK, Castellon R (2005). Oleuropein, a non-toxic olive iridoid, is an anti-tumour agent and cytoskeleton disruptor. Biochem. Biophys. Res. Commun. 334: 769–78.

Han J, Talorete TP, Yamada P, Isoda H (2009). Anti-proliferative and apoptotic effects of oleuropein and hydroxytyrosol on human breast cancer MCF-7 cells. Cytotechnology. 59: 45–53.

Hofman A, Ott A, Breteler MM, Bots ML, Slooter AJ, van Harskamp F, van Duijn CN, Van Broeckhoven C, Grobbee DE (1997). Atherosclerosis, Apolipoprotein E, and Prevalence of Dementia and Alzheimer's Disease in the Rotterdam Study. Lancet. 349: 151–54.

Jemai H, Bouaziz M, Fki I, El Feki A, Sayadi S (2008). Hypolipidimic and antioxidant activities of oleuropein and its hydrolysis derivative-rich extracts from Chemlali olive leaves. Chem. Biol. Interact. 176: 88–98.

Jemai H, El Feki A, Sayadi S (2009). Antidiabetic and antioxidant effects of hydroxytyrosol and oleuropein from olive leaves in alloxan-diabetic rats. J. Agric. Food Chem. 57 (19): 8798 -804.

Kaeidi A, Esmaeili-Mahani S, Sheibani V, Abbasnejad M, Rasoulian B, Hajializadeh Z, Afrazi S (2011). Olive (*Olea europaea* L.) leaf extract attenuates early diabetic neuropathic pain through prevention of high glucose-induced apoptosis: *in vitro* and *in vivo* studies. J. Ethnopharmacol. 136 (1): 188–96.

Khayyal MT, el-Ghazaly MA, Abdallah DM, Nassar NN, Okpanyi SN, Kreuter MH (2002). Blood pressure lowering effect of an olive leaf extract (*Olea europaea*) in L-NAME induced hypertension in rats. Arzneimittelforschung. 52 (11): 797–802.

Koca U, Süntar I, Akkol EK, Yilmazer D, Alper M (2011). Wound repair potential of Olea europaea L. leaf extracts revealed by *in vivo* experimental models and comparative evaluation of the extracts' antioxidant activity. J. Med. Food. 14 (1-2): 140–46.

Kiritsakis A (1998). Olive oil- Second Edition, From the tree to the table. Food and Nutrition. Press, Inc.; Trumbull, Connecticut, USA. p. 006611.

Lasserre B, Kaiser R, Huu Chanh P, Ifansyah N, Gleye J, Moulis C (1983). Effects on rats of aqueous extracts of plants used in folk medicine as antihypertensive agents. Naturwissenschaften. 70: 95–96.

Le Tutour B, Guedon D (1992). Antioxidant activities of *Olea europaea* leaves and related phenolic compounds. Phytochemistry. 31: 1173–78.

Lee OH, Lee BY, Lee J, Lee HB, Son JY, Park CS, Shetty K, Kim YC (2009). Assessment of phenolics-enriched extract and fractions of olive leaves and their antioxidant activities. Bioresour. Technol. 100: 6107–13.

Lee-Huang S, Zhang L, Chang YY, Huang PL (2003). Anti-HIV activity of olive leaf extract (OLE) and modulation of host cell gene expression by HIV-1 infection and OLE treatment. Biochem. Biophys. Res. Commun. 307: 1029–37.

Loizzo MR, Said A, Tundis R, Rashed K, Statti GA, Hufner A, Menichini F (2007). Inhibition of angiotensin converting enzyme (ACE) by flavonoids isolated from *Ailanthus excelsa* (Roxb) (Simaroubaceae). Phytother. Res. 21: 32–36.

Lopez-Lazaro M (2009). Distribution and biological activities of the flavonoid luteolin. Mini. Rev. Med. Chem. 9: 31–59.

Ma X, Li YF, Gao Q, Ye ZG, Lu XJ, Wang HP, Jiang HD, Bruce IC, Xia Q (2008). Inhibition of superoxide anion-mediated impairment of endothelium by treatment with luteolin and apigenin in rat mesenteric artery. Life Sci. 83:110–17.

Manna C, Migliardi V, Golino P, Scognamiglio A, Galletti P, Chiariello M, Zappia V (2004). Oleuropein prevents oxidative myocardial injury induced by ischemia and reperfusion. J. Nutr. Biochem. 15: 461–68.

Medina E, Brenes M, Romero C, García A, de Castro A (2007). Main antimicrobial compounds in table olives. J. Agric. Food Chem. 55 (24): 9817–23.

Mene P, Punzo G (2008). Uric acid: bystander or culprit in hypertension and progressive renal disease? J. Hypertens. 26: 2085–82.

Menendez JA, Vazquez-Martin A, Colomer R, Brunet J, Carrasco-Pancorbo A, Garcia-Villalba R, Fernandez-Gutierrez A, Segura-Carretero A (2007). Olive oil's bitter principle reverses acquired autoresistance to trastuzumab (Herceptin™) in HER2-overexpressing breast cancer cells. BMC. Cancer. 7: 80.

Menendez JA, Vazquez-Martin A, Garcia-Villalba R, Carrasco-Pancorbo A, Oliveras-Ferraros C, Fernandez-Gutierrez A, Segura-Carretero A (2008a). Anti-HER2 (*erb*B-2) oncogene effects of phenolic compounds directly isolated from commercial Extra-Virgin Olive Oil (EVOO). BMC. Cancer. 8: 377.

Menendez JA, Vazquez-Martin A, Oliveras-Ferraros C, Garcia-Villalba R, Carrasco-Pancorbo A, Fernandez-Gutierrez A, Segura-Carretero A (2008b). Analyzing effects of extra-virgin olive oil polyphenols on breast cancer-associated fatty acid synthase protein expression using reverse-phase protein microarrays. Int. J. Mol. Med. 22 (4): 433–39.

Menendez JA, Vazquez-Martin A, Oliveras-Ferraros C, Garcia-Villalba R, Carrasco-Pancorbo A, Fernandez-Gutierrez A, Segura-Carretero A (2009). Extra-virgin olive oil polyphenols inhibit HER2 (erbB-2)-induced malignant transformation in human breast epithelial cells: relationship between the chemical structures of extra-virgin olive oil secoiridoids and lignans and their inhibitory activities on the tyrosine kinase activity of HER2. Int. J. Oncol. 34 (1): 43–51.

Micol V, Caturla N, Perenz-Fons L, Mas L, Perez L, Estepa A (2005). The olive leaf extract exhibits antiviral activity against viral haemorrhagic septicaemia rhabdovirus (VHSV) Antivir. Res. 66: 129–36.

Miles EA, Zoubouli P, Calder PC (2005). Differential anti-inflammatory effects of phenolic compounds from extra virgin olive oil identified in human whole blood cultures. Nutrition. 21: 389–94.

Mohagheghi F, Bigdeli MR, Rasoulian B, Hashemi P, Pour MR (2011). The neuroprotective effect of olive leaf extract is related to improved blood-brain barrier permeability and brain edema in rat with experimental focal cerebral ischemia. Phytomedicine. 18 (2-3): 170–75.

Mulinacci N, Innocenti M, La Marca G, Mercalli E, Giaccherini C, Romani A, Erica S, Vincieri FF (2005). Solid olive residues: insight into their phenolic composition. J. Agric.Food Chem. 53 (23): 8963–69.

Muzzalupo I, Stefanizzi F, Perri E, Chiappetta AA (2011). Transcript levels of CHL P gene, antioxidants and chlorophylls contents in olive (*Olea europaea* L.) pericarps: a comparative study on eleven olive cultivars harvested in two ripening stages. Plant. Foods. Hum. Nutr. 66 (1): 1–10.

Obied HK, Allen MS, Bedgood DR, Prenzler PD, Robards K, Stockmann R (2005). Bioactivity and analysis of biophenols recovered from olive mill waste. J. Agric. Food Chem. 53 (4): 823–37.

Obied HK, Bedgood DR Jr, Prenzler PD, Robards K (2007a). Bioscreening of Australian olive mill waste extracts: biophenol content, antioxidant, antimicrobial and molluscicidal activities. Food Chem. Toxicol. 45 (7): 1238–48.

Obied HK, Bedgood DR Jr, Prenzler PD, Robards K (2008). Effect of processing conditions, prestorage treatment, and storage conditions on the phenol content and antioxidant activity of olive mill waste. J. Agric. Food Chem. 56 (11): 3925–32.

Obied HK, Karuso P, Prenzler PD, Robards K (2007b). Novel secoiridoids with antioxidant activity from Australian olive mill waste. J. Agric. Food Chem. 55 (8): 2848–53.

Omar SH (2010). Oleuropein in olive and its pharmacological effects. Sci. Pharm. 78 (2): 133–54.

Osim EE, Mbajiorgu EF, Mukarati G, Vaz RF, Makufa B, Munjeri O, Musabayane CT (1999). Hypotensive effect of crude extract *Olea africana* (Oleaceae) in normo and hypertensive rats. Cent. Afr. J. Med. 45 (10): 269–74.

Owen RW, Giacosa A, Hull WE, Haubner R, Würtele G, Spiegelhalder B, Bartsch H (2000). Olive oil consumption and health: the possible role of antioxidants. Lancet Oncol. 1: 107–112.

Owen RW, Haubner R, Würtele G, Hull E, Spiegelhalder B, Bartsch H (2004). Olives and olive oil in cancer prevention. Eur. J. Cancer. Prev. 13 (4): 319–26.

Perrinjaquet-Moccetti T, Busjahn A, Schmidlin C, Schmidt A, Bradl B, Aydogan C

(2008). Food supplementation with an olive (*Olea europaea* L.) leaf extract reduces blood pressure in borderline hypertensive monozygotic twins. Phytother. Res. 22 (9): 1239–42.

Petkov V, Manolov P (1978). Pharmacological studies on substances of plant origin with coronary dilatating and antiarrhythmatic action. Comp. Med. East West. 6: 123–30.

Petroni A, Blasevich M, Salami M, Papini N, Montedoro GF, Galli C (1995). Inhibition of platelet aggregation and eicosanoid production by phenolic components of olive oil. Thromb. Res. 78: 151–60.

Poudyal H, Campbell F, Brown L (2010). Olive leaf extract attenuates cardiac, hepatic, and metabolic changes in high carbohydrate-, high fat-fed rats. J. Nutr. 140 (5): 946–53.

Puel C, Mardon J, Agalias A, Davicco MJ, Lebecque P, Mazur A, Horcajada MN, Skaltsounis AL, Coxam V (2008). Major phenolic compounds in olive oil modulate bone loss in an ovariectomy/inflammation experimental model. J. Agric. Food. Chem. 56 (20): 9417–22.

Puel C, Mathey J, Agalias A, Kati-Coulibaly S, Mardon J, Obled C, Davicco MJ, Lebecque P, Horcajada MN, Skaltsounis AL, Coxam V (2006). Dose-response study of effect of oleuropein, an olive oil polyphenol, in an ovariectomy/inflammation experimental model of bone loss in the rat. Clin. Nutr. 25 (5): 859–68.

Puel C, Quintin A, Agalias A, Mathey J, Obled C, Mazur A, Davicco MJ, Lebecque P, Skaltsounis AL, Coxam V (2004). Olive oil and its main phenolic micronutrient (oleuropein) prevent inflammation-induced bone loss in the ovariectomised rat. Br. J. Nutr. 92 (1): 119–27.

Qian LB, Wang HP, Chen Y, Chen FX, Ma YY, Bruce IC, Xia Q (2010). Luteolin reduces high glucose-mediated impairment of endothelium-dependent relaxation in rat aorta by reducing oxidative stress. Pharmacol. Res. 61 (4): 281–87.

Raederstorff D (2009). Antioxidant activity of olive polyphenols in humans: a review. Int. J. Vitam. Nutr. Res. 79 (3): 152–65.

Ribeiro Rde A, de Melo MM, Fiuza, De Barros F, Gomes C, Trolin G (1986). Acute antihypertensive effect in conscious rats produced by some medicinal plants used in the state of Sao Paulo. J. Ethnopharmacol. 15: 261–69.

Roche M, Dufour C, Loonis M, Reist M, Carrupt PA, Dangles O (2009). Olive phenols efficiently inhibit the oxidation of serum albumin-bound linoleic acid and butyrylcholine esterase. Biochim. Biophys. Acta. 1790 (4): 240–48.

Rodríguez G, Lama A, Jaramillo S, Fuentes-Alventosa JM, Guillén R, Jiménez-Araujo A, Rodríguez-Arcos R, Fernández-Bolaños J (2009). 3,4-Dihydroxyphenylglycol (DHPG): an important phenolic compound present in natural table olives. J. Agric. Food Chem. 57 (14): 6298–304.

Saenz MT, Garcia MD, Ahumada MC, Ruiz V (1998). Cytostatic activity of some compounds from the unsaponifiable fraction obtained from virgin olive oil. Farmaco. 53: 448–49.

Saija A, Uccella N (2001). Olive biophenols: functional effects on human well-being. Trends. Food Sci. Technol. 11: 357–63.

Sato H, Genet C, Strehle A, Thomas C, Lobstein A, Wagner A, Mioskowski C, Auwerx J, Saladin R (2007). Anti-hyperglycemic activity of a TGR5 agonist isolated from *Olea europaea*. Biochem. Biophys. Res. Commun. 362: 793–98.

Scheffler A, Rauwald HW, Kampa B, Mann U, Mohr FW, Dhein S (2008). *Olea europaea* leaf extract exerts L-type Ca $^{(2+)}$ channel antagonistic effects. J. Ethnopharmacol. 120: 233- 40.

Servili M, Settanni L, Veneziani G, Esposto S, Massitti O, Taticchi A, Urbani S, Montedoro GF, Corsetti A (2006). The use of *Lactobacillus pentosus* 1MO to shorten the debittering process time of black table olives (Cv. Itrana and Leccino): a pilot-scale application. J. Agric. Food Chem. 54 (11): 3869–75.

Soler-Rivas C, Espin JC, Wichers HJ (2000). Oleuropein and related compounds. J. Sci. Food Agric. 80: 1013–23.

Somova LI, Shode FO, Ramnanan P, Nadar A (2003). Antihypertensive, anti atherosclerotic and antioxidant activity of triterpenoids isolated from *Olea europaea*, subspecies africana leaves. J. Ethnopharmacol. 84 (2-3): 299–305.

Sousa A, Casal S, Bento A, Malheiro R, Oliveira MB, Pereira JA (2011). Chemical characterization of "alcaparras" stoned table olives from northeast Portugal. Molecules. 16 (11): 9025–40.

Stamatakis G, Tsantila N, Samiotaki M, Panayotou GN, Dimopoulos AC, Halvadakis CP, Demopoulos CA (2009). Detection and isolation of antiatherogenic and antioxidant substances present in olive mill wastes by a novel filtration system. J. Agric. Food Chem. 57 (22): 10554–64.

Süntar IP, Akkol EK, Baykal T (2010). Assessment of anti-inflammatory and antinociceptive activities of *Olea europaea* L. J. Med. Food. 13 (2): 352–356.

Tassou CC, Nychas GJE, Board RG (1991). Effect of phenolic compounds and oleuropein on the germination of *Bacillus cereus* T spores. Biotech. Appl. Biochem. 13: 231–37.

Tassou CC, Nychas GJE (1994). Inhibition of *Staphylococcus aureus* by olive phenolics in broth and in a model food system. J. Food Prot. 57: 120–24.

Tassou CC, Nychas GJE (1995). Inhibition of *Salmonella enteritidis* by oleuropein in broth and in a model food system. Lett. Appl. Microbiol. 20: 120–24.Tranter HS, Tassou SC, Nychas GJ (1993). The effect of the olive phenolic compound, oleuropein, on growth and enterotoxin B production by. Staphylococcus aureus. J. Appl. Bacteriol. 74: 253–59.

Tripoli E, Giammanco M, Tabacchi G, Di Majo D, Giammanco S, La Guardia M (2005). The phenolic composition of olive oil: structure, biological activity, and beneficial effects on human health. Nutr. Res. Rev. 18: 98–112.

USDA (2012). National Nutrient Database for Standard Reference, Release 25.

Visioli F, Bellomo G, Galli C (1998a). Free radical-scavenging properties of olive oil polyphenols. Biochem. Biophys. Res. Commun. 247: 60–64.

Visioli F, Bellosta S, Galli C (1998b). Oleuropein, the bitter principles of olives, enhances nitric oxide production by mouse macrophages. Life Sci. 62: 541–46.

Visioli F, Bogani P, Galli C (2006). In: Healthful properties of olive oil minor components, in Olive Oil, Chemistry and Technology. Boskou D, editor. AOCS Press. Champaign, IL. pp. 173–90.

Visioli F, Caruso D, Galli C, Viappiani S, Galli G, Sala A (2000). Olive oil rich in natural catecholic phenols decrease isoprostane excretion in humans. Biochem. Biophys. Res. Commun. 278: 797–99.

Visioli F, Galli C (2001). Antiatherogenic components of olive oil. Curr.Atheroscler. Rep. 3 (1): 64–67.

Visioli F, Galli C, Galli G, Caruso D (2002 a). Biological activities and metabolic fate of olive oil phenols. Eur. J. Lipid Sci. Technol. 104: 677–84.

Visioli F, Poli A, Gall C (2002 b). Antioxidant and other biological activities of phenols from olives and olive oil. Med. Res. Rev. 22: 65–75.

Walker M (1996). Olive leaf extract. The new oral treatment to counteract most types of pathological organisms. Explore: The Journal of Science and Healing. 7: 31.

Walter WM, Jr, Flemming HP, Etchells JL (1973). Preparation of antimicrobial compounds by hydrolysis of oleuropein from green olives. Appl. Microbiol. 26: 773–76.

Zarzuelo A, Duarte J, Jimenez J, Gonzalez M, Utrilla MP (1991). Vasodilator effect of olive leaf. Planta. Med. 57: 417–19.

Chapter 20
Honey

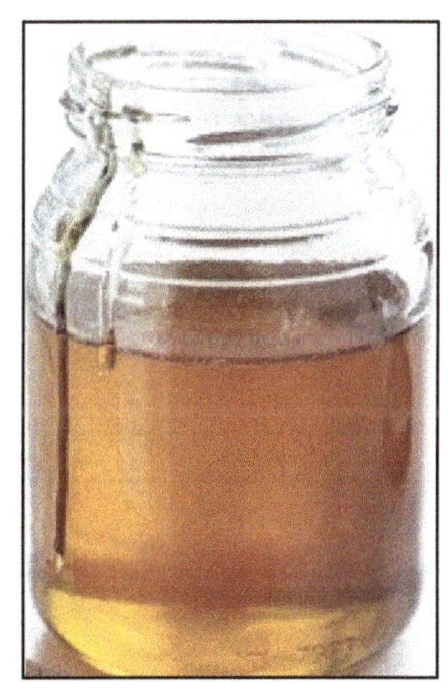

Honey is a natural highly nutritious product that has been widely used in folk medicine for a number of therapeutic purposes. Apart from ancient Egyptians and Greeks, populations all over the world used natural unprocessed honeys from different sources to treat a broad spectrum of wounds (Molan, 1999). Moreover, Honey is believed to be traditional, acceptable, accessible, natural and safe.

Varieties of Honey

Several varieties of honey are available throughout the world. Some of them are, Trigona carbonaria honey, from Australia, Tualang honey, Apis mellifera honey, Italian Castanea, Thymus, Arbutus, honeydew honeys, Tanzanian honey, RevamilH source (RS) honey and manuka honey.

Chemical and Nutritional Components of Honey

The nutritional and health relevant components of honey are carbohydrates, mainly fructose and glucose along with 25 different oligosaccharides. Honey is comparable to sugar in its nutritive value. Its composition on an average is 17.1 per cent water, 82.4 pe rcent total carbohydrate and 0.5 per cent proteins, amino acids, vitamins and minerals. The average carbohydrate content is mainly fructose (38.5 per cent) and glucose (31 per cent). The remaining 12.9 per cent of carbohydrates is made up of maltose, sucrose and other sugars (National Honey Board, 2003). Although honey is a high carbohydrate food, its glycemic index varies within a wide range from 32 to 85, depending on the botanical source. It also contains small amounts of proteins, enzymes, amino acids, minerals, trace elements, vitamins, aroma compounds and polyphenols (Bogdanov *et al.*, 2008).

Buratti *et al.* (2007) observed the composition of honey and beehive products to differ qualitatively and quantitatively depending on the regional plant ecology. Oddo *et al.* (2008) on analyses of Trigona carbonaria honey found the flavonoid content to be 10.02 ± 1.59 mg of quercetin equivalents/100 g of honey, and polyphenol contents of 55.74 ± 6.11 mg of gallic acid equivalents/100 g of honey. The antioxidant activity, expressed as percentage of 2,2'-azinobis-(3-ethylbenzothiazoline-6-sulfonic acid) cation decolourization, was 233.96 ± 50.95 µM Trolox equivalents, and free radical 1,1-diphenyl-2-picrylhydrazyl depletion was 48.03 ± 12.58 equivalents of ascorbic acid.

The physicochemical properties of honey harvested from popular honey-producing areas in Tanzania were investigated by Gidamis *et al.* (2004). Honey from Shibe-Dodoma had the highest values of specific gravity, total acidity, free fatty acid content, diastatic number, overall acceptability, and lowest hydroxymethyl-furfural (HMF) level as compared to honey samples from other areas. There was no significant difference in terms of HMF in the honey samples from Tanga, Morogoro, Same, Arusha, and Tabora. HMF levels in all honey samples were far below the maximum acceptable level of 40 mg/kg as recommended by the Codex Alimentarius Commission Standards prior to storage for 6 months. Fresh honey has low amounts of HMF—less than 15 mg/kg—depending on pH-value, temperature and age. The Standards established by Codex Alimentarius Commission (2003) requires that honey has less than than 40 mg/kg HMF to guarantee that the honey has not undergone heating during processing, except for tropical honeys which must be below 80 mg/kg. The physiological effects attributed to honey are supported by experimental and clinical observations.

Nutritional Value per 100 g

Nutrient	*Amount*	*Nutrient*	*Amount*
Energy (kcal)	304.0	Carbohydrates (g)	82.4
Dietary fiber (g)	0.2	Protein (g)	0.3
Calcium (mg)	6	Iron (mg)	0.42
Magnesium (mg)	2.0	Phosphorus (mg)	4.0
Potassium (mg)	52.0	Sodium (mg)	4.0
Zinc (mg)	0.22	Riboflavin (mg)	0.038
Niacin (Vit. B3) (mg)	0.121	Vitamin B6 (mg)	0.024
Folate (Vit. B9) (µg)	2.0	Vitamin C (mg)	0.5

USDA (2012).

Traditional Uses of Honey

Honey is the most common and popular remedy recommended by grand-parents for their grand-children. Honey is said to facilitate better physical performance and resistance to fatigue, particularly for repeated effort; it also promotes higher mental efficiency. Traditionally, ayurvedic system of medicine in India, use honey predominantly as a vehicle for faster absorption of various drugs such as herbal extracts. Secondarily, it is also thought to support the treatment of several more specific ailments, particularly those related to respiratory irritations and infections, mouth sores and eye cataracts. It is administered with hot water and lemon juice. Traditional and Complementary healthcare Approach reported that honey is used by 29 per cent parents for their children. For cough 19.5 per cent Nigerians reported the use of honey with lemon. For ear infections 17 per cent plugged the ear with cotton wool previously dipped in honey, or alcohol (Oyejide and Oke, 1995). The therapeutic value of honey has been partly attributed to its antioxidant properties (Aljadi and Kamaruddin 2004; The National Honey Board, 2003; Gheldof and Engeseth, 2002). Honey is sometimes used as a sugar substitute to limit the exposure to sucrose.

Honey possesses several health benefits due to its antioxidant, antibacterial and antifungal activities and hence considered valuable especially for children and sportsmen.

Antioxidant Properties of Honey

Oxidative damage is implicated in the etiology of cancer, aging, neurological degeneration, cardiovascular disease, inflammatory and other degenerative disorders. The protective effect of antioxidants against coronary heart diseases, has led to the quest for foods rich in antioxidants. Recent nutritional research has focused on the antioxidant potential of foods as the current dietary recommendations insist on increased intake of antioxidant-rich foods rather than supplement specific nutrients (Phillips. *et al.*, 2009). Thus recently many scientists have been concentrating on the antioxidant property of honey.

Tualang honey found in the Malaysian rain forest has been used traditionally for the treatment of various diseases, where its therapeutic value has partly been attributed to its antioxidant properties. Van den Berg *et al.* (2008) reported American buckwheat honey to be most effective in reducing ROS levels amongst other honey samples tested and the authors reported that the major antioxidant properties in buckwheat honey are derived from its phenolic constituents, which are present in relatively large amounts. Kishore *et al.* (2011) confirmed that the elevated free-radical scavenging and antioxidant activity of Tualang honey is due to the increased level of phenolic compounds. Khalil *et al.* (2011) opined that in addition to phenolic compounds, flavonoid in Tualang honey might have contributed to its free radical-scavenging activities.

Khalil *et al.* (2012) evaluated the effects of evaporation, gamma irradiation and temperature on the total polyphenols, flavonoids and 1,1-diphenyl-2-picrylhydrazyl radical-scavenging activities of Tualang honey samples (n = 14) following storage over three, six or twelve months. They found the gamma irradiated honey samples had higher antioxidant potential while evaporation and temperature had minor effects on antioxidant potential although, Mohamed *et al.* (2009) observed the antioxidant properties of gamma irradiated Tualang honey to be similar to other types of honeys reported in the literature, confirming in fact that there is no untoward effect of irradiation on the antioxidant potential of honey.

Honey as Antimicrobial Agent

Honey is increasingly valued for its antibacterial activity which has been known since even before bacteria were discovered. It has been shown to be active against a diverse range of micro-organisms and reports of its inhibitory effect on specific micro-organisms have been extensively documented (Alnaqdy *et al.*, 2005; Al-Waili *et al.*, 2005; Adebolu, 2005; Davis, 2005). Mohapatra *et al.* (2011) proved that honey's bacteriostatic and bactericidal effect are similar to antibiotics, against Gram-positive bacteria (*S. aureus, B. subtilis, B. cereus, E. faecalis,* and *M. luteus*) and Gram-negative bacteria (*E. coli, P. aeruginosa,* and *S. typhi*) organisms and provide alternative therapy against certain bacteria. Brudzynski and Lannigan (2012) demonstrated that bacteriostatic effect of honeys on methicillin-resistant *S. aureus* and vancomycin-resistant *E. faecium* was dose-dependently related to generation of •OH from honey H_2O_2.

Mechanism of Action

Among the possible mechanisms are the presence of inhibitory factors such as flavonoids (Havsteen, 1983) and hydrogen peroxide (Wahdan, 1998; White *et al.*, 1963), low pH and high osmolarity due to its sugar concentration (Willix *et al.*, 1992). Nassar *et al.* (2012) demonstrated more inhibition of bacterial growth, viability, and biofilm formation than artifical honey which contained the same amount of sugars highlighting the potential antibacterial properties of natural honey and suggesting that the antimicrobial mechanism of natural honey is not solely due to its high sugar content.

The good control of infection is attributed to the high osmolarity, but honey can have additional antibacterial activity because of its content of hydrogen peroxide and unidentified substances from certain floral sources. Canadian honeys exhibited antibacterial activity, with higher selectivity against *E. coli* than *B. subtilis*, and that these antibacterial activities were correlated with hydrogen peroxide production in honeys. Thus, Brudzynski (2006) reported that hydrogen peroxide level in honey is a strong predictor of its antibacterial activity.

The non-peroxide antibacterial activity of manuka honey at a concentration of 1.8 per cent (v/v) inhibited the growth of S. aureus during incubation for 8 h. But the growth of seven major wound-infecting species of bacteria tested by the authors was completely inhibited by honeys with and without non-peroxide antibacterial activity at concentration below 11 per cent (v/v) (Willix *et al.*, 1992).

The antibacterial effects of honey were explained subsequently by other scientists. Boukraâ and Amara (2008) speculated that the amylase present in honey hydrolyzed the starch chains of the media to dextrin and maltose which increased the osmotic effect of the media and consequently increased the antibacterial effects. *In vitro*, the antibacterial effect of honey was found to be more pronounced on *E. coli* than on *S. typhimurium* by Badawy *et al.* (2004). Water content, pH value, HMF and the presence of H_2O, all played an important role in the potency of honey as an antibacterial agent. They also reported lower mortality due to infections among mice treated with honey.

Recently, Kwakman *et al.* (2011) attributed the effect to the high sugar concentration, hydrogen peroxide and low pH in honey and more recently, they identified methyl glyoxal and antimicrobial peptide bee defensin-1 as important antibacterial compounds.

Varietal Differences

Paulus *et al.* (2011) reported the differences between the two medical honeys. Revamil H source (RS) honey killed *B. subtilis*, *E. coli* and *P. aeruginosa* within 2 hours, whereas manuka honey had such rapid activity only against B. subtilis. After 24 hours of incubation, both honeys killed all tested bacteria, including methicillin-resistant *S. aureus*. But manuka honey retained activity up to higher dilutions than RS honey. Methylglyoxal was a major bactericidal factor in manuka honey, but after neutralization of this compound manuka honey retained bactericidal activity due to several unknown factors. RS and manuka honey have highly distinct compositions of bactericidal factors, resulting in large differences in bactericidal activity.

Australia has unique native flora and produces honey with a wide range of different physicochemical properties. Irish *et al.* (2011) analysed 477 honey samples and found potentially therapeutically useful antibacterial activity level in 57 per cent of the honey samples, with exceptional activity in samples derived from marri (Corymbia calophylla), jarrah (Eucalyptus marginata) and jellybush (Leptospermum polygalifolium). They attributed the antibacterial activity to hydrogen peroxide produced by the bee-derived enzyme glucose oxidase. Non-hydrogen peroxide activity was detected in 80 (16.8 per cent) samples, and was most consistently seen in honey produced from *Leptospermum* spp.

Voidarou *et al.* (2011) studied the antimicrobial activity of sixty samples of honey of various botanical origins against 16 clinical pathogens and their respective reference strains. All honey samples, despite their origin (coniferous, citrus, thyme or polyfloral), showed antibacterial activity against the pathogens and their respective reference strains at variable levels. Coniferous and thyme honeys showed the highest activity with an average minimum dilution of 17.4 and 19.2 per cent (w/v) followed by citrus and polyfloral honeys with 20.8 and 23.8 per cent respectively.

Fangio *et al.* (2007) found that honeys from the southeast region of Buenos Aires province are active against *E. coli* at 25 and 50 per cent (w/v) concentrations. A reduction of microbial growth of 96 per cent in Mueller-Hinton broth and of 90 per cent in Mac Conkey broth by honey solutions containing 50 per cent and 25 per cent (w/v) respectively was observed.

Tualang honey has a bactericidal as well as bacteriostatic effect. It is used in the dressings as it is easier to apply and is less sticky compared to Manuka honey. Nasir *et al.* (2010) reported that Tualang honey is not as effective as other products such as silver-based dressing or medical grade honey dressing for Gram positive bacteria. Though Tualang honey exhibited variable activities against different microorganisms, they were within the same range as those for Manuka honey. On this basis, Tan *et al.*

(2009) suggested that Tualang honey could potentially be used as an alternative therapeutic agent against certain microorganisms, particularly *A. baumannii* and *S. maltophilia*.

Oral Infections

Honey has been proved to be effective against oral bacterial infections. Badet and Quero (2011) who worked on oral bacteria found Manuka honey to be able to reduce oral pathogens within dental plaque and also to be able to control dental biofilm deposit. Elbagoury and Rasmy (1993) on testing two samples of natural Honey for their antibacterial effect on Bacteroides, mainly the pathogenic black pigmented *B. melaninogenicus* isolated from ten cases of dental infections (dental abscesses and chronic osteomyelitis) observed that the inhibitory effect of honey was not due to its high sugar content or to its acidic pH, when using Schaedler's broth adjusted to the same pH as control.

GI Infections

According to Haffejee and Moosa (1985) honey shortens the duration of bacterial diarrhoea, does not prolong the duration of non-bacterial diarrhoea, and may safely be used as a substitute for glucose in an oral rehydration solution containing electrolytes. Klein *et al.* (2000) confirms that honey has proven antimicrobial activity.

Honey has also been used to treat adult and neo-natal post-operative infections, burns, boils, necrotizing fasciitis, venous ulcers and diabetic foot ulcers (Al-waili *et al.*, 2011).

Wound Healing

Chronically infected wounds are a costly source of suffering, and the widespread existence of unhealed wounds, ulcers, and burns has a great impact on public health and economy. Many interventions, including new medications and technologies, are being used to help achieve significant wound healing and to eliminate infections.

Honey has been used as a wound treatment for more than 2,000 years. The potential role for honey as a topical agent to manage surgical site or wound infections is increasingly acknowledged (Gethin *et al.*, 2008). Greater scientific understanding of how it works, particularly as an antibacterial agent, has led practitioners to reconsider the therapeutic value of honey. Honey is a broad spectrum antimicrobial agent which can enhance wound healing. Honey which is a natural, non-toxic, and an inexpensive product has activity against the *P. aeruginosa* isolated from infected wounds may make it an alternative topical choice in the treatment of wound infections (Shenoy *et al.*, 2012).

Honey contains different enzymes, including glucose-oxidase that generates hydrogen peroxide and gluconic acid in the presence of glucose and water. The viscosity and the hygroscopic qualities of honey permit it to be evenly spread on the wound bed, creating a favourable environment for wound healing.

An important factor in the failure of a sore to heal is the presence of multiple species of bacteria, living cooperatively in highly organized biofilms. The biofilm protects the bacteria from antibiotic therapy and the patient's immune response. Honey has been used as a wound treatment for millennia. Alandejani *et al.* (2009) used a previously established biofilm model to assess antibacterial activity of honey against 11 methicillin-susceptible SA (MSSA), 11 methicillin-resistant SA (MRSA), and 11 PA isolates. Honeys were tested against both planktonic and biofilm-grown bacteria and were found to be effective in killing 100 percent of the isolates in the planktonic form. The bactericidal rates for the Sidr and Manuka honeys against MSSA, MRSA, and P. aeruginosa biofilms were 63-82 percent, 73-63 percent, and 91 percent, respectively. These rates were significantly higher ($P<0.001$) than those seen with single antibiotics commonly used against and S.aureus.

As early as 2000, Dunford *et al.*, found that specific, sterilised honeys intended for wound care will provide a safe natural product to manage colonised or infected wounds that would otherwise remain unresponsive to treatment. Van der Weyden (2003) found in addition to healing of wounds, the antibacterial activity of honey had a deodorizing effect on the wounds and its anti-inflammatory actions helped reduce the level of pain.

Honey promotes moist wound healing and stimulates immune responses within a wound (Lusby *et al.*, 2002). Honey has also been used to treat adult and neo-natal post-operative infection, burns, boils, necrotizing fasciitis, venous ulcers and diabetic foot ulcers (Al-Waili *et al.*, 2011).

Al-Waili *et al.* (2011) demonstrated that the wound healing properties of honey include stimulation of tissue growth, enhanced epithelialization, and minimized scar formation. These effects are ascribed to honey's acidity, hydrogen peroxide content, osmotic effect, nutritional and antioxidant contents, stimulation of immunity, and to unidentified compounds. Prostaglandins and nitric oxide play a major role in inflammation, microbial killing, and the healing process. Honey was found to lower prostaglandin levels and elevate nitric oxide end products. These properties might help to explain some biological and therapeutic properties of honey, particularly as an antibacterial agent or wound healer.

Topical honey treatment has been shown to possess antimicrobial properties, promote autolytic debridement, stimulate growth of wound tissues to hasten healing, and to start the healing process in dormant wounds, stimulating anti-inflammatory activity that rapidly reduces pain, oedema and exudate production. Bittmann *et al.* (2010) by reviewing several studies emphasized the use of honey as a form of complementary and alternative medicine in paediatric wound management.

Merckoll *et al.* (2009) reinforced the reintroduction of honey, as a conventional wound treatment may help improve individual wound care, prevent invasive infections, eliminate colonization, interrupt outbreaks and thereby preserve current antibiotic stocks.

Radiation-induced tissue injury and wounds with radiation-impaired healing are traumatic for patients and challenging for their caregivers. Robson and Cooper (2009) treated patients with honey and found complete healing in 2.5 weeks (with honey and paraffin) and 6 weeks (with honey-soaked hydrofiber rope), respectively. No adverse events were reported. Honey as an adjunct to conventional wound/skin care post radiation therapy shows promise for less painful healing in these chronic wounds.

Honey, prednisolone and even disulfiram also have some value in preventing the formation of free radicals released from the inflamed tissues (Bilsel *et al.*, 2002). Salomon *et al.* (2010) confirms that honey with its high concentration of sugar is an efficient treatment of chronic wounds of the lower leg and also of abdominal wounds.

Wound Dressing

Honey dressing enhances wound contraction in fresh wounds which is one of the key features of wound healing. Also honey dressing causes increased granulation tissue formation in wounds dressed with honey compared to control group (Osuagwu *et al.*, 2004). Due to anti microbial property, honey-based wound dressings (which were used world-wide since ancient times) received US Federal Drug Administration (USFDA) approval in 2007, making it an option for wound care (Pieper, 2009). Sare (2008) treated chronic leg ulcer patient with medical honey and reported a reduction in the incidence of infection, reduction in pain and the provision of comfort. Antibacterial medical honey should therefore be considered as a dressing option when assessing and managing chronic wounds.

Burns

Burn injury is associated with a high incidence of death and disability; yet, its management remains problematic and costly. Malik *et al.* (2010) demonstrated greater efficacy of honey over silver sulphadiazine cream for treating superficial and partial-thickness burns.

On burns, it has an initial soothing and later rapid healing effects. It has been used as wound barrier against tumour implantation in laparoscopic oncological surgery. No infection has been reported from the application of honey to open wounds. It has a potential therapeutic role in the treatment of gingivitis and periodontal disease (Khan *et al.*, 2007).

A systematic review by Bardy *et al.* (2008) of 43 studies on use of honey in relation to wounds (n = 19), burns (n = 11), skin (n = 3), cancer (n = 5) and others (n = 5) revealed that majority of studies noted the efficacy of honey in clinical use. But he feels that these studies had been generally poor in quality because of small sample sizes, lack of randomization and absence of blinding.

According to Song and Salcido (2011) use of honey in minor burns and prevention of radiation mucositis appear to be two areas where honey shows therapeutic promise.

Honey-based wound dressings have been used worldwide since ancient times. A honey product received US Federal Drug Administration approval in 2007, making this dressing an option for wound care. Honey has been found to exert anti-inflammatory and antibacterial effects without antibiotic resistance, promote moist wound healing, and facilitate debridement (Pieper, 2009).

Honey and Cough

Cough is a symptom of upper respiratory infections (URIs) prevalent especially among most children. Honey has been used as a treatment for curing cough since ancient times. The use of honey and lozenges to soothe upper respiratory tract irritation is common, inexpensive, and potentially more effective in treating the symptoms than pharmacological interventions. Kapil *et al.* (1990) studied the locally prevalent traditional dietary beliefs. 'Cold' foods like curd, butter milk were restricted during an episode of cough while 'hot' foods like tea, ginger with honey, were preferred.

Just a teaspoon or two of honey with its antimicrobial activity suppresses cough (Moyad 2009). There is as yet no reliable treatment to control URIs and their related cough. However, drugs such as dextromethorphan (DM) and diphenhydramine (DPH) are now mainly used in the world. Dealleaume *et al.* (2009) recommend Dextromethorphan (DM) for adults and honey for children to provide some relief. Although data from acute studies suggest a potential role for honey in relieving cough, Mulholland and Chang (2009) do not recommend these treatments when managing very young children.

Interestingly, parents rated honey as compared to DM most favourably for symptomatic relief of their child's nocturnal cough and sleep difficulty due to upper respiratory tract infection. Hence Paul *et al.* (2007) did not find any significant differences in symptom improvement or cough frequency while comparing honey with DM but reported that honey may be a preferable treatment for the cough and sleep difficulty associated with childhood upper respiratory tract infection as there is a decrease in frequency and severity of cough compared with DM or no treatment.

Two randomized controlled trials were performed on children by Micheal *et al.* (2011). to study the effect of a night-time dose of honey in comparison to dextromethorphan or diphenhydramine on coughing episodes. In both the trials it was found that honey was superior in treating pediatric cough when compared to dextromethorphan, diphenhydramine or no treatment.

Again, Oduwole and his coworkers (2010) also, extracting data from selected studies reported that honey was more effective than no treatment in reducing frequency of cough and sleep quality of the child and the effect was on par with that of Dextromethorphan. But a superior effect of honey over DM and DPH was reported by Shadkam *et al.* (2010) at a dose of 2.5-ml before sleep in alleviating URI-induced cough.

Honey has good anti-Rubella activity and therefore Zeina *et al.*, (1996) justified the continuing use of honey in traditional medicines from different ethnic communities worldwide and in some modern medications such as cough syrups.

Weight Management

Honey with lime and warm water is believed to help in weight management. Chepulis (2007) observed overall percentage weight gain was significantly lower in honey-fed rats than those fed sucrose or mixed sugars, despite a similar food intake.

The explanation given by Zaid *et al.* (2010) for the role of honey in weight management is the reduction in total food intake after consumption of honey, as honey is a highly concentrated source of energy (313 calories per 100 g) which helps in reducing food intake. Certain bioactive compounds in Tualang honey might have prevented the gain in weight of ovariectomised rats. They also observed the total food intake in ovariectomised Tualang honey-treated rats was significantly lower than ovariectomised non-honey treated rats. This was also shown to prevent uterine atrophy, vaginal epithelium atrophy, promote increased bone density and suppress the increased of body weight seen in menopausal state.

Larson-Meyer *et al.* (2010) found honey consumption to delay the postprandial appetite hormone (ghrelin) response and blunted the glucose response compared with consumption of the sucrose-containing meal. Meal-induced insulin response, hunger ratings, thermo genesis, and subsequent ad libitum food intake, however, did not differ between diet treatments. Thus, they explained that the alterations in meal-induced responses of ghrelin but not the meal-induced thermogenesis to be responsible in part for the potential "obesity protective" effect(s) of honey consumption. A blunted glycemic response may be beneficial for reducing glucose intolerance.

A mild reduction in body weight (1.3 per cent) and body fat (1.1 per cent), total cholesterol (3 per cent), LDL-C (5.8), triacylglycerol (11 per cent), Fasting Blood Glucose (4.2 per cent), C Reactive Proteins (CRP) (3.2 per cent); and increase in HDL-C (3.3 per cent) in subjects with normal values was demonstrated by Yaghoobi *et al.* (2008). Whereas in patients with elevated variables, honey caused reduction in total cholesterol by 3.3 per cent, LDL-C by 4.3 per cent, triacylglycerol by 19 per cent, and CRP by 3.3 per cent. It is thus proved that consumption of natural honey reduces cardiovascular risk factors, particularly in subjects with elevated risk factors, and it does not increase body weight in overweight or obese subjects.

Nemoseck *et al.* (2011) observed that in comparison with sucrose, honey reduces weight gain. Body weight gain was 14.7 per cent lower (P d".05) for rats fed honey, corresponding to a 13.3 per cent lower (P d".05) consumption of food/energy, whereas food efficiency ratios were nearly identical. Epididymal fat weight was 20.1 per cent lower for rats fed honey. Thus the authors suggest that in comparison with sucrose, honey may reduce weight gain and adiposity, presumably due to lower food intake, and promote lower serum triglycerides but higher non-high-density lipoprotein cholesterol concentrations.

Honey as Cardioprotective

It has been found that honey ameliorates cardiovascular risk factors in healthy individuals as well as in patients with elevated risk. Many chronic diseases are associated with increased oxidative stress caused by an imbalance between free-radical production and the antioxidant level. The composition and source of honey greatly dictates its biochemical properties. Antioxidants, which are abundant in natural honey, are free-radical scavengers that either reduce the formation of or neutralize free radicals. Kishore *et al.* (2011) observed that the elevated free-radical scavenging and antioxidant activity of tualang honey is due to the increased level of phenolic compounds.

Rakha *et al.* (2008) reported that the possible mechanism of natural wild honey in exerting cardio protective and therapeutic effects against epinephrine-induced cardiac disorders and vasomotor dysfunction is via its very pronounced total antioxidant capacity and/or indirectly, the enhancement of the endothelium-derived relaxing factor nitric oxide release through the influence of ascorbic acid. They praise the great wealth of both enzymatic and nonenzymatic antioxidants of honey besides its substantial quantities of minerals such as magnesium, sodium, and chlorine which make natural wild honey to involve in cardiovascular defense mechanisms.

But the effect on honey on cholesterol need further work to decide its definitive role. The only study conducted specifically on the effect of honey on cholesterol by Münstedt *et al.* (2009) reported that neither honey nor sugar solution significantly influenced cholesterol or triglyceride values in both sexes although in women, the LDL cholesterol value was found to increase in the group fed sugar solution but not in the women taking honey.

Honey on Diabetes

It is believed that honey is better than sugar for diabetic patients. A number of studies have focused on the glycemic index of honey. The glycemic index of honey varies from 32 to 91 depending on botanical origin (Bogdanov, 2010). Robert and Ismail (2009) tested two varieties of honey (Malaysian and Australian) for their Glycemic index. The mean area under control for the two were 174+/-19 and 158+/-16 mmolxmin/l, respectively, and were significantly less than that after glucose intake, 259+/-15 mmolxmin/l ($P<0.001$). The mean GI of Malaysian wild honey was 65+/-7, and that of Australian honey was 59+/-5. Deibert *et al.* (2010) found glycaemic index of five of the eight German honey grades differing in their floral source and carbohydrate composition was below 55; for six of the eight tested varieties, the glycaemic load was lower than 10 (portion size of 20 g honey).

Investigation on streptozotocin-induced diabetic rats on the effect of honey as an adjunct to diabetic drugs like glibenclamide or metformin on the glycemic control revealed that honey in combination with drugs, significantly reduced the blood glucose levels and fructose-amine levels. Also, the combination significantly reduced the elevated levels of creatinine, bilirubin, TGs and VLDL cholesterol, thus providing additional metabolic benefits (Erejuwa *et al.*, 2011). Honey supplementation significantly reduced fasting blood glucose and lipid peroxidation along with restoration of superoxide dismutase activity. Histopathological examination of kidneys revealed that mesangial matrix expansion and thickening of glomerular basement membrane were reduced in honey-treated diabetic rats (Omotayo *et al.*, 2010).

Comparing the relative tolerance to honey and glucose of subjects with impaired glucose tolerance or mild diabetes, Agrawal *et al.* (2007) noted the plasma glucose levels in response to honey peaked at 30-60 minutes and showed a rapid decline as compared to that to glucose. The high degree of tolerance to honey in subjects with diabetes indicated lower glycemic index of honey.

The mean glycemic index of four US honey varieties namely, clover, buckwheat, cotton, and tupelo in 12 healthy adult men and women ranged between 69.2+/-8.1, and 74.1+/-8.2. However, no statistically significant differences were apparent between the honeys, nor was a relationship between glycemic index and the fructose-to-glucose ratio detected, indicating that small differences in fructose-to-glucose ratio do not substantially impact glycemic index of honey (Ischayek and Kern 2006). Glucose response was significantly lower in the natural honey consumers at all time points (P < 0.005) compared to the simulated honey consumers and D-Glucose consumers. Natural honey stabilizes physiological glycemic response with rebound recovery of plasma glucose level (Ahmed *et al.*, 2008).

Makhdoom *et al.* (2009) observed excellent results in treating diabetic wounds with dressings soaked with natural honey. The disability of diabetic foot patients was minimized by decreasing the rate of leg or foot amputations and thus enhancing the quality and productivity of individual life.

Bahrami *et al.* (2009) demonstrated that 8-week consumption of honey can provide beneficial effects on body weight and blood lipids of diabetic patients. However, an increase in the hemoglobin A (1C) level upon consumption of honey, cautions diabetics of its regular intake.

There is always a great concern on the recommendation of honey for diabetics. Oral administration of pure small or large-bee honeys in 5 ml/kg/doses could not produce a significant (P greater than 0.05) increase in glucose levels in normal and alloxan-diabetic rabbits (Akhtar and Khan 1989).

As compared to sucrose, honey may reduce weight gain and adiposity, presumably due to lower food intake. Shambaugh *et al.* (1990) compared Honey with fructose and sucrose on blood sugar levels. Fructose showed minimal changes in blood sugar levels, consistent with other studies. Sucrose gave higher blood sugar readings than honey at every measurement, producing significantly greater glucose intolerance. Honey provided the fewest subjective symptoms of discomfort. Given that honey has a gentler effect on blood sugar levels on a per gram basis, and tastes sweeter than sucrose so that fewer grams would be consumed, it would seem prudent to recommend honey over sucrose. Samanta *et al.* (1985) suggested that though honey may prove to be a valuable sugar substitute in diabetics, both the glycemic Index as well as Peak Incremental Index should be used in the analysis of food.

Honey in Ulcers

The therapeutic value of honey in healing oral mucosal ulcers in comparison with Glyceroloxytriester (TGO) tested on 30 wistar rats showed that there was no significant difference between the two with regard to biopsy specimens and hydroxy pyroline levels (Yilmaz *et al.*, 2009).

Gethin and Cowman. (2009) reported Manuka honey to be effective in desloughing thus improving healing outcomes in 108 patients with venous leg ulcers having >or=50 per cent wound area covered in slough.

Honey in Cancer:

Cancer is one of the deadly diseases that burden the society since long and is diagnosed in approximately 11 million people and is responsible for almost 8 million deaths worldwide every year. Although chemotherapy is well-advanced, it is still not able to prevent the cancer death by hundred percent. Honey has been found to be effective in the management of radiation-induced mucositis in patients receiving head and neck radiotherapy (Motallebnejad *et al.*, 2008).

Fauzi *et al.* (2011) showed that Tualang honey (TH) has significant anticancer activity against human breast and cervical cancer cells as there was an increase in lactate dehydrogenase leakage from the cell membranes indicating that TH is cytotoxic to all the cancer cells with effective concentrations of 2.4-2.8 per cent.

Ehrlich ascites carcinoma is a spontaneous murine mammary adenocarcinoma adapted to ascites form and carried in outbred mice by serial intraperitoneal (i/p) passages. Jagannathan's team (2010) showed that honey containing higher phenolic content significantly inhibit the growth of Ehrlich ascites carcinoma and therefore suggested honey and eugenol (one of the phenolic constituents of honey) to be promising candidates in cancer chemoprevention. Again, Jaganathan *et al.* (2011b) demonstrated molecular mechanism of eugenol-induced apoptosis in human colon cancer cells and thus reinforced eugenol as a potential chemopreventive agent against colon cancer.

Honey may cause cell death in the human renal cancer cell lines (ACHN), in which apoptosis plays an important role. Most of the drugs used in the cancer treatment are apoptotic inducers, hence apoptotic nature of honey is considered vital. Samarghandian *et al.* (2011) prepared cell cultures in Dulbecco's modified Eagle's medium with 10 per cent fetal bovine serum treated with different concentrations of honey for 3 consecutive days. Cell viability was quantified by the 3-(4,5-Dimethylthiazol-2-yl)-2,5-diphenyltetrazolium bromide assay. Apoptotic cells were determined using Annexin-V-fluorescein isothiocyanate (FITC) by flow cytometry. They found a decrease in the cell viability in the malignant cells with honey in a concentration–and time-dependent manner.

Honey was found to be a suitable alternative for wound healing, burns and various skin conditions and to potentially have a role within cancer care. Bardy *et al.* (2008) opined that in the cancer setting, honey may be used for radiation-induced mucositis, radiotherapy-induced skin reactions, hand and foot skin reactions in chemotherapy patients and for oral cavity and external surgical wounds.

Honey applied topically to the oral mucosa of patients undergoing radiation therapy appears to provide a distinct benefit by limiting the severity of mucositis (Khanal. *et al.*, 2010). Rashad *et al.* (2009) confirmed the prophylactic use of pure natural honey as effective in reducing mucositis resulting from radiochemotherapy in patients with head and neck cancer.

But when the effect of active Manuka honey was assessed on radiation-induced mucositis in 131 patients (diagnosed with head and neck cancer and undergoing radiotherapy) by Bardy *et al.* (2011), Manuka honey was not found to improve mucositis. But both the honey and the syrup seemed to be associated with a reduction in bacterial infections. It is presumed by the authors that poor compliance after the onset of mucositis, may have affected the findings.

In the case of oral squamous cell carcinomas (OSCC) and human osteosarcoma (HOS) the treatment includes surgery and/or radiotherapy which often lead to reduced quality of life. Ghashm *et al.* (2010) proved that Tualang honey has antiproliferative effect on OSCC and HOS cell lines by inducing early apoptosis. Tomasin and Gomes-Marcondes (2011) also confirmed that honey can modulate tumour growth by reducing cell proliferation and increasing apoptosis susceptibility.

One of the major stumbling blocks for cancer chemotherapy is multidrug resistance (MDR) developed by cancer cells. Since ancient times, honey has been used successfully for the treatment of a broad spectrum infections with no risk of resistance development. MDR in nosocomial pathogens is a continually evolving and alarming problem in health care units. Majtan *et al.* (2011) proved that Honeydew honey with strong antibacterial activity could be used as a potential agent to eradicate multi-drug resistant clinical isolates as Slovak honeydew honey showed exceptional antibacterial activity against multi-drug resistant S. maltophilia isolates and was more efficient than manuka honey.

Jagannathan (2011a) promulgates honey with common flavonoids like chrysin, genistein, biochanin, quercetin, kaempferol, and naringenin as a potential candidate for reversing MDR. He foresees that honey, a novel chemo sensitizer, can reduce the huge amount invested in developing new chemo sensitizers to overcome the burden of chemo-resistance. Moreover honey is readily available, affordable and well accepted by patients making it useful for improving the quality of life in irradiated patients.

Shoma *et al.* (2010) investigated whether the addition of pentoxifylline (PTX) alone or in combination with topical honey is effective in its management compared to the standard measures. Group A received standard burn treatment (control group). Group B received additionally 400 mg PTX twice daily. Group C received the same treatment as Group B with adding topical purified honey ointment. The addition of honey was associated with marked pain relieving effect and rescue of proper motion. Honey was also associated with shorter duration of treatment as 74 per cent of group C patients completely recovered after 12 weeks, compared to only 54 per cent and 36 per cent of groups B and A respectively. Thus it is proved that combination of PTX and honey is an ideal measure for treatment of radiation-induced burn following breast conservative surgery.

Honey and Hormones

On administration of Tualang honey at all doses, for 2 weeks in female adult ovariectomised rats, a model for menopausal symptoms, Zaid *et al.* (2010) found significant lack of atrophy of the vaginal epithelium. The uterine endometrium maintained the thickness in non-ovariectomised rats. They also noted vacuolation of the vaginal epithelial cells implying increase in mucopolysacharide (glycogen) content. Thus Tualang honey was shown to prevent uterine atrophy, vaginal epithelium atrophy, promote increased bone density and suppress body weight gain seen in menopausal state. Clinical trials are required to see if these benefits could be translated to post menopausal women. If inferred to human, such finding may be of benefit to women who experience vaginal dryness after menopause and thus honey could be considered an alternative to Hormone Replacement Therapy.

According to Buratti *et al.* (2007) and Willix *et al.* (1992) the improvement of uterus and vagina atrophy is due to the presence of biologically active estrogen-like molecules or phytoestrogens in honey. Further, flavonoids, present in honey could retard biologically destructive chemical reactions in living organisms through their ability to scavenge oxidants and free radicals. Flavonoids particularly kaempferol and quercetin have been shown to have weak estrogenic activity.

Honey for the Skin

As per the reports of Al-Waili (2001), all the patients with skin problems responded markedly with application of honey. Itching was relieved and scaling disappeared within one week. Skin lesions were healed and disappeared completely within 2 weeks. In addition, patients showed subjective improvement in hair loss. None of the patients treated with honey application once weekly for six months showed relapse while the patients who had no prophylactic treatment with honey experienced a relapse of the lesions 2-4 months after stopping treatment. Thus the author concluded that crude honey could markedly improve seborrheic dermatitis and associated hair loss and prevent relapse when applied weekly.

Honey as a Preservative

Due to the bactericidal property of hydrogen peroxide present in honey in combination of various sugars, can be used as a preservative for milk samples (Krushna *et al.*, 2007).

Paulus *et al.* (2011) showed that the food spoilage bacterium *B. subtilis* is highly susceptible to Manuka honey, and also *Bacillus cereus* is effectively killed by honey. Since manuka honey retains bactericidal activity against food-spoiling bacilli up to very high dilution, this honey has better potential than Revamil source honey for food preservation.

Other Benefits of Honey

Patients with protein-energy malnutrition (PEM) have delayed gastric emptying time (GET) which may affect nutritional rehabilitation. Honey supplementation increased GET in PEM patients with positive effect on the improvement in the anthropometric measurements and serum albumin Shaaban *et al.*, 2010). PEM is also associated with a significant impairment of cell-mediated immunity and complement system, which may be responsible for the high incidence of infections among these patients. Honey, as a natural substance, increased the level of 50 per cent complement hemolytic activity (CH50) in patients with PEM (Abdulrehman *et al.*, 2011).

Cooper *et al.* (2010) noticed presence of lower level of risk factors of vascular and other diseases among 41 men eating honey than the 624 men who had not consumed honey. Mortality due to all causes was considerably lower in the men who had consumed honey, the hazard ratio, adjusted for a number of possible confounding factors, being 0.44.

5-Hydroxymethyl-2-furfural (5HMF) has been found to bind specifically with intracellular sickle hemoglobin (HbS). Preliminary *in vivo* studies using transgenic sickle mice showed that orally administered 5HMF inhibits the formation of sickled cells in the blood (Abdulmalik *et al.*, 2005).

In an inflammatory model of colitis, intra rectal honey administration is as effective as prednisolone treatment. Honey, prednisolone and even disulfiram also have some value in preventing the formation of free radicals released from the inflamed tissues (Bilsel *et al.*, 2002).

Safety Issues

There is a vast research studies on the use of honey-based products in wound care, demonstrating their efficacy, cost-effectiveness and excellent record of safety. This has resulted in a variety of new honey-based wound products into the market (Evans and Flavin, 2008). Certainly, for the purposes of wound management it has to be 'medical grade', i.e it has been sterilized by gamma irradiation and has a standardized antibacterial activity.

Medihoney™ has been one of the first medically certified honeys licensed as a medical product for professional wound care in Europe and Australia (Molan and Betts, 2004; Molan, 2006). A honey product received US Federal Drug Administration approval in 2007, making this dressing an option for wound care. Health officials currently advise limiting honey use because of the risk of botulism. Honey allergy is a very rare condition which shows a clinical picture ranging from cough to anaphylaxis after ingestion (Karakaya and Fuat Kalyoncu, 1999).

Another promising area where honey has a promise is its use as a carbohydrate source for athletes. Encouraging results of the three double-blind, placebo-controlled studies on honey for athletes conducted at the University of Memphis Exercise and Sport Nutrition Laboratory, led by Dr. Richard Kreider were presented at the annual meetings of Experimental Biology, the American College of Sports Medicine and the National Strength and Conditioning Association.

Conclusions

Thus, the numerous research studies published on health benefits of honey proves the traditional beliefs on its merits. But the role of honey on weight reduction and as hypocholesterolemic agent has not been conclusive. Future research may need to focus on these aspects.

References

Abdulmalik O, Safo MK, Chen Q, Yang J, Brugnara C, Ohene-Frempong K, Abraham DJ, Asakura T (2005). 5-hydroxymethyl-2-furfural modifies intracellular sickle haemoglobin and inhibits sickling of red blood cells. British Journal of Haematology.128 (4): 552–61.

Abdulrehman MA, Nassar MF, Mostafa HW, El-Khayat ZA, El Naga MW (2011). Effect of honey on 50 per cent complement hemolytic activity in infants with protein energy malnutrition: a randomized controlled pilot study. J. Med. Food. 14 (5): 551–55.

Adebolu TT (2005). Effect of natural honey on local isolates of diarrhea- causing bacteria in South Western Nigeria. Afri. J. Biotech. 4 (10): 1172–74.

Agrawal OP, Pachauri A, Yadav H, Urmila J, Goswamy HM, Chapperwal A, Bisen PS, Prasad GB (2007) Subjects with impaired glucose tolerance exhibit a high degree of tolerance to honey. J. Med. Food. 10 (3): 473- 78.

Ahmad A, Azim MK, Mesaik MA, Khan RA (2008). Natural honey modulates physiological glycemic response compared to simulated honey and D-glucose. J. Food Sci. 73 (7): H165–67.

Akhtar MS, Khan MS (1989). Glycaemic responses to three different honeys given to normal and alloxan-diabetic rabbits. J. Pak. Med. Assoc. 39 (4): 107–13.

Alandejani T, Marsan J, Ferris W, Slinger R, Chan F (2009). Effectiveness of honey on Staphylococcus aureus and Pseudomonas aeruginosa biofilms. Otolaryngol Head Neck Surg. 141 (1): 114–18.

Aljadi AM, Kamaruddin MY (2004). Evaluation of the phenolic contents and antioxidant capacities of two Malaysian floral honeys. Food Chemistry. 85: 513–18.

Alnaqdy A, Al-Jabri A, Al Mahrooqi Z, Nzeako B, Nsanze H (2005). Inhibitory effect of honey on the adherence of *Salmonella* to intestinal epithelial cells *in vitro*. Int. J. Food Microbiol. 103: 347–51.

Al-Waili NS (2001). Therapeutic and prophylactic effects of crude honey on chronic seborrheic dermatitis and dandruff. Eur J Med Res. 6 (7): 306–308.

Al-Waili NS, Akmal M, Al-Waili FS, Saloom KY, Ali A (2005). The antimicrobial potential of honey from United Arab Emirates on some microbial isolates. Med. Sci. Monitor. 11 (12): BR 433–38.

Al-Waili N, Salom K, Al-Ghamdi AA (2011). Honey for wound healing, ulcers, and burns; data supporting its use in clinical practice. Scientific World Journal. 1: 766–87.

Badawy OF, Shafii SS, Tharwat EE, Kamal AM (2004). Antibacterial activity of bee honey and its therapeutic usefulness against Escherichia coli O157:H7 and Salmonella typhimurium infection. Rev. Sci. Tech. 23 (3): 1011–22.

Badet C, Quero F (2011). The *in vitro* effect of manuka honeys on growth and adherence of oral bacteria. Anaerobe. 17 (1): 19–22.

Bahrami M, Ataie-Jafari A, Hosseini S, Foruzanfar MH, Rahmani M, Pajouhi M (2009). Effects of natural honey consumption in diabetic patients: an 8-week randomized clinical trial. Int. J. Food Sci. Nutr. 60 (7): 618–26.

Bardy J, Molassiotis A, Ryder WD, Mais K, Sykes A, Yap B, Lee L, Kaczmarski E, Slevin N. (2011) A double-blind, placebo-controlled, randomised trial of active manuka honey and standard oral care for radiation-induced oral mucositis. Br. J. Oral Maxillofac. Surg. 2011 May 31. [Epub ahead of print].

Bardy J, Slevin NJ, Mais KL, Molassiotis A (2008). A systematic review of honey uses and its potential value within oncology care. J. Clin. Nurs. 17 (19): 2604–623.

Bilsel Y, Bugra D, Yamaner S, Bulut T, Cevikbas U, Turkoglu U (2002). Could honey have a place in colitis therapy? Effects of honey, prednisolone, and disulfiram on inflammation, nitric oxide, and free radical formation. Dig. Surg. 19 (4): 306–311.

Bittmann S, Luchter E, Thiel M, Kameda G, Hanano R, Längler A (2010). Does honey have a role in paediatric wound management? Br. J. Nurs. 19 (15): S19–20, S22, and S24.

Bogdanov S, Jurendic T, Sieber R, Gallmann P (2008). Honey for nutrition and health: a review. J. Am. Coll. Nutr. 27 (6): 677–89.

Bogdanov S (2010). Nutritional and functional properties of honey.Vopr. Pitan.79 (6): 4–13.

Boukraâ L, Amara K (2008). Synergistic effect of starch on the antibacterial activity of honey. J. Med. Food. 11 (1): 195–98.

Brudzynski K (2006). Effect of hydrogen peroxide on antibacterial activities of Canadian honeys. Can. J. Microbiol. 52 (12): 1228–37.

Brudzynski K, Lannigan R (2012). Mechanism of Honey Bacteriostatic Action Against MRSA and VRE Involves Hydroxyl Radicals Generated from Honey's Hydrogen Peroxide. Front. Microbiol. 3: 36.

Buratti S, Benedetti S, Cosio MS (2007). Evaluation of the antioxidant power of honey, propolis and royal jelly by amperometric flow injection analysis. Talanta. 71 (3): 1387–92.

Chepulis LM (2007). The effect of honey compared to sucrose, mixed sugars, and a sugar-free diet on weight gain in young rats. J. Food Sci. 72 (3): S224–29.

Codex Alimentarius Commission (2003) Joint FAO/WHO Food Standards Programme. Viale. Delle. Terme. Di. Caracalla. 00100 ROME.

Cooper RA, Fehily AM, Pickering JE, Erusalimsky JD, Elwood PC (2010). Honey, health and longevity. Curr. Aging Sci. 3 (3): 239–41.

Davis C (2005). The use of Australian honey in moist wound management. Rural industries research and development corporation report. 1–18.

Dealleaume L, Tweed B, Neher JO (2009). Do OTC remedies relieve cough in acute URIs? J. Fam. Pract. 58(10): 559 a-c.

Deibert P, König D, Kloock B, Groenefeld M, Berg A (2010). Glycaemic and insulinaemic properties of some German honey varieties. Eur. J. Clin. Nutr. 64 (7): 762–64.

Dunford C, Cooper R, Molan P, White R (2000). The use of honey in wound management. Nurs. Stand. 15 (11): 63–68.

Elbagoury EF, Rasmy S (1993). Antibacterial action of natural honey on anaerobic bacteroides. Egypt. Dent. J. 39 (1): 381–86.

Erejuwa OO, Sulaiman SA, Wahab MS, Sirajudeen KN, Salleh MS, Gurtu S (2011). Glibenclamide or metformin combined with honey improves glycemic control in streptozotocin-induced diabetic rats. Int. J. Biol. Sci. 7 (2): 244–52.

Evans J, Flavin S (2008). Honey: a guide for healthcare professionals. Br. J. Nurs. 17 (15): S24, S26, S28–30.

Fangio MF, Iurlina MO, Fritz R (2007). [Antimicrobial activity of honey the southeast of Buenos Aires Province against *Escherichia coli*]. Rev. Argent. Microbiol. 39 (2): 120–23.

Fauzi AN, Norazmi MN, Yaacob NS (2011). Tualang honey induces apoptosis and disrupts the mitochondrial membrane potential of human breast and cervical cancer cell lines. Food Chem. Toxicol. 49 (4): 871–78.

Gethin G, Cowman S (2008). Bacteriological changes in sloughy venous leg ulcers treated with manuka honey or hydrogel: An RCT. (246-7). J. Wound Care. 17: 241–434.

Gethin G, Cowman S (2009). Manuka honey vs. hydrogel—a prospective, open label, multicentre, randomised controlled trial to compare desloughing efficacy and healing outcomes in venous ulcers. J. Clin. Nurs. 18 (3): 466–74.

Ghashm AA, Othman NH, Khattak MN, Ismail NM, Saini R (2010). Antiproliferative effect of Tualang honey on oral squamous cell carcinoma and osteosarcoma cell lines. BMC. Complement. Altern. Med. 14 (10): 49.

Gheldof N, Engeseth NJ (2002). Antioxidant capacity of honeys from various floral sources based on the determination of oxygen radical absorbance capacity and inhibition of *in vitro* lipoprotein oxidation in human serum samples. J. Agric. Food Chemistry. 50: 3050–55.

Gidamis AB, Chove BE, Shayo NB, Nnko SA, Bangu NT (2004). Quality evaluation of honey harvested from selected areas in Tanzania with special emphasis on hydroxymethyl furfural (HMF) levels. Plant. Foods Hum. Nutr. 59 (3): 129–32.

Haffejee IE, Moosa A (1985). Honey in the treatment of infantile gastroenteritis. Br. Med. J. (Clin. Res. Ed). 290 (6485): 1866–67.

Havsteen B (1983). Flavonoids, a class of natural products of high pharmacological potency. Biochem. Pharmacol. 32: 1141–48.

Irish J, Blair S, Carter DA (2011). The antibacterial activity of honey derived from Australian flora. PLoS. One. 6 (3): e18229.

Ischayek JI, Kern M (2006). US honeys varying in glucose and fructose content elicit similar glycemic indexes. J. Am. Diet. Assoc. 106 (8): 1260–62.

Jagannathan SK (2011a). Can flavonoids from honey alter multidrug resistance? Med. Hypotheses. 76 (4): 535–37.

Jagannathan SK, Mazumdar A, Mondhe D, Mandal M (2011b). Apoptotic effect of eugenol in human colon cancer cell lines. Cell. Biol. Int. 35 (6): 607–615.

Jagannathan SK, Mondhe D, Wani ZA, Pal HC, Mandal M (2010). Effect of honey and eugenol on Ehrlich ascites and solid carcinoma. J. Biomed. Biotechnol. 989163.

Kapil U, Sood AK, Gaur DR (1990). Maternal beliefs regarding diet during common childhood illnesses. Indian Pediatr. 27 (6): 595–99.

Karakaya G, Fuat Kalyoncu A (1999). Honey allergy in adult allergy practice. Allergol Immunopathol. (Madr). 27 (5): 271–72.

Khalil MI, Alam N, Moniruzzaman M, Sulaiman SA, Gan SH (2011). Phenolic acid composition and antioxidant properties of Malaysian honeys. J. Food Sci. 76 (6): C921-C928.

Khalil MI, Sulaiman SA, Alam N, Moniruzzaman M, Bai'e S, Man CN, Jamalullail SM, Gan SH (2012). Gamma irradiation increases the antioxidant properties of Tualang honey stored under different conditions. Molecules. 17 (1): 674–87.

Khan FR, Ul Abadin Z, Rauf N (2007). Honey: nutritional and medicinal value. Int. J. Clin. Pract. 61 (10): 1705–707.

Khanal B, Baliga M, Uppal N (2010). Effect of topical honey on limitation of radiation-induced oral mucositis: an intervention study. Int. J. Oral. Maxillofac. Surg. 39 (12): 1181–85.

Kishore RK, Halim AS, Syazana MS, Sirajudeen KN (2011). Tualang honey has higher phenolic content and greater radical scavenging activity compared with other honey sources. Nutr. Res. 31 (4): 322–25.

Klein C, Sato T, Meguid MM, Miyata G (2000). From food to nutritional support to specific nutraceuticals: a journey across time in the treatment of disease. J. Gastroenterol. 35 Suppl. 12: 1–6.

Krushna NS, Kowsalya A, Radha S, Narayanan RB (2007). Honey as a natural preservative of milk. Indian J. Exp. Biol. 45 (5): 459–64.

Kwakman PH, Zaat SA (2011). Antibacterial components of honey, IUBMB Life. Nov. 17. doi: 10.1002/iub.578.

Larson-Meyer DE, Willis KS, Willis LM, Austin KJ, Hart AM, Breton AB, Alexander BM (2010). Effect of honey versus sucrose on appetite, appetite-regulating hormones, and postmeal thermogenesis. J. Am. Coll. Nutr. 29 (5): 482–93.

Lusby PE, Coombes A, Wilkinson JM (2002). Honey: a potent agent for wound healing? J. Wound Ostomy. Continence. Nurs. 29 (6): 295–300.

Majtan J, Majtanova L, Bohova J, Majtan V (2011). Honeydew honey as a potent antibacterial agent in eradication of multi-drug resistant Stenotrophomonas maltophilia isolates from cancer patients. Phytother. Res. 25 (4): 584–87.

Makhdoom A, Khan MS, Lagahari MA, Rahopoto MQ, Tahir SM, Siddiqui KA (2009). Management of diabetic foot by natural honey. J. Ayub. Med. Coll. Abbottabad. 21 (1): 103–105.

Malik KI, Malik MA, Aslam A (2010). Honey compared with silver sulphadiazine in the treatment of superficial partial-thickness burns. Int. Wound. J. 7 (5): 413–17.

Merckoll P, Jonassen TØ, Vad ME, Jeansson SL, Melby KK (2009). Bacteria, biofilm and honey: a study of the effects of honey on 'planktonic' and biofilm-embedded chronic wound bacteria. Scand. J. Infect. Dis. 41 (5): 341–47.

Mohamed M, Sirajudeen K, Swamy M, Yaacob NS, Sulaiman SA (2009). Studies on the antioxidant properties of Tualang honey of Malaysia. Afr J Tradit. Complement. Altern. Med. 7 (1): 59–63.

Mohapatra DP, Thakur V, Brar SK (2011). Antibacterial efficacy of raw and processed honey. Biotechnol. Res. Int. 2011: 917505.

Molan PC (1999). Why honey is effective as a medicine. 1. Its use in modern medicine. Bee. World. 80: 80–92.

Molan PC (2006). The evidence supporting the use of honey as a wound dressing. Int. J. Low. Extrem. Wounds. 5: 40–54.

Molan PC, Betts JA (2004). Clinical usage of honey as a wound dressing: an update. J. Wound. Care. 13: 353–56.

Motallebnejad M, Akram S, Moghadamnia A, Moulana Z, Omidi S (2008). The effect of topical application of pure honey on radiation-induced mucositis: a randomized clinical trial. J. Contemp. Dent. Pract. 9: 40–47.

Moyad MA (2009). Conventional and alternative medical advice for cold and flu prevention: what should be recommended and what should be avoided? Urol. Nurs. 29 (6): 455–58.

Mulholland S, Chang AB (2009). Honey and lozenges for children with non-specific cough. Cochrane. Database. Syst. Rev. 15 (2): CD007523.

Münstedt K, Hoffmann S, Hauenschild A, Bülte M, von Georgi R, Hackethal A (2009). Effect of honey on serum cholesterol and lipid values. J. Med. Food. 12 (3): 624–28.

Nasir NA, Halim AS, Singh KK, Dorai AA, Haneef MN (2010). Antibacterial properties of tualang honey and its effect in burn wound management: a comparative study. BMC Complement. Altern. Med. 10: 31.

Nassar HM, Mingyun Li, Richard L. Gregory (2012). Effect of Honey on *Streptococcus mutans* Growth and Biofilm Formation. Appl. Environ. Microbiol. 78 (2): 536–40.

National Honey Board (2003), Honey-Health and therapeutic qualities. 390, Lashley street, Longmont. www.nhb.org.

Nemoseck TM, Carmody EG, Furchner-Evanson A, Gleason M, Li A, Potter H, Rezende LM, Lane KJ, Kern M (2011). Honey promotes lower weight gain, adiposity, and triglycerides than sucrose in rats. Nutr. Res. 31 (1): 55–60.

Oddo LP, Heard TA, Rodríguez-Malaver A, Pérez RA, Fernández-Muiño M, Sancho MT, Sesta G, Lusco L, Vit P (2008). Composition and antioxidant activity of Trigona carbonaria honey from Australia. J. Med. Food. 11 (4): 789–94.

Oduwole O, Meremikwu MM, Oyo-Ita A, Udoh EE (2010). Honey for acute cough in children. Cochrane Database Syst. Rev. 20 (1): CD007094.

Omotayo EO, Gurtu S, Sulaiman SA, Ab Wahab MS, Sirajudeen KN, Salleh MS (2010). Hypoglycaemic and antioxidant effects of honey supplementation in streptozotocin-induced diabetic rats. Int. J. Vitam. Nutr. Res. 80 (1): 74–82.

Osuagwu FC, Oladejo OW, Imosemi IO, Aiku A, Ekpos OE, Salami AA, Oyedele OO, Akang EU (2004). Enhanced wound contraction in fresh wounds dressed with honey in Wistar rats (Rattus Novergicus). West. Afr. J. Med. 23 (2): 114–18.

Oyejide CO, Oke EA (1995). An ethnographic study of acute respiratory infections in four local government areas of Nigeria. Afr. J. Med. Sci. 24 (1): 85–91.

Paul IM, Beiler J, McMonagle A, Shaffer ML, Duda L, Berlin CM Jr (2007). Effect of honey, dextromethorphan, and no treatment on nocturnal cough and sleep quality for coughing children and their parents. Arch. Pediatr. Adolesc. Med. 161 (12): 1140–46.

Paulus H. S. Kwakman, Anje A. te Velde, Leonie de Boer, Christina M. J. E. Vandenbroucke-Grauls, Sebastian A. J. Zaat (2011) Two Major Medicinal Honeys Have Different Mechanisms of Bactericidal Activity. PLoS. ONE. 6 (3): 1–7. e17709.

Phillips KM, Carlsen MH, Blomhoff R (2009). Total antioxidant content of alternatives to refined sugar. J. Am. Diet. Assoc. 109 (1): 64–71.

Pieper B (2009). Honey-based dressings and wound care: an option for care in the United States, J. Wound Ostomy. Continence. Nurs. 36 (1): 60–66.

Rakha MK, Nabil ZI, Hussein AA (2008). Cardioactive and vasoactive effects of natural wild honey against cardiac malperformance induced by hyperadrenergic activity. J. Med. Food. 11 (1): 91–98.

Rashad UM, Al-Gezawy SM, El-Gezawy E, Azzaz AN (2009). Honey as topical prophylaxis against radiochemotherapy-induced mucositis in head and neck cancer. J. Laryngol. Otol. 123 (2): 223–28.

Robert SD, Ismail AA (2009). Two varieties of honey that are available in Malaysia gave intermediate glycemic index values when tested among healthy individuals. Biomed. Pap. Med. Fac. Univ. Palacky. Olomouc. Czech. Repub. 153 (2): 145–47.

Robson V, Cooper R (2009). Using leptospermum honey to manage wounds impaired by radiotherapy: a case series. Ostomy.Wound Manage. 55 (1): 38–47.

Salomon D, Barouti N, Rosset C, Whyndham-White C (2010). [Honey: from Noe to wound care]. Rev. Med. Suisse. 6 (246): 871–74.

Samanta A, Burden AC, Jones GR (1985). Plasma glucose responses to glucose, sucrose, and honey in patients with diabetes mellitus: an analysis of glycaemic and peak incremental indices. Diabet. Med. 2 (5): 371–73.

Samarghandian S, Afshari JT, Davoodi S (2011). Honey induces apoptosis in renal cell carcinoma. Pharmacogn. Mag. 7 (25): 46–52.

Sare JL. (2008) Leg ulcer management with topical medical honey. Br. J. Community. Nurs. 13 (9): S22, S24, S26 passim.

Shaaban SY, Abdulrehman MA, Nassar MF, Fathy RA (2010). Effect of honey on gastric emptying of infants with protein energy malnutrition. Eur. J. Clin. Invest. 40 (5): 383–87.

Shadkam MN, Mozaffari-Khosravi H, Mozayan MR (2010). A comparison of the effect of honey, dextromethorphan, and diphenhydramine on nightly cough and sleep quality in children and their parents. J. Altern. Complement. Med. 16 (7): 787–93.

Shambaugh P, Worthington V, Herbert JH (1990). Differential effects of honey, sucrose, and fructose on blood sugar levels. J Manipulative Physiol Ther. 13 (6): 322–25.

Shenoy VP, Ballal M, Shivananda P, Bairy I (2012). Honey as an antimicrobial agent against pseudomonas aeruginosa isolated from infected wounds. J. Glob. Infect. Dis. 4 (2): 102–105.

Shoma A, Eldars W, Noman N, Saad M, Elzahaf E, Abdalla M, Eldin DS, Zayed D, Shalaby A, Malek HA (2010). Pentoxifylline and local honey for radiation-induced burn following breast conservative surgery. Curr. Clin. Pharmacol. 5 (4): 251–56.

Simon Arne, Kirsten Traynor, Kai Santos, Gisela Blaser, Udo Bode and Peter Molan (2009). Medical Honey for Wound Care—Still the 'Latest Resort'? eCAM 6 (2): 165–73.

Song JJ, Salcido R (2011). Use of honey in wound care: an update. Adv. Skin. Wound. Care. 24 (1): 40–44.

Tan HT, Rahman RA, Gan SH, Halim AS, Hassan SA, Sulaiman SA, Kirnpal-Kaur B (2009). The antibacterial properties of Malaysian tualang honey against wound and enteric microorganisms in comparison to manuka honey. BMC. Complement. Altern. Med. 9: 34.

Tomasin R, Gomes-Marcondes MC (2011). Oral administration of Aloe vera and honey reduces Walker tumour growth by decreasing cell proliferation and increasing apoptosis in tumour tissue. Phytother. Res. 25 (4): 619–23.

USDA (2012). National Nutrient Data base for standard reference, release 25.

van den Berg AJ, van den Worm E, van Ufford HC, Halkes SB, Hoekstra MJ, Beukelman CJ (2008). An *in vitro* examination of the antioxidant and anti-inflammatory properties of buckwheat honey. J. Wound. Care. 17 (4):172–74, 176–78.

Van der Weyden EA (2003). The use of honey for the treatment of two patients with pressure ulcers. Br. J. Community Nurs. 8 (12): S14–20.

Voidarou C, Alexopoulos A, Plessas S, Karapanou A, Mantzourani I, Stavropoulou E, Fotou K, Tzora A, Skoufos I, Bezirtzoglou E (2011). Antibacterial activity of different honeys against pathogenic bacteria. Anaerobe. Apr. 16. [Epub ahead of print].

Wahdan HA (1998). Causes of the antimicrobial activity of honey. Infection. 26: 26–31.

White JW, Jr, Subers MH, Schepartz AI (1963). The identification of inhibine, the antibacterial factor in honey, as hydrogen peroxide and its origin in a honey glucose-oxidase system. Biochim. Biophys. Acta. 73: 57–70.

Willix DJ, Molan PC, Harfoot CG (1992) A comparison of the sensitivity of wound-infecting species of bacteria to the antibacterial activity of manuka honey and other honey. J. Appl. Bacteriol. 73(5): 388–94.

Yaghoobi N, Al-Waili N, Ghayour-Mobarhan M, Parizadeh SM, Abasalti Z, Yaghoobi Z, Yaghoobi F, Esmaeili H, Kazemi-Bajestani SM, Aghasizadeh R, Saloom KY, Ferns GA (2008). Natural honey and cardiovascular risk factors; effects on blood glucose, cholesterol, triacylglycerole, CRP, and body weight compared with sucrose. Scientific. World. Journal. 8: 463–69.

Yýlmaz N, Nisbet O, Nisbet C, Ceylan G, Hoþgör F, Ö.Doðu Dede (2009). Biochemical evaluation of the therapeutic effectiveness of honey in oral mucosal ulcers. Bosnian. Journal of Basic Medical Sciences. 9 (4): 295 – 95.

Zaid. Siti SM, Sulaiman Siti A, Kuttulebbai NM Sirajudeen, Nor H Othman (2010). The effects of tualang honey on female reproductive organs, tibia bone and hormonal profile in ovariectomised rats–animal model for menopause. BMC. Complementary and Alternative Medicine. 10: 82.

Zeina B, Othman O, al-Assad S (1996). Effect of honey versus thyme on Rubella virus survival *in vitro*. J. Altern. Complement. Med. 2 (3): 345–48.

Glossary

Adaptogen – Substance that improves the body's ability to adapt to stress.

Adrenergic – sympathomimetic amines which exert their effects on adrenergic receptors of effector cells

Akt signaling – Akt, also known as Protein Kinase B (PKB), is a serine/threonine-specific protein kinase that plays a key role in multiple cellular processes such as glucose metabolism, apoptosis, cell proliferation, transcription and cell migration

Amenorrhoea – The absence of a menstrual period in a woman of reproductive age

Analgesiometer – An analgesiometer was used to measure the pain threshold by applying pressure around the ventral midline of the abdomen. This reading was taken as the baseline pain threshold.

Antiapoptotic – An agent that prevents apoptosis. Apoptosis is a type of cell death in which a series of molecular steps in a cell leads to its death.

Antiautophagic property – inhibition of intracellular degradation system

Antiemetic–An agent that prevents or arrests vomiting

Antimutagenic agent — any substance that reduces the rate of spontaneous mutations or counteracts or reverses the action of a mutagen

Antispasmodic effect – An agent that prevents or arrests vomiting

Antitussive (Cough suppressant) effect – Cough suppressant

Antiurolithiatic effect – an agent that prevents urinary stones

Aphrodisiac effect – an agent that arouses sexual desire

Atonic dyspepsia – Dyspepsia with impaired tone in the muscular walls of the stomach

Carminative — A drug or agent that induces the expulsion of gas from the stomach or intestines.—antiflatulent

Carminative – is an agent that either prevents formation of gas in the gastrointestinal tract or facilitates the expulsion of said gas, thereby combating flatulence.

DPPH – A chemical compound 2,2-diphenyl-1-picrylhydrazyl

Dysmenorrhoea – Dysmenorrhea is the occurrance of painful cramps during menstruation.

Galactogogue – an agent that promotes the secretion of milk—called also *lactagogue*

Hemostatic agent – an agent used to reduce bleeding from small blood vessels by speeding up the clotting of blood or by the formation of an artificial clot.

Lumbago – A painful condition of the lower back

Muscarinic – pertaining to the transmission of nerve impulses mediated by muscarinic receptors; these may be adrenergic or cholinergic

Phytochemicals – A nonnutritive bioactive plant substance, such as a flavonoid or carotenoid, considered to have a beneficial effect on human health

TBARS – Thiobarbituric acid reactive substances which are formed as a byproduct of lipid peroxidation and used as markers of oxidative stress.

Wnt signaling pathway – is a network of proteins that passes signals from receptors on the surface of the cell through the cytoplasm and ultimately to the cell's nucleus where the signaling cascade leads to the expression of target genes.

Index

www.ingramcontent.com/pod-product-compliance
Ingram Content Group UK Ltd.
Pitfield, Milton Keynes, MK11 3LW, UK
UKHW021009290726
14059UKWH00001BA/42